ABORIGINAL HEALTH IN CANADA: HISTORICAL, CULTURAL, AND EPIDEMIOLOGICAL PERSPECTIVES

Numerous studies, inquiries, and statistics accumulated over the years have demonstrated the poor health status of Aboriginal peoples relative to the Canadian population in general. This state of affairs has led to charges of neglect, indifference, and even genocide against the federal government and Canadian society by Aboriginal groups and their supporters. The debate on Aboriginal health services has focused on their current availability, adequacy, accessibility, effectiveness, and sensitivity to community needs. While there are several books on particular aspects of Aboriginal health and health care in Canada, a comprehensive historical review which is national in scope and combines the methodologies and perspectives of epidemiology, history, and anthropology has not been available until now.

Aboriginal Health in Canada is about the complex web of physiological, psychological, spiritual, historical, sociological, cultural, economic, and environmental factors that contribute to health and disease patterns among the Aboriginal peoples of Canada. The authors explore the evidence for changes in patterns of health and disease prior to and since European contact up to the present. They discuss medical systems and the place of medicine within various Aboriginal cultures and trace the relationship between politics and the organization of health services for Aboriginal people. They also examine popular explanations for Aboriginal health patterns today, and emphasize the need to understand both the historical-cultural context of health issues and the diversity of circumstances that give rise to variations in health problems and healing strategies in Aboriginal communities across the country. An overview of Aboriginal peoples in Canada provides a very general background for the non-specialist. Finally, contemporary Aboriginal healing traditions, the issue of self-determination and health care, and current trends in Aboriginal health issues are examined.

JAMES B. WALDRAM is a professor in the Department of Native Studies, University of Saskatchewan. He is editor, with N. Dyck, of *Anthropology, Public Policy and Native Peoples in Canada*. D. ANN HERRING is an associate professor, Department of Anthropology, McMaster University. She is editor, with Leslie Chan, of *Strength in Diversity: A Reader in Physical Anthropology*. T. KUE YOUNG is a professor in the Department of Community Health Sciences, Faculty of Medicine, University of Manitoba. He is author of *The Health of Native Americans* and *Health Care and Cultural Change*.

JAMES B. WALDRAM, D. ANN HERRING,
AND T. KUE YOUNG

Aboriginal Health in Canada: Historical, Cultural, and Epidemiological Perspectives

UNIVERSITY OF TORONTO PRESS
Toronto Buffalo London

ISBN 0-8020-5956-2 (cloth)
ISBN 0-8020-6887-1 (paper)

∞

Printed on acid-free paper

Canadian Cataloguing in Publication Data

Waldram, James B. (James Burgess)
    Aboriginal health in Canada: historical, cultural, and epidemiological
    perspectives

Includes index.
ISBN 0-8020-5956-2 (bound)   ISBN 0-8020-6887-1 (pbk.)

    1. Native peoples – Canada – Health and hygiene – History.*   2. Native
    peoples – Canada – Medical care – History.*   3. Native peoples – Canada
    – Medicine.*
    I. Herring, Ann, 1951–   .   II. Young, T. Kue.
    III. Title.

RA449.W35 1995   362.1'089'97071   C95-930971-3

University of Toronto Press acknowledges the financial assistance to its
publishing program of the Canada Council and the Ontario Arts Council.

This book has been published with the help of a grant from the Social Science
Federation of Canada, using funds provided by the Social Sciences and
Humanities Research Council of Canada.

Contents

Figures and tables

TABLES

Preface

The state of health and health care for Canada's Aboriginal peoples has often been the subject of controversy. Numerous studies, inquiries, and statistics accumulated over the years have demonstrated the poor health status of Aboriginal peoples relative to the Canadian population in general. Based on this evidence, charges of neglect, indifference, and even genocide have been made against the federal government and the larger Canadian society by Aboriginal groups and their supporters. Speaking in their own defence, government agencies responsible for health care often point to the extensive network of health facilities in the remotest corners of the country and the high level of health expenditures allocated to Aboriginal communities. The discrepancy in perception has at times led to confrontation between the users and the providers of health services, instances of which have attracted considerable media and public attention.

Much debate on Aboriginal health services to date has focused on their current availability, adequacy, accessibility, effectiveness, comprehensiveness, quality, and sensitivity to community needs and aspirations. The current system, however, did not come about spontaneously, but has been shaped over the years by policies and practices reflecting the social and political realities of the time and influenced by changing demographic and epidemiological conditions.

While there is an extensive literature on Aboriginal health and health care in Canada, it is scattered in the biomedical and social science literatures. Many documents belong to the 'grey literature,' which is difficult to access. Only a handful of books devoted exclusively to various Aboriginal health issues have been published. Kue Young's *Health Care and Cultural Change* (University of Toronto Press 1988) is a regional study of the Cree-Ojibwa in the Canadian Subarctic and is concerned with the linkages between health status, health services, and social change. This is followed by *The Health of Native Americans* (Oxford University Press 1994), which is concerned with the distribution, risk factors, and preventive strategies of selected diseases prevalent among Aboriginal peoples in Canada and the United States. Books on contemporary Aboriginal healing practices in Canada include Wolfgang Jilek's *Indian Healing* (Hancock House 1982) and David Young, Grant Ingram, and Lise Swartz's *Cry of the Eagle* (University of Toronto Press 1989). Dara Culhane Speck's *An Error in Judgement* (Talonbooks 1987) is a case study of the conflict between a British Columbia coastal community and the medical establishment. Thus, while there are several books on particular aspects of Aboriginal health and health care in Canada, a comprehensive historical review which is national in scope and combines the methodologies and perspectives of epidemiology, history, and anthropology has not been available. It is our intention to fill this gap.

This book's broad, interdisciplinary perspective on the topic of Aboriginal health reflects the diverse backgrounds of the authors and the need to present as comprehensive a picture as possible. To this end it is important for the reader to be aware of the academic backgrounds of the authors and their specific involvement in the book. Dr James Waldram is a medical anthropologist who has undertaken research among both northern and urban Aboriginal peoples, and with Aboriginal offenders. As a cultural anthropologist, he brings a broad understanding of Aboriginal health matters from a cultural perspective. He is responsible primarily for chapters 1, 5, 6, 7, 9, and 10. Dr Ann Herring, also a medical anthropologist, approaches her research from the perspective of biological anthropology. Her work in historical epidemiology, as evident in chapters 2 and 3, is informed by her expertise in assessing the effects of past disease processes from archaeological remains and historical sources. Dr Kue Young, a community health physician, contributes both a 'medical' perspective and that of contemporary epidemiology to the book in chapters 4 and 8. He has worked extensively as a practitioner, administrator, and researcher in various Aboriginal communities in northern Canada, as well as internationally in the circumpolar zone. It should be stated at the outset that none of the authors is of Aboriginal ancestry, and this book in no way pretends to offer an 'Aboriginal' perspective on issues of health and health care. The authors are committed sociocultural and biomedical scientists who have done extensive research in the areas covered in this book, and it is from these perspectives that the book is offered.

While individual authors are responsible for specific chapters, as indicated above (with the exception of chapter 11, which is jointly written by all three authors), we have reviewed and critiqued each other's work extensively in an attempt to avoid duplication and achieve a logical progression of ideas and a consistent prose style.

While we have not taken a strictly chronological approach, we try to cover the major issues and events from the time of early contact with Europeans to the 1990s. We strive for national coverage wherever possible, recognizing the cultural diversity of the Aboriginal peoples in Canada. We also consciously include data and materials, where available, from status and non-status Indians, Métis and Inuit, and from both urban and rural areas. While we deal with issues of both health status and health care, we do not claim to have provided exhaustive coverage of our topic.

Many individuals assisted us in the preparation of this book. We are indebted to Virgil Duff of the University of Toronto Press for maintaining his interest in this project, to the anonymous reviewers whose suggestions we have tried to incorporate into the final product, and to the copy editor, Margaret Allen. Several colleagues read parts or all of the draft and offered useful suggestions and friendly criticisms. Trudy Nicks at the Royal Ontario Museum; Shelley Saunders, Anne Keenleyside, and Wayne Warry at McMaster University; Jerry Cybulski at the Museum of Civilization; Ralph Pastore at Memorial University of Newfoundland; Brian Postl, Linda Garro, and John O'Neil at the University of Manitoba; David Young at the University of Alberta; and Winona Stevenson at the University of Saskatchewan. James Waldram received financial support from the University of Saskatchewan for his research on several aspects of the project. Some research support was provided by the Northern Health Research Unit of the University of Manitoba and by McMaster University.

A NOTE ON TERMINOLOGY

Given the variety of terms that continue to emerge regarding the first peoples of this country, it is necessary to be able to identify the relevant groups clearly. Taking our lead from the Constitution of Canada, we will use the term 'Aboriginal' to refer to all peoples of Indian, Inuit, and Métis heritage, including non-status Indians. When the discussion pertains to only one group, such as the registered Indians, that fact will be indicated. Similarly, where it is necessary or possible to identify specific cultural groups, such as 'Blackfoot' or 'Cree,' we will do so. To avoid confusion, other terms which are currently in usage, such as 'Native' or 'First Nations peoples' will not be used. However, quotations in this book taken from other sources will demonstrate a variety of terms.

We will use the upper case for the term 'Aboriginal' in keeping with current trends within the field of Native studies. Regardless of the terms used, readers should be aware that the selection and discarding of terms in a volume such as this invariably leads to some inconsistency and confusion (for example, where we refer to 'Aboriginal' peoples, some of our sources may use 'Native' peoples). Our governing aim has been, at all times, to employ terms that are both accurate and respectful of those they refer to.

With respect to non-Aboriginal peoples, we generally use the term 'Euro-Canadian,' as well as 'non-Aboriginal' where appropriate. We realize that there are many Canadians whose origins are not in Europe; however, the European colonization of Canada remains the single most important historical fact in our analysis, and the institutions which govern the country (and indeed the people who govern it) are primarily of European heritage.

ABORIGINAL HEALTH IN CANADA:
HISTORICAL, CULTURAL, AND
EPIDEMIOLOGICAL PERSPECTIVES

1

An overview of the Aboriginal peoples of Canada

This book is about health, the fundamental human condition. It takes as axiomatic that the health of any human population is the product of a complex web of physiological, psychological, spiritual, historical, sociological, cultural, economic, and environmental factors. In Canada, one of the most telling examples of how these factors interact can be found in the health of the country's Aboriginal peoples. Long considered to be the most disadvantaged group in an otherwise affluent society, Aboriginal peoples today experience the kinds of health problems most closely associated with poverty, yet they also suffer from problems linked to their historical position within the Canadian social system. This book seeks to explain the current health problems being experienced by Aboriginal peoples, to provide an overview of health and health care from a historical perspective, and to look to the future as fundamental changes to the health care system attempt to grapple with the most pressing problems.

According to the 1991 census, slightly more than one million people in Canada consider themselves to have some Aboriginal ancestry, slightly less than 4 per cent of the total Canadian population.[1] The growth in the Aboriginal population in Canada since the beginning of this century is shown in Figure 1, and it is clear that the period between 1951 and 1981 is characterized by a marked increase in population size. The complexities of Aboriginal Canada seem to grow by leaps and bounds, as events rapidly alter existing perspectives and understandings. It is essential for readers to be aware of these complexities in order to understand properly the many issues dealt with in this book. The aim of this first chapter, therefore, is to provide readers with some background information that helps to explain current conditions.

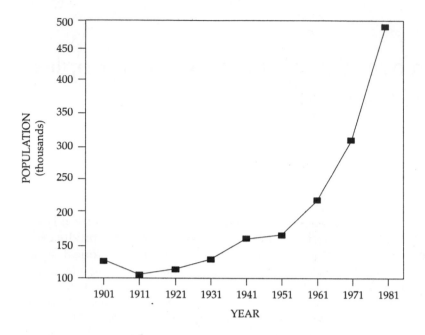

Figure 1
Increase in Aboriginal population in Canada according to the census, 1901–1981

SOURCE: Based on data in Norris (1990) and Leacy (1983)

WHO ARE THE ABORIGINAL PEOPLES?

There are three broad dimensions to understanding the Aboriginal peoples of Canada, with particular reference to health and health care. These
are the biological, cultural, and legal dimensions. The cultural dimension
is the most complex of the three and pertains to both the pre-contact
cultural formations and the *degree* of orientation to Aboriginal or Euro-
Canadian cultures of present-day individuals. We will therefore deal
separately with the two distinct aspects of the cultural dimension.

THE BIOLOGICAL DIMENSION

Archaeologists, linguists, and physical anthropologists have developed
a body of evidence that indicates to them that the earliest ancestors of
contemporary Aboriginal peoples came to the Americas from Asia via a

now-submerged land bridge in the Bering Strait (Beringia or the Bering Land Bridge) (Greenberg, Turner, and Zegura 1986). Geological evidence shows that the Bering Land Bridge was exposed during periods of glaciation when the sea level dropped by about fifty metres, uniting the two continents and allowing the movement of plants, animals, and people between northeast Siberia and Alaska from around 60,000 to 11,000 years ago (Hoffecker, Powers, and Goebel 1993). Currently, disagreement centres on whether population expansion over this prairie-like region occurred very early or whether it was a relatively recent phenomenon, on the order of 12,000 to 14,000 years ago (see Zegura 1985).

Several lines of biological evidence strongly support the theory of the Asian origins of Aboriginal Americans, among them phenotypic characteristics such as dental morphology (Turner 1985) and skeletal features (Szathmary and Ossenberg 1978), as well as a host of genetic characteristics (see Szathmary 1985, 1993 for excellent reviews). Studies of mitochondrial DNA among living populations of Aboriginal Americans suggest that there may have been three or four major waves of migration (Williams et al. 1985; Ward et al. 1992; Wallace, Garrison, and Knowler 1985; Wallace and Torroni 1992; Gibbons 1993; Pollitzer 1994), but others argue that it is difficult to recognize particular migrations from the data at hand (Szathmary 1993). In any event, it is generally agreed that the ancestors of contemporary Indians and Inuit entered North America from Asia. Thereafter, they increasingly differentiated in biological and social dimensions, giving rise to unique societies and civilizations, but maintained unity through intergroup gene flow.

Aboriginal peoples have their own views of how they came to be, and these invariably involve a 'creation' in areas more or less identical to where they live today. Their rich oral traditions link the existence of peoples with specific territories, and define both secular and spiritual places. Their sense of place and of relationships to the land and animals is invariably rooted in these traditions. 'Well-being,' as broadly understood, is a product of this connectedness in the eyes of many Aboriginal people.

THE PRE-CONTACT CULTURAL DIMENSION

Prior to the arrival of Europeans on this continent, there were thousands of autonomous Aboriginal bands, tribes, or 'nations,' as many are referred to today, living in what would become Canada. Linguists have identified within this diversity eleven different language families – that is, groupings of related, though separate, languages. In descending order in terms of the numbers of current language speakers, these families are: Algonquian, Athapaskan, Eskimo-Aleut, Haida, Tlingit, Siouan, Tsimshian, Wakashan, Salishan, Kutenai, and Iroquoian. Figure 2 presents data from the 1991 Aboriginal Peoples Survey of Statistics Canada on the number of speakers of some of these languages. There were as many as fifty or sixty different languages in Canada at the time of European contact in the fifteenth century; today, many of these languages are considered 'threatened' or in danger of disappearing. The Cree, Ojibwa, and Inuktitut languages, which have the largest number of speakers and are spoken across much of Canada, may well be the only ones that are truly safe, for the time being. Many Aboriginal groups are working diligently to save their languages, however, and the process of language loss may ultimately be reversed.

It is important to realize just how different Aboriginal languages are, both from English or French and from each other. The latter point is often misunderstood by Anglophones and Francophones. The structural differences between, say, Cree and Mohawk (both found in Quebec) are much greater than those between French and English! There are also regional and local dialect differences which are detectable by speakers of a particular language.

Out of a concern for the development of typologies, anthropologists initially grouped Aboriginal peoples into 'culture areas.' This concept has been defined by Harold Driver as follows: 'A culture area is a geographical area occupied by a number of peoples whose cultures show a significant degree of similarity with each other and at the same time a significant dissimilarity with the cultures of the peoples of other such areas' (Driver 1969:17). The culture areas which have been identified for Canada are: Arctic, Western Subarctic, Eastern Subarctic, Northeastern Woodlands, Plains, Plateau, and Northwest Coast. Of course, many attributes are combined when anthropologists seek to develop such areas; the concept implies only significant *similarities*, and not identical traits. What is striking is the fact that these culture areas correspond to a great extent to the boundaries of the language families, most of which correspond well to natural geographic features, such as vegetation patterns. Furthermore, it has become more common recently to speak of patterns of adaptation, rather than culture areas, an approach that emphasizes the manner in which human groups exploited available resources. Hence, for instance, the pre-contact Cree, Ojibwa, and Inuit of the Subarctic and Arctic culture

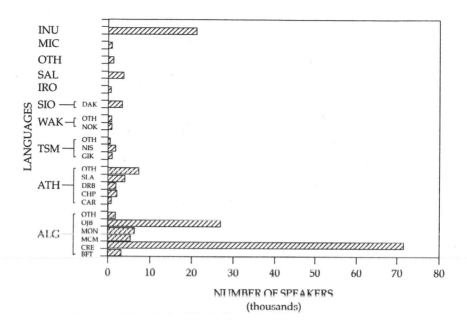

Figure 2
Speakers of Aboriginal languages in Canada according to the 1991 Aboriginal Peoples
Survey

Note: Because of the large number of Aboriginal individuals and communities who declined to participate in the 1991 Census and the Aboriginal Peoples Survey, the numbers
presented here should be regarded with caution. For example, the number of Iroquoian
speakers is probably grossly underestimated, as most Iroquoian reserves in Ontario and
Quebec were not enumerated. These reserves could account for as many as 12,000 residents, although not all of them were speakers of an Iroquoian language.

ABBREVIATIONS

INU   Inuktitut   (language spoken by Inuit)

MIC   Michif   (language spoken by Métis)

OTH   Other Aboriginal languages   (not elsewhere specified, including
                                         Haida, Kutenai, Tlingit)

SAL   Salishan languages   (e.g., Halkomelem, Shuswap,
                                         Thompson, Okanagan, Bella Coola,
                                         Squamish, Sechelt)

Continued on next page

Figure 2 – *Continued*

IRO	Iroquoian languages			(e.g., Mohawk, Oneida)
SIO	Siouan languages	Dak	Dakota	
WAK	Wakashan languages	Nok	Nootka	
		Oth	Other (e.g., Kwakiutl, Haisla, Heilt-suk)	
TSM	Tsimshian languages	Nis	Nishga	
		Gik	Gitksan	
		Oth	Other (e.g., Coast Tsimshian)	
ATH	Athapaskan languages	Sla	Slavey	
		Drb	Dogrib	
		Chp	Chipewyan	
		Car	Carrier	
		Oth	Other (e.g., Beaver, Kutchin, Chicotin, Tutchone, Hare, Sekani, Tahltan, Sarcee)	
ALG	Algonquian languages	Ojb	Ojibwa	
		Mon	Montagnais-Naskapi	
		Mcm	Micmac	
		Cre	Cree	
		Bft	Blackfoot	
		Oth	Other (e.g., Malecite)	

SOURCE: Statistics Canada (1993b)

areas can be thought of as hunter-gatherers (although this still does not imply that the cultures were identical). The ecological base of Aboriginal cultures is easily established, and the role of language as a cultural marker is self-evident.

Given the variability of the environmental zones found in Canada, from the tundra in the north to the woodlands in the east and the mountains in the west, it is not surprising that Aboriginal cultures developed in a diverse manner. But it is also true that the sharing of certain ecological zones, combined with cultural diffusion, resulted in similarities among neighbouring groups.

What did these cultures look like at the time of contact? Through anthropological and ethnohistorical inquiry, we have been able to develop some profiles for this period. However, the reader is cautioned that the evidence for pre-contact cultural formations is fragmented, and that there was extensive cultural diversity even within ecological zones.[2]

It is evident that for much of Canada, including the Arctic and Subarctic areas, Aboriginal peoples lived primarily by hunting small and large game and by gathering plant foods, berries, lichens, nuts and other seasonally available land foods. Peoples such as the Cree, the Ojibwa, the Chipewyan, and the Inuit covered large territorial ranges on foot, hunting and fishing on a seasonal basis at known locales. The primary social unit, the 'band,' was relatively small, often consisting of only fifty to one hundred people. When resources were plentiful, a number of these bands might temporarily join together into a larger entity, the 'regional band'; however, during times of hardship, the band might break up into its constituent parts, nuclear and extended families. Hence, each family existed within a delicate balance, containing all of the essential skills to exist, at least for short periods.

These northern hunters can be contrasted with the peoples of other areas, whose environments allowed for greater aggregates of people and hence greater cultural complexity. The peoples of the Eastern Woodlands, for instance, were horticulturalists, producing a variety of crops (including maize or corn, beans, and squash) as the staple of their diet. Greater certainty in food supply allowed peoples such as the Huron and the Five Nations of the Iroquois (Mohawk, Seneca, Cayuga, Oneida, and Onondaga) to establish permanent villages, and areas of southern Ontario and Quebec are dotted with the ancestral remains of many of these. In the Plains region, Aboriginal peoples such as the Plains Cree, Saulteaux, Assiniboine, and the nations of the Blackfoot Confederacy (Blackfoot, Blood, and Peigan) developed a reliance on the bison as a staple, a reliance that became even more significant as horses, introduced by the Spanish in the sixteenth century in the southern part of the continent, began to make their way onto the northern plains by the mid-eighteenth century. Iroquoian villages often numbered in the high hundreds, and even thousands, while Plains Indian groups often spent the summer bison-hunting season in equally large encampments. Unlike the Iroquoians, however, the Plains Indians tended to split into smaller units – bands – for the harsher winter months.

The Aboriginal peoples of the Northwest Coast, such as the Haida, Tlingit, Kwakiutl, and Gitksan, lived in permanent villages along the coastal areas, or inland along the many rivers, and survived primarily by hunting sea mammals and by fishing. Their societies were perhaps the most diverse and complex of all the northern Aboriginal peoples, and their impressive artistic traditions are perhaps the best recognized throughout the world.

In contrast to these Aboriginal groups, the Métis are a post-contact phenomenon. With roots in both the northern Aboriginal (Cree, Ojibwa, Chipewyan) and European cultures (especially French), the Métis were the product of intermarriage between Aboriginal peoples and fur traders throughout the seventeenth, eighteenth, and nineteenth centuries. Out of these relationships, a distinctive Aboriginal culture emerged.

THE LEGAL DIMENSION

The cultural context of contemporary Aboriginal Canada is complicated by Canadian government legislation and other policies. We can identify two broad legal categories of Aboriginal peoples: those with Indian 'status,' and those without. 'Status' or 'registered' Indians are those individuals legally recognized by the federal government to be 'Indians' for purposes of the *Indian Act*. First passed in 1876, the *Indian Act* was designed to facilitate the administration of programs to Indians, as well as the assimilation of Indians into mainstream Canadian society. It included definitions of who was an 'Indian,' and how such status could be gained or lost. Those Aboriginal peoples who were culturally 'Indian' but who for a variety of reasons lost legal status (or who never gained it in the first place), are often referred to as 'non-status Indians.' Every status Indian in Canada has a unique registration number; this facilitates the gathering of social, economic, and health data for this population, and for this reason much of the contemporary data referred to in this book pertains to them.

Some of the Aboriginal peoples of Canada signed treaties with the British and Canadian governments. These individuals are often referred to as 'treaty Indians.' The intent of the treaties, which cover much of western Canada, including northern Ontario but excluding most of British Columbia, was to remove the Indians' title to the lands, and to remove the Indians themselves, to allow for settlement and exploitation of the natural resources by European immigrants. There are many controversial issues regarding the signing of the treaties, and many treaty Indians believe that the promises made to them in return for their surrender of the land have not been fulfilled. Some Indian peoples believe they did not even agree to surrender the land, but rather agreed to share it. Chapter

7 of this book examines the treaty promises in the area of health care.

A 'treaty Indian' is always a status or registered Indian. However, the converse is not always true: there are many registered Indians in Canada who are not 'treaty.' The federal government is responsible for both the registered and the treaty Indians under the *Indian Act*, including areas related to their health. However, much of the federal responsibility has centred on registered Indians on reserves. Reserves are parcels of land held by Canada on behalf of Indian bands. In practice, in many areas the federal government does not take responsibility for Indians who move off the reserves to live elsewhere, but leaves them to seek services under provincial or municipal jurisdiction.

The Inuit are separate from the registered Indians, and there is no legislation comparable to the *Indian Act* defining them. The federal government has nevertheless assumed primary responsibility for these peoples, and provides services to them as if they were registered Indians.

The Métis and non-status Indians have a legal status which is, essentially, no different from that of non-Aboriginal Canadians. The provinces or territories in which they live deliver programs to these people as part of their obligations to all their citizens, although some special 'Native' programs may also be developed in recognition of their special needs or circumstances. Only the province of Alberta has set aside tracts of land for the exclusive use of Métis people. Nonetheless, there exists a string of Métis communities across the central and northern parts of the prairie provinces as well as in the Northwest and Yukon Territories.

There is often confusion over the differences between Métis and non-status Indians. Indeed, in many Aboriginal communities, one may find a reserve and an adjacent Métis or non-status Indian community. The term 'Métis' is more likely to be heard in such circumstances, despite the fact that the people are more culturally 'Indian' than anything else. The Métis National Council, a political organization which represents the interests of the Métis, argues that only individuals with ancestral ties to the historic Métis populations in Red River (now Winnipeg) and Saskatchewan can claim to be 'Métis.'

Currently, the Indian, Inuit, and Métis peoples are recognized as 'aboriginal peoples' under Section 35 of the Constitution, and their 'existing aboriginal and treaty rights [are] recognized and affirmed.' While the courts and politicians continue to wrangle with the legal implications of this section, clearly the Constitution establishes the Aboriginal peoples as unique with special status within Canada.

CONTEMPORARY CULTURAL ORIENTATION

There have been a great many changes to Aboriginal cultures since the time of first contact. As a result of legislated attempts to destroy these cultures, combined with the effects of residential schools and more subtle pressures which result from contact between cultures, Aboriginal peoples today display a range of cultural orientations. There are still many individuals, especially on reserves and in communities in rural and remote areas, who, though fluent in their Aboriginal language, may speak little or no English or French, and may have had little formal education. Their contact with the larger, Euro-Canadian society will have been minimal. In contrast, there are also many Aboriginal people who have little or no knowledge of their heritage cultures. These individuals may have been adopted into Euro-Canadian families at a young age (an all-too-common phenomenon in Canada until recently) or have spent large portions of their formative years in Euro-Canadian foster homes or residential schools. Even where they may have had sustained contact with their Aboriginal parents, they may not have been exposed to their Aboriginal language or culture to any great extent, perhaps as a result of conscious efforts by their parents to prepare them for the 'White' world. Yet others are effectively bilingual, able to speak both their Aboriginal language and English or French, and bicultural, with extensive experience in both worlds.

Much social and medical scientific research has lumped Aboriginal peoples together into a 'Native' category, to be contrasted with the Canadian population according to a variety of dimensions. The preceding, and necessarily brief, discussion of the cultural and legal complexity of Aboriginal Canada brings the legitimacy of this practice into question. The reader should keep this fact in mind throughout this book. While a work of this nature must necessarily generalize, we are mindful of the problems inherent in so doing.

ABORIGINAL-EUROPEAN POST-CONTACT HISTORY

When Aboriginal and European peoples first encountered each other in what would become North America, the 'first peoples' of the continent exhibited a wide variety of political entities which, at the time, were construed by Europeans to be 'nations.' These nations of Aboriginal peoples had been here for a very long time.

Although the earliest contacts between Aboriginal peoples and Europeans occurred along the eastern coasts and were related to the fishery, for most of Canada the history of contact is linked to the development of the fur trade and to missionary activities. In these endeavours, the British and the French gained ascendancy over the other European powers, such as the Dutch, Portuguese, and Spanish, who were also carving out stakes in the New World.

When in 1604 the beaver felt hat became a popular fashion item in Europe, the vast fur resources of the Canadian wilderness beckoned. In 1670, the 'Company of Adventurers Trading into Hudson Bay,' or 'Hudson's Bay Company' (HBC), was formed. Under a charter granted to the company by King Charles II of England, the HBC was granted a monopoly to trade in all the territory drained by the rivers which emptied into Hudson Bay, an enormous expanse of land the boundaries of which were not even known in 1670. Initially, the HBC showed little inclination to explore, and preferred to establish posts or 'factories' along the coasts of Hudson Bay and James Bay. The Indians brought their furs to the posts via a vast network of trade involving coastal and interior groups. However, it was not long before other European and eastern Canadian interests saw the lucrative profits to be made in the fur trade, and many defied the charter to establish rival operations in the interior. Indeed, it was many of the traders of these other companies, most notably the North West Company (NWC), who charted much of the interior of Canada during the search for new sources of furs.

The Aboriginal peoples became involved in the fur trade because it was to their benefit. They were able to exchange a common commodity – beaver pelts – for items of European manufacture – such as knives, pots, and guns – which greatly improved their livelihoods. In the early years of the trade, little disruption of their traditional lifestyles ensued, since it was their skills in the bush as hunters which also made them successful in the fur trade. But over successive generations, they became increasingly and irreversibly dependent on European technologies. This posed little real problem as long as there were various companies and 'free' traders competing for their furs, a strong European market, and plenty of animals. However, when in 1821 the HBC and the NWC amalgamated to form a new, leaner HBC, the position of the Indians engaged in the fur trade deteriorated dramatically.

When Canada was formed in 1867, a legislative basis for dealing with the Indian peoples as 'nations' already existed. The Royal Proclamation of 1763, a piece of British legislation, had referred to the 'Nations or Tribes of Indians,' and implied fairly clearly that they had some form of land title recognizable by British law. The Royal Proclamation established the basis by which the Crown could secure that title by purchase or cessation, to allow for settlement. The *British North America Act* in 1867 granted to Canada jurisdiction over 'Indians and the lands reserved for Indians,' which bound Canada to the Royal Proclamation's notion of Indian title and the need to obtain proper surrender of Indian lands. Hence was born the treaty process.

Treaties are normally thought of as international agreements, signed between 'nations.' Between 1871 and 1930, treaties and 'adhesions' were signed between Canada and the Indian peoples over much of the country. There is still argument today about whether or not Canada was explicitly recognizing Indian bands and tribal groupings as 'nations' in this international sense (that is, as entities with all the rights, privileges, and powers of nations in the regular sense). The government's intent in signing treaties was clear: to secure title to the land and resources. While the Indians made efforts to negotiate good deals, the evidence suggests that they were at a distinct disadvantage. For instance, by the time the so-called numbered treaties commenced in the west in 1871, the Indians were becoming destitute and ever-mindful of encroaching settlement that appeared to be accelerating even without the treaties. Indians in the west were often presented with a pre-written treaty by a treaty commissioner whose instructions were not to alter the provisions in any way. Treaty commissioners frequently threatened to move on without signing the treaty if the Indian bands continued to dissent. In fact, one of the few treaties where it is clear that the Indians were able to have new clauses inserted was Treaty Six, signed in 1876 in central Saskatchewan and Alberta. In this instance, the clause referred to a 'medicine chest' and government assistance in the event of 'famine or pestilence,' two allusions to health care which are discussed in chapter 7.

During the period of the fur trade, some Indians found work around the trading posts, hunting or doing other chores for the traders. Eventually, greater numbers of Indians began to establish more or less permanent residences around the posts. These people became known as the 'Homeguard,' and their dependence on the European traders for both technology and wages dramatically increased. The legacy of the Homeguard is still with us today. Many northern Aboriginal communities can be found at the sites of old fur trade posts such as Nelson House, York Factory, and Cumberland House. Perhaps more significant is that these historic permanent Indian populations allowed for extensive intermarriage with the French, English, and Scottish traders. Out of these unions came mixed-blood children, and eventually an entirely new population, the Métis.

The Métis developed essentially as a labouring class in the fur trade. Able to speak both Indian and European languages (typically, a combination of Cree, Ojibwa, French, and English out of which eventually a synthesis language, called 'Michif,' developed), they were equally able to function in the bush and at the posts. Some began to work their way into southern areas, particularly into what would become Manitoba, and by the early 1800s there was a sizeable population there involved in wage labour, farming, fishing, and bison hunting.

The missionaries also had a profound influence on the Aboriginal peoples of the New World. The desire of European powers to save the Indians' 'souls' through conversion to Christianity was a dominant theme in the post-contact historical period. Indeed, the seizing of Indian lands and resources and the attempts at forced assimilation were often couched in humanitarian, Christian terms. Simply put, the Indians were understandably unfamiliar with the Christian God, Jesus, the Holy Sacraments, and so on, and therefore by definition were considered 'savages'; they required careful, paternalistic care until they could become 'civilized.' Of course this meant being assimilated into Euro-Canadian cultural patterns and belief systems.

While the early efforts of the missionaries met with mixed results (due, in part, to Indian views that their own religious systems were better), progress was made throughout Canada as many Indians began to experience the poverty that accompanied the declining of the fur trade after 1821. With their populations eroded by European-introduced diseases, and their economies declining (both the beaver and the bison were seriously depleted in many areas by the third quarter of the nineteenth century), Indian people were less able to resist the efforts of the missionaries. The greatest effects of missionization came after the formation of Canada, in 1867, when the churches were given control of Indian education.

Many Aboriginal people today express the view that the church-run residential schools did serious damage to their lives and cultures. Historian J.R. Miller (1989) has documented that the roots of the post-Confederation 'residential-school syndrome' can be found in Upper Canada in the 1840s, when the shift from day schools to residential schools was first noted. The Methodists were among the first Christian denominations to participate in these new institutions, but they were ultimately joined by many other groups. The goals of these schools included education and technical training, but they were, in effect, instruments of assimilation. However, as Miller (1989:107–8) argues, 'What the missionaries and administrators responsible for this extension of residential schooling sometimes forgot was that Indian resistance to the assimilationist purpose

of these schools appeared almost immediately in the 1840s and 1850s.'
The fact remains, however, that the residential schools caused irreversible
changes within Aboriginal societies.

The treaties in western Canada included promises that education
would be provided to the Indians; indeed, the Indian leaders at the time
recognized that their children required new skills to adapt to the changing
political and economic realities in the west. Hence the 1880s saw the
development of residential schools. As Miller (ibid. 196) notes, the assimilationist underpinnings of the new schooling system required that the
children be separated from their families and, therefore, their cultures;
the Catholic, Anglican, Methodist, and Presbyterian churches took the
lead in this regard. Although only a minority of children ever experienced
these schools (ibid. 198), and although Indian resistance to their operation
was extensive, many children in effect became 'deculturized,' losing both
their ability to be culturally 'Indian' and the ability to provide good
parental role models to their own children as they reached adulthood.
This last problem has been particularly troublesome, and even though
the last true residential schools closed in the 1960s, the 'residential school
syndrome' remains a legacy of these institutions.

The missionaries were active in other ways as well. In 1884, the Northwest Coast feasting ceremonial system known as the 'potlatch' was
banned, largely at the insistence of the missionaries. In 1886, the 'Sun
Dance' of the Plains Indians was effectively banned as well. Both these
ceremonies included practices considered by missionaries and government administrators to be essentially heathen and repugnant, and therefore roadblocks to civilization (J.R. Miller 1989:193; Dickason 1992:286).
The ultimate effect of such laws was to drive these and other religious
(and related healing) practices underground. They have survived, in altered forms, until today, but one legacy of these oppressive acts has been
to make Aboriginal people very secretive about what were once public
activities. There are many Aboriginal people today, for instance, who feel
that Euro-Canadians should not be taught about their traditional medicine.

The history of the Inuit people reflects that of the Indians to the south,
although extensive contact with Europeans occurred later, as did federal
government administration programs. However, social change, when it
did begin to accelerate in the 1950s and 1960s, came rapidly and caused
many social problems.

The Inuit were active in the fur trade, and some were also involved in
commercial whaling for many years. But by the 1950s, neither industry

was actively supporting the Inuit. Some groups were still hunting extensively, especially in the interior, and although many had been missionized, at least marginally, there were still many bands living more or less as they had in the past (Brizinski 1989:327).

In 1939, the Supreme Court of Canada ruled that the Inuit were included in the more general term 'Indian' for purposes of federal government jurisdiction, although they were not to be classified as 'Indians' under the *Indian Act*. In an effort to provide administrative services (including health services) to these peoples, in 1941 the government began attempts to register the Inuit in a manner similar to that for registered Indians; special 'disks' with identification numbers stamped on them were issued to some people, and these were to be worn at all times. Since most Euro-Canadians could not pronounce Inuit names (and made no effort to learn), the 'disk list' system provided a convenient bureaucratic means of identifying individuals. However, the system was not widely accepted by the Inuit, and soon fell into disuse (Smith 1993). Nevertheless, the federal government has continued to develop policies for the Inuit which resemble those for registered Indians.

The post-Confederation years were ones of great change for the Indians, Inuit and Métis of Canada. There were occasional flourishes of concerted resistance by some, most notably in Red River in 1869–70 and in Saskatchewan in 1885, events which galvanized Canadian opinion about the French-speaking Métis in particular. As the Indians were settled on reserves, the Métis were pushed farther and farther from their 'homeland' in Manitoba, through Saskatchewan and Alberta, with some even making new homes for themselves in the Territories. The Inuit stayed mostly outside the public eye until the 1950s and the onset of the Cold War, when government turned its attention northward. Government attempts to assimilate Aboriginal peoples continued unabated, and met with some success. Nevertheless, the resistance of Aboriginal peoples throughout this era, although relatively passive, ensured that some elements of language and culture would remain intact.

While periodic wage-labour activities were available (for instance, the Plains Indians were noted agricultural workers and the Indians of British Columbia were actively involved in the commercial fishery in the early years of the settlement of the west), these Aboriginal groups slowly became more economically and socially marginalized. For northern Indians and Inuit, hunting, fishing, and trapping activities continued. The Iroquoian peoples in southern Ontario and Quebec started to become more involved in the economies of surrounding Euro-Canadian communities.

Indians and Métis on the western Plains continued to participate to some degree in the agricultural economy, although as a result of problems with government agricultural policies, their own operations were often marginal (N. Dyck 1986; Carter 1990). And out on the Northwest Coast, salmon and other river and ocean resources remained the staples of many local economies. But times were changing, and widespread poverty became the norm. By 1945, it seemed as though Aboriginal peoples in Canada had all but disappeared from the national conscience.

It was in the 1960s that Aboriginal peoples in Canada began once again to be heard. The seminal event which launched what is known today as the Aboriginal-rights movement was the federal government's White Paper on Indian policy (Weaver 1981).[3] This 1969 policy statement proposed, among other things, to make Indians 'equal' to other Canadians by terminating the *Indian Act*, and therefore their separate legal distinction, as well as eliminating reserves and turning over administrative jurisdiction of Indian programs to the provincial governments. In general, the Indians reacted angrily to these proposals. Cree author Harold Cardinal perhaps summarized the Indian viewpoint best when he wrote, 'The *Indian Act* is a lever in our hands and an embarrassment to the government, as it should be ... We would rather continue to live in bondage under the inequitable *Indian Act* than surrender our sacred rights' (1969:140). What was at issue was not the question of the oppressive nature of federal administration of Indians (the Indians agreed with this), but rather Indian fears that this form of 'termination' without recognition of their special rights and unique status would lead to even greater assimilation and oppression by the provinces.

The federal government never formally adopted the White Paper on Indian policy, but the legacy of that failed effort was to shape Indian-federal relationships for more than two decades. Many Aboriginal people grew increasingly suspicious of Canada's motives whenever any new programs were announced. Fears that inherently assimilationist policies would be developed, perhaps under the rhetoric of 'equality,' remained constant.

An opportunity to entrench the rights of Aboriginal peoples within the Canadian federation came when Canada attempted to patriate the Constitution. Prior to the early 1980s, Canada's Constitution was actually the *British North America Act*. When it became evident that then-Prime Minister Pierre Trudeau was going to be successful in developing a new, 'made in Canada' Constitution, the Aboriginal peoples realized the opportunity was at hand to have their 'Aboriginal' rights recognized as well.

After a great deal of political activity, they were actually able to secure these ill-defined rights in the 1982 *Constitution Act*. Section 35 (1) states: 'The existing aboriginal and treaty rights of the aboriginal peoples of Canada are hereby recognized and affirmed.' And according to Section 35 (2), 'the aboriginal peoples of Canada' were to include 'the Indian, Inuit and Metis peoples of Canada.' This represented a major coup for the Métis in particular, who until that time were not really considered to be an 'Aboriginal' people on a par with the Indians and the Inuit. However, the question of what these specific 'aboriginal and treaty rights' were was not defined at the time; this was to be left for a subsequent First Ministers Conference (FMC).

In fact, between 1983 and 1987, four FMCs were held, attended by provincial premiers and the prime minister, their aides, and representatives of four major Aboriginal organizations: the Assembly of First Nations (status and treaty Indians), the Métis National Council (Métis), the Native Council of Canada (non-status Indians and off-reserve Indians), and the Inuit Tapirisat (Inuit). The conferences came to focus primarily on 'self-government' as the key Aboriginal and treaty right. The FMCs proved to be relatively fruitless exercises, with many of the first ministers refusing to entrench Aboriginal self-government in the Constitution in the absence of an agreed-upon working definition. Aboriginal groups insisted that this right be recognized as inherent, that is, a right they have always had and never surrendered; in contrast, most of the premiers seemed to support, at most, a policy of delegated authority, from federal and/or provincial governments to Aboriginal governments. Aboriginal leaders rejected this notion, and the talks ended with no agreement and much bitterness (Brizinski 1989:253).

In the wake of the collapse of the FMCs, the federal government continued to pursue its own agenda with regard to Aboriginal self-government, predicated on the notion of delegated powers and the creation of municipal-style Indian governments. In 1975, the *James Bay and Northern Quebec Agreement* had been signed between the Cree and Inuit of northern Quebec and the federal and Quebec governments. The subsequent *Cree-Naskapi (of Quebec) Act* of 1984 gave these northern Aboriginal peoples the authority to govern a wide variety of areas, such as education and health, although only as a result of delegated powers. Some hailed the agreement as a model; others condemned it as simply Aboriginal management of federal and provincial programs.

By 1986, the Sechelt Band in British Columbia had devised its own model of self-government, and had obtained federal government approval via Bill C-93. The bill allowed the band to take over many of the powers that the federal government had under the *Indian Act*, including obtaining fee-simple ownership of reserve lands and the ability to control education, health and social services, taxation, public order and safety, utilization of natural resources, and infrastructure developments. Again, this model was criticized in some quarters as being insufficient, since the federal government still, in effect, maintained legislative control over the band.

The 1980s saw the federal government develop many joint ventures with Indian bands, and many bands took delegated control of areas such as social services, education, and health under 'transfer' programs. In some instances, these programs involved the cooperation of provincial governments. However, the major national Indian organization, the Assembly of First Nations, in conjunction with the Métis National Council, the Native Council of Canada, and the Inuit Tapirisat, continued to lobby for constitutional recognition of the inherent right to self-government. The so-called Charlottetown Accord, rejected by the Canadian electorate in a referendum in October of 1992, contained within it just such a recognition amid a myriad of other items, most of which pertained to other constitutional matters. The fact that most Aboriginal people apparently voted against the accord came as a shock to some analysts and leaders. The complex notion of Aboriginal self-government is still years away from being sorted out.

In contrast to registered Indians, the Inuit have recently gained a form of public self-government with the approval to create a new territory in the eastern Arctic, to be known as Nunavut. By virtue of their demographic majority, the Inuit will be able to exercise political will over the territory. The Métis, on the other hand, continue to struggle to develop a form of self-government, hampered by the fact that they lack a land base and are scattered throughout the various western provinces.

CURRENT SOCIO-ECONOMIC CONDITIONS

The 1991 Aboriginal Peoples Survey (APS) (Statistics Canada 1993a, 1993b, 1993c) provides a snapshot of the general conditions of life for Aboriginal peoples; characteristically, such data are very general. To understand the health issues which currently face these peoples, and the prospects for change in health and health care, one must appreciate the significance of various factors.

Demographically, the Aboriginal population is quite young: 38 per cent were under the age fifteen, giving a dependency ratio of only 1.6

adults per child. In terms of education, and despite many new initiatives, it is evident that Aboriginal peoples have not yet attained educational levels on a par with other Canadians. For instance, in the fifteen to forty-nine age bracket, only 50 per cent of those in the survey reported having completed secondary school, with only 3 per cent having completed a university degree. Some 17 per cent had not completed grade 9. While 33 per cent of the Aboriginal people surveyed reported at least some post-secondary education experience, the figure for Canadians nationally was 51 per cent.

There is a relatively high unemployment rate among Aboriginal people. In Canada overall, the unemployment rate for Aboriginal people was almost 25 per cent, compared to around 10 per cent for Canadians in general; the labour force participation rate for Aboriginal people was only 57 per cent, compared to 68 per cent nationally. The highest unemployment rates were noted for Newfoundland (44.3 per cent) and the Yukon (35.4 per cent); the lowest for Ontario (17.1 per cent) and Alberta (23.8 per cent). However, these data mask the consequences of living in rural and remote areas. For instance, in some northern Aboriginal communities, the unemployment rate reaches as high as 90 per cent at various times throughout the year. In many communities, seasonal employment in wage labour or activities such as commercial fishing or trapping is often followed by long periods of unemployment.

Not surprisingly, reported income levels are lower for Aboriginal people. For instance, while 54 per cent of the Aboriginal respondents reported an annual income in 1990 of less than $10,000, only 35 per cent of Canadians as a whole did likewise (this includes individuals who reported earning no income). And while 15 per cent of Canadians reported an income in excess of $40,000, only 5 per cent of Aboriginal people did as well. But, as is the case for most socio-economic variables, there are significant discrepancies when we examine specific Aboriginal categories. For instance, on-reserve Indians and Inuit exhibit the highest proportion of income earners reporting less than $10,000 in annual income (65 per cent and 57 per cent, respectively); the proportion is lower among off-reserve Indians (50 per cent) and Métis (49 per cent).

Data such as these mask the effects of regional differences and other relevant conditions of life for Aboriginal peoples. In general, for those Indians living on reserves, lower educational levels and higher unemployment rates than the national Aboriginal standards are reported in the 1991 survey. Similar results are found for various infrastructure variables.

Housing and infrastructure problems are invariably related to many of the health problems people experience. In general, the housing and living conditions of Aboriginal people have consistently been poor and below national standards. Despite many initiatives by both federal and provincial governments to provide electricity, proper sewage disposal, potable water, and better quality housing, discrepancies still exist. The 1991 APS (Canada, DNHW 1994) reported a higher average number of persons per dwelling and persons per room in Aboriginal households than in households nationally. While 32 per cent of homes nationally required either minor or major repairs, 49 per cent of Aboriginal households were in need of repair. Residents of Indian reserves, in particular, experience poor housing conditions, with 68 per cent of homes requiring minor or major repairs.

Most Aboriginal homes obtain water from municipal sources, but for 20 per cent of these the available water is considered undrinkable. Some people still draw their water from lakes and rivers, or have it trucked to their residences. While 89 per cent of Aboriginal homes have flush toilets and 6 per cent use outhouses, for reserve homes the figures are 75 per cent and 22 per cent respectively. Overall, 93 per cent of Aboriginal homes have electricity and 94 per cent have heating systems. On these indicators, reserve residents appear not to be disadvantaged. However, while wood is used as a source of heat in 18 per cent of homes overall, it is used in 43 per cent of reserve homes.

CONCLUSIONS

This introductory overview of the Aboriginal peoples in Canada has been necessarily brief. It has not been possible to examine individual cultures, or major historical processes, to any great extent. Such an understanding is nevertheless important for those who wish to understand current health issues affecting Aboriginal peoples. We would direct your attention to the literature referred to in this chapter for more comprehensive treatment of these issues. What we have established here is that the Aboriginal peoples of Canada are exceptionally diverse, culturally, linguistically, socially, economically, and in other ways. The recognition and acceptance of such diversity is essential to an accurate understanding of developments in the health care field and to an appreciation of the myriad processes that have affected the health status of Aboriginal peoples in both the pre-contact and the post-contact periods. The remainder of this book will examine these aspects in greater detail.

2

Health and disease in the pre-contact period

One of the important questions to be addressed in any history of health and disease among Aboriginal Canadians concerns the extensive period of time before sustained European contact. Scholars investigating this problem depend on a body of mostly fragmentary material evidence that has been pieced together by physical anthropologists and palaeopathologists from surviving tissue in the form of bone, teeth, and mummified remains in an archaeological context. What this evidence means is then interpreted in the light of current theories and methods in these fields, with reference to contemporary thinking about disease, and by comparison to the health experience of Aboriginal populations elsewhere in the world.

By and large, such studies have depicted the people of the Americas as relatively healthy and disease-free prior to European contact. The image of good health appears to be particularly compelling when contrasted, as it often is, to the post-contact period (popularly defined as AD 1492 and onward), when new diseases from Eurasia and Africa produced epidemics that dramatically altered the social and biological structure of Aboriginal communities. Henry Dobyns (1983) wrote in *Their Number Become Thinned*: 'Aside from *verruga* and some form of venereal disease, almost the only biological weapons Native Americans possessed were severe forms of intestinal parasites ... The near absence of lethal pathogens in the aboriginal New World allowed the native peoples to live in almost a paradise of well-being that contrasted with their historic purgatory of disease' (35).

The idea of a kind of pre-contact Eden finds expression in frequently cited quotations about the extraordinary health and physical fitness of Aboriginal Americans at contact (see T.K. Young 1988:32). It is buttressed by the concept of an Arctic disease filter which is hypothesized to have transformed the microbiological flora and fauna of migrants from Asia to the Americas (Stewart 1973:19–20). These ideas are linked, in turn, to the impression of a special vulnerability to introduced infection, owing to this lack of experience with pathogens common elsewhere in the world, as in Wherrett's (1965:57) observation that 'The Indian seems to have lacked the natural resistance [to tuberculosis] of white people.' Further support comes from recollections of Aboriginal people of the time before European contact, when: 'There was then no sickness; they had no aching bones; they then had no high fever ... no smallpox; ... no burning chest; ... no abdominal pain; ... no consumption; ... no headache' (Crosby 1972:36, cited in Merbs 1992:4).

Ecological and demographic arguments have also served to bolster the view that infectious diseases were rare prior to sustained European contact. It has been suggested that there are four major factors that historically led infectious diseases to gain prominence in human populations: sufficiently large population sizes to enable some infections to become established and others to be amplified; social conditions, such as crowding and poor hygiene, which increased the opportunity for diseases to be spread from person to person; undernutrition, which increased overall susceptibility to disease; and close contact with animals, domesticated or not, which were reservoirs for micro-organisms (McKeown 1988:48).

In the case of the Americas, it is generally agreed that the lack of domestic animals, such as cows, sheep, pigs, ducks, and chickens, which are reservoirs of viral and bacterial infection and potential sources of infection for humans, reduced the range of infectious diseases which had the potential to afflict pre-contact populations. Likewise, the general absence within Canada[1] of the large and dense populations usually associated with large-scale agriculture (see Cohen 1989:38–54) suggests that acute community infections, such as measles, could not have been sustained in the small, dispersed social groups which typified most societies in the Subarctic and Arctic.

These are the central premises upon which the vision of a relatively disease-free pre-contact Aboriginal life is based. Yet, as more evidence has accumulated through the work of epidemiologists, physical anthropologists, and archaeologists (see Verano and Ubelaker 1992; Larsen and Milner 1994), it has become increasingly difficult to support the disease-free view which is 'partly conjecture, and partly myth' (Merbs, 1992:4). That infectious disease loads grew substantially with sustained European contact is undisputed, but there is no reason to believe that transmissible diseases were absent in the pre-contact period or that they did not take a substantial toll of human life from time to time in various communities (Merbs 1992; Saunders, Ramsden, and Herring 1992; Herring 1992; Larsen 1994). What appears to be emerging is a new approach to the epidemiology of the pre-contact Americas that stresses diversity in the experience of disease, and at the same time attempts to understand local patterns of morbidity and mortality within the social and ecological contexts that may have given rise to them.

CONSTRUCTING IMAGES OF PRE-CONTACT DISEASE

It is no easy task to construct a coherent picture of pre-contact health and disease. The project in fact is acknowledged to be largely inferential, based on limited information and analytic methods (Johansson 1982:134–5). The reconstruction of prehistoric disease patterns depends extensively on the careful weighing and patching together of several lines of evidence by various researchers working independently on diverse questions, rather than on a single grand synthesis by a lone researcher. To appreciate the pitfalls in the endeavour and to develop a healthy respect for its limitations, it is necessary to be fully aware of the problems facing investigators of pre-contact disease patterns.

Chief among these is the daunting time span over which health and disease must be appraised over the huge geographical expanse of present-day Canada.[2] If a new generation is produced every twenty to thirty years, a truly comprehensive survey of health and disease must be based on archaeological evidence for some 600 to 1,000 generations of people who lived at different times and places, in a variety of social and environmental circumstances. After all, there is no reason to suppose that pre-contact American societies were any less complex, dynamic, diverse, or subject to social change than societies elsewhere in the world, even if they have often been represented as static and unchanging until European contact (Dobyns 1983:25).

It is obviously unrealistic to expect such a fine degree of texture and historical detail, so broad generalizations about disease over time and space are often made out of necessity. They remain generalizations, nonetheless, and care must be taken to avoid according the status of dogma to provisional assessments and to refrain from assuming that broad regional or time trends have been replicated at the community level. It also is worth recalling that archaeological work is not spread evenly across the country. Some regions have longer and more extensive records than others, either because of preservation conditions, length of time of occupation, a history of archaeological interest in the area, the pace of urban development, or just plain luck. Legitimate concerns by Aboriginal groups about the removal, study, and reburial of Aboriginal human remains has effectively limited pre-contact skeletal research in some provinces, such as Ontario.

The dearth of material from which information about health and disease can be inferred further complicates the creation of plausible pre-contact scenarios. The evidence generally falls into two categories: material remains from the past and studies of living populations undergoing recent or new contact with developing and developed societies.

MAKING INFERENCES ABOUT PRE-CONTACT HEALTH

The clearest available signs of pre-contact health and disease come from autopsies of intentionally or accidentally mummified human remains. Just such an examination led to the identification of acid-fast bacilli of *Mycobacterium tuberculosis*, the micro-organism associated with tuberculosis, in the lungs of a young Peruvian boy whose death is estimated to have occurred in the eighth century, some 800 years before European contact (Allison, Mendoza, and Pezzia 1973). Many other infectious and non-infectious diseases, antigens, and evidence of medical treatment have been identified from autopsies of pre-contact mummies (see Allison 1976).

Preserved human faeces, also known as coprolites, provide information on pre-contact parasitic infestations. Roundworms have been found in archaeological sites in the Colorado Plateau dating from 1100 BC to AD 200 (Fry 1974), and pinworms come from many other sites as well (Rheinhard, Ambler, and McGuffie 1985). Hookworms may have debilitated people from the American Southeast prior to 200 BC (Rheinhard 1992). Parasite burdens, however, tend to decrease with increasing latitude and thus were probably less of a threat north of 40° North. On the other hand, consumption of animal food tends to increase with latitude, heightening the risks of meat-borne parasitic infections (Cohen 1989:98). In all likelihood, roundworms, trematodes, and tapeworms of domestic dogs and wolves were transmitted to pre-contact Alaskans (Fortuine 1989:60) and, presumably, to other Arctic dwellers (see chapter 4, pages 81–2).

Lest worm infestations be taken lightly, Riley (1993) points out that roundworm larvae can infect the lungs, producing pneumonia or symptoms of asthma; they can also lodge in and cause damage to the central nervous system. Adult roundworms inhabit the lumen of the alimentary tract, inducing nausea, vomiting, and sleeplessness; they produce abdominal distension in children and inhibit normal growth. Hookworm infections provoke iron-deficiency anaemia in both adults and children and can compromise the immune system's ability to cope with other infections. In other words, these are seriously debilitating parasites that not only afflicted past Aboriginal populations, but may even have been treated with *Chemopodium* (goosefoot or lamb's-quarters) in some societies (Riley 1993).

Mummified human remains and coprolites are quite rare in the Canadian context. More often than not, skeletal and dental remains provide the best clues to past diseases. Much of the skeletal evidence is non-specific in nature, showing up as general inflammations of bone like osteomyelitis and periostitis. Aspects of dental form and structure, tooth wear, dental caries, periodontal disease, and developmental defects help skeletal biologists reconstruct past lifestyles (Mayhall 1992:75). In fact, dental pathology is considered to be a reliable general marker of disease loads and nutritional stress. Evidence of shifts in the frequency of dental pathology over time and space allows valuable inferences to be made about episodic or altered disease stress and malnutrition, but it is difficult nonetheless to take such observations to a more precise level of disease specificity. It may be necessary to turn to epidemiological studies of dental disease in living people to sort out the impact of cultural differences and change on pre-contact peoples (Skinner and Goodman 1992:169)

Because of the scarcity and non-specific nature of most of the skeletal and dental evidence, only the barest epidemiological outlines can be sketched for the pre-contact period – what Ortner (1992:5) calls 'probabilities, possibilities, and impossibilities.' It is virtually impossible to outline a clearly defined suite of specific diseases for particular times and places, let alone determine what the leading causes of illness and death were or the magnitude of disease loads. Acute infectious diseases rarely leave signs on bone, so their effects must be deduced from other indirect clues, such as unusual age profiles in skeletal samples (Jackes 1983; Larocque 1991), or from bone-tissue responses to the presence of infection (Stuart-Macadam 1992).

The diagnostic process is made even more complex because different micro-organisms produce similar effects on bone. The similarities between osseous lesions resulting from tuberculosis and those produced by pathogenic fungi, for instance, led Shadomy to dub their associated micro-organisms 'the great mimics' (Shadomy 1981:25). Knowledge of the contemporary geographic distribution of micro-organisms and their ecological affinities also assists with the detective process (see Long and Merbs 1981; Pfeiffer 1984:188).

There is also a very marked bias in the kinds of infectious conditions which are expressed and detectable in bone. Most lesions stem from chronic *bacterial* infections which have followed a protracted course that, ironically, the individual survived owing to adequate immunological resistance. In other words, there is a paradoxical tendency for the evidence for disease, infectious or otherwise, to come from the remains of *healthier* individuals (see Wood et al. 1992). There is some optimism that antibodies to viral diseases may eventually be extractable from archaeological bone and thus expand the array of identifiable diseases in the past, but the results so far are mixed. Measles, smallpox, scarlet fever, and influenza, to name a few, are important infectious diseases which cannot be detected in bone.[3]

Because the symptoms and soft-tissue evidence needed to make provisional diagnoses are not observable in bone, investigators essentially must evaluate a distinctive *patterning* of bone lesions throughout the skeleton to narrow down the range of possible underlying conditions. This is particularly important, for instance, for distinguishing leprosy from yaws and syphilis (Steinbock 1976). Comparison of the patterns of distribution of osteoarthritis in some pre- and post-contact skeletal remains from the Americas suggests that activity and work patterns changed after European contact (Larsen 1994:140).

Here the issues of completeness, preservation, and sample sizes of skeletal populations come to the fore. Depending on the conditions of deposition, a skeleton, or more frequently *parts* of a skeleton, may survive the effects of climate, moisture, soil conditions, plant roots, farmers' ploughs, rodent gnawing, animal scavenging, or any other post-mortem environmental factor which may distort or destroy skeletal remains. The surface and microstructure of the bones may be well preserved, permitting detailed analysis, or they may be so worn or pitted that they cannot be studied. Sometimes post-mortem disturbances by plants and animals create the illusion of pathogenic processes. Henderson (1987) describes a misdiagnosis of syphilis made on the basis of cranial lesions that were produced by post-mortem chewing by beetles!

The small size of many skeletal samples lowers the statistical probabilities of detecting the presence of a disease in bone. Tuberculosis is a case in point. If tuberculosis is manifest in bones and joints in from 1 per cent (T.M. Daniel 1981) to 7 per cent of cases (Steinbock 1976), then the chances of finding it in a skeletal sample are low, even if the disease was prevalent when the population was living. Indeed, while large skeletal samples increase the odds of finding examples of pathological lesions, there is still the difficulty of translating their presence into meaningful statements about a community's experience of the disease. In her study of the pre-contact Uxbridge ossuary (1490 +/− AD 80) from southern Ontario, for instance, Pfeiffer (1984) identified a minimum of 8 children and 18 adults with tubercular lesions out of a possible 457 individuals. These people represent a population that lived over many years. However, because the age structure of mortality from tuberculosis changes over time (Frost 1939) as the population experiences the epidemic wave (Grigg 1958; Bates 1982), we can only speculate about what these results might mean in terms of the Uxbridge peoples' history of exposure to and death from tuberculosis.

Sampling problems also influence our understanding of non-infectious conditions in the prehistoric past. Because no large skeletal samples have been excavated in the Cree-Ojibwa territory, we cannot ascertain whether congenital dislocation of the hip was as common in the pre-contact period as the unusually high prevalence of 6 per cent suggests for the region in the twentieth century (Pfeiffer 1991:14). Clearly, the calculation of basic epidemiological measures such as prevalence and incidence is difficult, if not impossible, for the pre-contact period, as is the charting of epidemics.

Although the issues of sample size and representativeness are troubling (see Saunders and Herring 1995), advances in the analysis of bone tissue at the microscopic and molecular levels may help circumvent some of the problems associated with morphological assessments of skeletal pathology (see Rothschild 1992). The tantalizing possibilities inherent in immunological approaches, which involve recognizing specific antibodies in bone, are also just beginning to be realized. The identification in present-day Indiana of treponemal disease[1] in a Pleistocene bear via antisyphilis antisera (Rothschild and Turnbull 1987), though controversial, has generated great enthusiasm about the prospect for immunological techniques to solve long-standing debates about pre-contact disease. However, other attempts at identifying specific diseases immunologically have been stymied by technical problems and by antigenic cross-reactions between micro-organisms (Rothschild 1992:137). These approaches, along with research into DNA extraction, nonetheless represent the wave of the future in terms of differential diagnosis of disease in archaeological bone. DNA from *Mycobacterium tuberculosis* (Salo et al. 1994) and from *Trepo-*

nema (Rogan and Lentz 1994) have been extracted from pre-contact mummies from South America, for example, and research along these lines is multiplying rapidly.

Other sophisticated methods for going beyond surface marks on bone to cellular and chemical levels have further expanded the amount of information that can be gleaned from human remains. Microscopic analysis of thin sections of bone, for instance, makes it possible to compare adult bone mass and cortical bone density between populations and, hence, the risks of fracture (Pfeiffer 1991; Southern 1990). Evaluation of the chemical constituents and trace elements offers a means of assessing diet and nutritional stress. The introduction of maize into the Great Lakes region of southern Ontario, for instance, has been well documented through the analysis of stable carbon isotopes (Schwarcz et al. 1985), and attempts have been made to link this dietary change to specific disease indicators (Katzenberg 1992). It should be evident nevertheless that a true 'palaeo-epidemiology' of the Americas has yet to be developed and that it may never be possible to discuss fully the dynamics, determinants, and distribution of prehistoric diseases:

We can never know what specific physiological, immunologic, or genetic characteristics prevailed in earlier human populations which may have influenced the invasiveness, virulence, or pathogenicity of infectious agents. Similarly, we do not know what specific physiological or genetic characteristics prevailed in prehistoric bacteria, viruses, or fungi which may have conditioned their effect on human hosts. Simply put, the specific nature and course of host-parasite relationships, as revealed and understood in modern clinical and epidemiological studies, may not be exactly the same as in the past. (Widmer and Perzigian 1981:100)

Despite these important caveats and limitations, a great deal has been learned about many facets of pre-contact disease in what has become present-day Canada. This is illustrated with examples drawn from three areas: southern Ontario Iroquoia, the Arctic, and the Northwest Coast.

PRE-CONTACT DISEASES IN CANADA

1 Southern Ontario Iroquoia

Southern Ontario Iroquoia encompasses an area of approximately 40,000 square miles between Lakes Ontario, Erie, and Huron. This is the area in which the Huron, Petun, and Neutral tribal groups lived when the first

Europeans visited the region in the early 1600s. Archaeological excavations in the region have produced some of the most extensively studied collections of Aboriginal skeletal remains in Canada.

While many of the sites have yielded relatively small and poorly preserved skeletal samples, others are ossuaries consisting of thousands of individual bones, representing the remains of hundreds of individuals (Anderson 1969; Pfeiffer 1986; Jackes 1994). Most of these sites were excavated more than twenty years ago, owing to a voluntary research moratorium in this region on all but salvage sites (Pfeiffer and Fairgrieve 1994). This extraordinary abundance of information has stimulated intense interest and analysis by a large cadre of skeletal biologists over several decades (Anderson 1969; Hartney 1981; Jackes 1986, 1988; Katzenberg 1989; Katzenberg et al. 1993; Molto and Melbye 1984; Patterson 1984; Pfeiffer 1984, 1986, 1991; Pfeiffer and King 1983; Saunders 1988; Saunders and Melbye 1990; Schwarcz et al. 1985; Southern 1990; Saunders et al. 1992).

Equally important to the enterprise is a strong and well-defined archaeological record which includes whole village plans, controlled dating of sites based on artifact and radiocarbon analyses, and detailed regional sequences. Without reasonably good appraisals of the socio-ecological context of the living population, it is difficult to evaluate its skeletal remains and develop hypotheses about prevailing diseases and causes of death. Fortunately, the archaeological sequence for southern Ontario is quite solid and offers insight into changes over time in subsistence activities, trade routes, population size and density, patterns of migration and other forms of interpersonal contact, village sanitation and relocation practices, seasonal resource availability, and the presence of reservoirs and possible vectors for the spread of infection (Starna et al. 1984; Fecteau et al. 1991). The accumulated evidence makes it clear that there were significant social, demographic, and health changes in the region well before European contact.

Of course, the question of what actually constitutes 'contact' needs to be addressed at this point. Even though AD 1492 has become a powerful metaphor for the cascade of processes set in motion as a result of the first contact between people from the western Mediterranean and the Americas, direct and regular contact between ethnically diverse groups of Europeans and North Americans began at different times, in different places. For southern Ontario, the onset of the beaver fur trade around AD 1580 essentially represents the point at which intense and habitual direct contact occurred between Europeans and Aboriginal groups. The pre-contact period for this region therefore ends in the last decades of the sixteenth century, although European influences reached the area before this time.

Much of the research on skeletal remains from pre-contact sites falls into three categories: identification of nutritionally mediated disease stress associated with the introduction of maize from the sixth to the fourteenth centuries, evaluation of time trends in the incidence of non-specific disease indicators such as caries and bone density, and detection and assessment of the impact of specific infectious diseases.

Considerable attention has been paid to the relationship between a nutritional shift towards higher carbohydrate consumption in the form of maize and changes in disease patterns over time (Katzenberg and Schwarcz 1986; Schwarcz et al. 1985; Katzenberg, Saunders, and Fitzgerald 1993). It is not known exactly when maize entered the diet or became a widely cultivated food source, but the combined results of carbon isotope[5] and archaeological analysis indicate that maize consumption increased significantly between AD 500 and 1200. Although it probably never made up more than 50 per cent of the pre-contact diet, maize nevertheless became a major food source between AD 900 and 1300 (Schwarcz et al. 1985). Over roughly the same period, the consumption of animal protein remained quite stable and the subsistence base of pre-contact Iroquoian villages involved mixed swidden horticulture, hunting, fishing, and collecting from the fifth century to the contact period.

The impact of the trend towards an increasingly large maize component in the diet on the health of pre-contact Iroquoian peoples is difficult to assess. There is a large anthropological literature that equates horticultural and agricultural societies with higher pathogen loads, largely because settled village life is associated with the accumulation of wastes, increased contact with domesticated animals, and higher population densities which enhance the opportunities for transmission of infectious diseases. Heavy reliance on cultigens, moreover, places a population at risk of starvation from periodic crop failures and from nutritional deficiencies, depending on the extent to which monoculture is practised and essential amino acids are missing from the diet (Cohen 1989). This sets up the well-known synergistic cycle of malnutrition–infectious disease–malnutrition so common in less developed countries today.

In this regard, the regular relocation of Iroquoian villages at twelve- to twenty-year intervals has been attributed to soil and other local resource depletion as well as to crop infestations; but deteriorating village conditions, dreams, and misfortune also may have contributed to the relocation cycle (Starna, Hamell, and Butts 1984; Fecteau et al. 1991). It cannot be denied, however, that pre-contact Iroquoian villages exploited a wide range of nutritional sources and never relied completely on cultivated crops. Katzenberg's (1992) stable isotope analysis suggests nonetheless that bone lesions from infections were highest when maize consumption was highest, although this may have been influenced by concomitant increases in population density which would have enhanced the chances of disease transmission.

Further support for a link between maize horticulture and infectious disease comes from the skeletal remains of twenty-nine individuals from the MacPherson Site, a pre-contact Ontario Neutral Iroquoian village site dated to AD 1530–80.[6] Two young children aged three to four years present the only known cases of circular caries detected so far among the southern Ontario skeletal remains (Katzenberg, Saunders, and Fitzgerald 1993). Circular caries is a defect in the enamel which develops during deciduous tooth formation; later, caries form in the portions of the tooth where the enamel is thin. Such lesions are particularly prevalent today in children from countries with less developed economies and are often a consequence of malnutrition following chronic diarrhoea. This has led Katzenberg and co-workers to hypothesize that the circular caries in the MacPherson children were the scars of nutritionally mediated infection during early postnatal development. The ratios of nitrogen isotopes indicate that the diet onto which these children were weaned was high in maize. Since high carbohydrate weaning diets may contribute to child mortality, the combination of nutritionally mediated infection and a high-carbohydrate weaning diet may have created insurmountable stress for these two children. However, like most of the data that bear on the question of pre-contact disease, this evidence, though persuasive, is still non-specific and indirect. There is no way to determine which infectious diseases might have afflicted the children, for how long, or how often.

Other indirect evidence for nutritionally related conditions in pre-contact southern Ontario Iroquoia is summarized by Pfeiffer (1991) and Pfeiffer and Fairgrieve (1994). One of the more intriguing conditions found at a number of pre- and post-contact adult Iroquoian sites is relatively thin childhood and adult cortical bone. This is significant because growth in cortical-bone thickness can be retarded during nutritional and disease stress. In fact, the density of bone among adult Iroquoians appears to have decreased over time and reached subnormal values by the late fifteenth century (Southern 1990). Although thin cortical bone has been interpreted as possible evidence for disease stress (Saunders, Ramsden, and Herring 1992), it is difficult to disentangle the relative contributions that diet, disease, nutrition-disease interaction, or other factors may have made to the phenomenon (Pfeiffer and Fairgrieve 1994). This is presumptive evidence, nonetheless, that health was declining in some groups in the region before European contact.

The identification of porotic hyperostosis in skeletal remains from a number of pre-contact sites constitutes additional presumptive evidence for the action of infectious disease. Porotic hyperostosis is a condition of the skull vault visible to the unaided eye as small holes of varying size on the surface of the bone. There is general agreement among skeletal biologists that it is most often a manifestation of acquired iron-deficiency anaemia. Until recently, the condition was considered to be an indication of nutritional stress, but a new perspective argues that the withholding of iron (hypoferrin) which porotic hyperostosis expresses is more properly viewed as successful adaptation to pathogen stress (Stuart-Macadam 1992). Regardless of the source of hematological stress, there is solid evidence of porotic hyperostosis from a number of pre-contact sites, with the Fairty ossuary sample showing an especially high prevalence of 38 per cent among juveniles (Pfeiffer and Fairgrieve 1994).

Although the discussion so far has emphasized *non-specific* indicators of disease, there is also clear evidence for the pre-contact presence of *specific* infectious diseases in southern Ontario. A great deal of attention has been paid to tuberculosis, whose presence has been identified by numerous investigators in sites from AD 100 to AD 1650 (Hartney 1981). This has led some to speculate that tuberculosis epidemics occurred in the region prior to European contact (Pfeiffer 1984). Several cases of treponemal disease have also been described (Molto and Melbye 1984; Saunders 1988).

Southern Ontario Iroquoia, especially just prior to direct European contact, appears to have been a particularly fertile ground for infectious disease. From the eighth to the seventeenth centuries there are clear trends to increasing population density, larger and more numerous villages, and increased population density within villages. Crowding within villages was quite high, and longhouses were rarely separated by more than three metres. Refuse dumps, consisting mostly of organic waste, dotted the villages, usually no more than eight metres from the longhouses (Warwick 1984). By the second half of the fifteenth century and certainly by the time that trade goods appear in Ontario Iroquoian sites, these socio-demographic changes had increased the opportunity for outbreaks of infectious disease (Saunders, Ramsden, and Herring 1992). It has been argued, moreover, from evidence from Huron ossuaries that fertility was not high enough to sustain the population in the face of the disastrous famines, wars, and epidemics that swept through Huronia between AD 1634 and AD 1650 (Jackes 1994).

2 The Arctic

In contrast to the relative wealth of skeletal information on pre-contact health and disease in southern Ontario Iroquoian populations, there is very little information about Arctic populations. Vanast claims, in fact, that 'scholars have almost completely avoided the medical aspects of arctic history' (Vanast 1991:76). What evidence there is comes from studies of Aleutian mummies and from skeletal remains from sites throughout the Arctic, but especially from Alaska and the Aleutian islands. Speculation based on climatic and demographic patterns, along with references to health and disease in early contact narratives, figure prominently in current reconstructions of pre-contact epidemiologic patterns in the Arctic.

The Arctic regions occupy a particularly important intellectual space in the thinking about pre-contact disease in the Americas. The idea of a disease-free America, in fact, is predicated upon the idea that a 'cold screen' filtered out Old World diseases during the peopling of the Americas via the Bering Land Bridge.[7] The concept, popularized by T. Dale Stewart in his influential book *The People of America*, depicted Beringia and the northern regions leading to and from it 'as a germ filter that served to hold back the diseases of the people who passed through it' (Stewart 1973:19). This ensured that 'the men who passed through this cold zone in effect passed through a germ filter, leaving behind whatever disease germs there were in the old world' and that 'only the fittest survived the harsh northern climate that existed over the whole distance' (Stewart 1973:20). In Stewart's vision, ice and glaciers acted as significant barriers to pathogens and prevented contact with Eurasian populations. The cold climate, moreover, was 'unfavourable to the spread and perpetuation of disease germs' (Stewart 1973:19). This depiction of the northern regions as inimical to infectious disease has some merit. Parasite burdens tend to decrease with increasing latitude, and the relatively simple Arctic ecosystem supports lower species diversity than tropical regions (Dunn 1968:226–7). Fewer viruses are found in temperate than tropical zones (van Rooyen 1968:548.) Diseases caused by parasites which spend part of their life cycle outside the host, like hookworms, are substantially less common in the north (Cohen 1989:98). Cold climates are inhospitable for many insect vectors and, hence, preclude infection with the pathogenic micro-organisms they harbour (Newman 1976:668).

Stewart's idealization of the health of Arctic peoples is not supported by current evidence, however, and it is clear that they were anything but disease-free prior to European contact. Robert Fortuine (1989), in particular, refutes many of the traditional contentions about a natural or genetic tendency to good health in the pre-contact Arctic. He draws attention to environmental hazards, such as toxic substances in water hemlock and other poisonous plants; the potential for paralytic shellfish poisoning; and the danger of ingesting environmental type E *Clostridium botulinum* in soil, associated with marine mammal butchering (Fortuine 1989: 53–6).

As for the purported lack of insect vectors, it is worth remembering that the necessary conditions for the reproduction of biting insects are created whenever surface water accumulates in tundra and taiga climates. Mosquitoes (*Culicidae*), black flies (*Simulidae*), snipe flies (*Leptidae*), punkies (*Heleidae cubicoides*), and house flies (*Tabanidae*) multiply profusely in the Arctic (van Rooyen 1968:548): 'No one who has passed a summer in Alaska has failed to notice – sometimes in unprintable language – the myriads of biting insects that swarm around any warm-blooded creature, including humans ... Mosquitoes, although present throughout Alaska, were a particular curse in the coastal areas ... Continuous scratching of bites usually led to skin infections such as impetigo, which could then be spread to other parts of the body or to other persons' (Fortuine 1989: 57). Lice and their eggs are commonly found in pre-contact Aleut mummies, and early contact narratives confirm that Arctic peoples sustained heavy infestations of head and body lice. The combination of crowded living and sleeping conditions, heavy fur clothing, and a shortage of water created 'almost perfect living conditions' for them (Fortuine 1989: 64).

Exposure to pathogenic micro-organisms also occurred simply because northern populations were in frequent and close contact with mammals (domestic and feral), birds, fish, and insects, as well as with their waste products (Cohen 1989). Bacterial diseases such as brucellosis (caribou reservoir), tularemia (probable muskrat reservoir), and salmonellosis (birds) found in Arctic wildlife today may have infected pre-contact communities. Although rabies has long been endemic in Arctic foxes and wolves, it is not yet possible to determine whether these animals acted as its reservoirs prior to European contact (Fortuine, 1989:62–3).

The heavy emphasis on animal foods in the diet of Arctic peoples also resulted in enhanced exposure to food-borne parasites, especially in uncooked meat. Trichinosis, roundworms, trematodes, and the tapeworms of domestic dogs and wolves can be acquired through eating ungulates like moose and caribou (Fortuine 1989:59). Not surprisingly, Eskimos have been observed to suffer from trichinosis and tapeworms (Cohen 1989:98). Careful autopsies of Aleutian mummies have confirmed the presence of a variety of infections, including trichinosis and fish trematode infestations, prior to European contact. Respiratory diseases, such as pneumonia and anthracosis,[8] and a possible case of the fungal infection associated with histoplasmosis, have also been identified. There are clear cases of chronic otitis media and mastoiditis as well (Zimmerman, Yeatman, Sprinz, and Titterington 1971; Zimmerman and Smith 1975; Zimmerman, Trinkaus, LeMay, et al. 1981; Zimmerman and Aufderheide 1984).

Early contact narratives from the Arctic also provide a glimpse of some of the health problems prevalent at the time. They contain many references to skin ulcers, sores, boils, carbuncles, and throat infections (Fortuine 1989:65–7). In contrast, diarrhoeal diseases receive scant mention, but 'the record of a brief or casual encounter with Alaska Natives would not be expected to include observations on the frequency or character of their stools' (Fortuine 1989:70). Of course, the brevity of such contacts and the heavy clothing of Arctic peoples would have hidden all but the most obvious signs of illness, so only particularly noticeable symptoms would have been mentioned. The very sick would have stayed behind in the village, further skewing the impressions of health and disease formed by early explorers (Fortuine 1971).

In any event, virtually none of the infections, infestations, or intoxications mentioned so far can be diagnosed in bone. This explains to a great extent why much of the skeletal research on pre-contact Arctic populations has emphasized more readily observable dental disease, trauma, cribra orbitalia / porotic hyperostosis, various lesions, and evidence for non-specific infections, treponemal disease, and tuberculosis (T.D. Stewart 1932, 1979; Merbs, Wilson, and Laughlin 1961; Merbs and Wilson 1960; Merbs 1963; Way 1978; Salter 1984). It fails to explain why there have been so few systematic skeletal analyses of temporal changes in the health of Arctic populations (Keenleyside 1993; an exception is Laughlin, Harper, and Thompson 1979). Schindler (1985) has taken the provocative stance that skeletal biologists working on Arctic material have been preoccupied with the antiquated and long-abandoned anthropological enterprise of race classification, instead of exploring the dynamic interaction between culture and biology. It should be noted, however, that most

Arctic skeletal remains date to the post-contact or late pre-contact periods, prior to which sample sizes are exceedingly small (Cybulski, personal communication).

In her analysis of osteological collections held at the Smithsonian Institution in Washington, Anne Keenleyside (1993, 1994) documents a number of health problems diagnosable in the skeletal remains of 193 Alaskan Aleuts and northern coastal Eskimos from five pre-contact sites. As one would expect, most of the infectious lesions were of non-specific origin, although active periostitis on the pleural surfaces of the ribs of one young adult male indicates some form of pre-contact respiratory infection. The presence of cribra orbitalia and porotic hyperostosis in the cranial remains was also noted, evidence of bone tissue response to pathogen load. Fractures of the crania, ribs, clavicles, hands, and feet were the most common type of trauma observed.

As other researchers have noted, and in contrast to southern Ontario Iroquoia, there is no conclusive evidence either for tuberculosis or for treponemal disease in the pre-contact Arctic. In fact, there is general agreement that both were likely to have been acquired by Arctic people recently, probably through contact with eighteenth-century Russian fur hunters and nineteenth-century European whalers (Keenleyside 1990:7–8; Holcomb 1940). The rarity of dental disease also stands in stark contrast to the situation found in pre-contact southern Ontario (Keenleyside 1993:4). This difference is likely explained by dietary differences between the two regions, with the higher carbohydrate diet associated with maize horticulture in southern Ontario resulting in greater nutritionally mediated dental disease.

Perhaps the most interesting feature of Keenleyside's work is the documentation and discussion of significant differences in health between the pre-contact Aleut and Eskimo samples. The Aleut skeletal remains showed significantly more trauma and infection than those of the Eskimos. The higher frequency of trauma among adult Aleut males may reflect their greater involvement in warfare, which is suggested by the archaeological record during this period and by Aleut oral tradition. Although there is probably a complex of factors that underlies the higher prevalence of infection among Aleuts, Keenleyside suggests that housing differences between Aleuts and Eskimos may have contributed to it. Since Aleuts lived in large, semi-subterranean dwellings estimated to have accommodated anywhere from 30 to 300 people, the opportunity for the spread of infection was substantially higher than that for the Eskimos, who occupied much smaller houses containing 8 to 12 individuals (Keenleyside 1993:5–6). In other words, it appears that differences in the pre-contact social contexts of the two groups produced divergences in their health profiles, just as one would expect.

3 The Northwest Coast

The early contact period for the Northwest Coast generally spans the late eighteenth to mid-nineteenth centuries. While it has been argued that introduced diseases diffused over large geographical expanses and infected Aboriginal groups who had no direct contact with Europeans (Dobyns 1983, 1992; Reff 1991), archaeological, historical, and Indian oral tradition sources indicate that this was not the case for the Northwest Coast. Old World diseases appear to have been introduced to this region quite late, after 1774 (Boyd 1992:249). The pre-contact period for this area, therefore, is not located in the distant past but hovers just three or four generations beyond living memory.

The best known Northwest Coast archaeological and osteological sequences come from coastal British Columbia (Cybulski 1994), developed from the results of systematic, controlled excavations carried out in the 1960s and 1970s (Cybulski 1990:55). The earliest human remains date to 3500 BC and coincide with the onset of shell-midden build-up that typifies most prehistoric sites in coastal British Columbia. There are thirty pre-contact sites where preservation and completeness are sufficient to allow analysis of 759 skeletal individuals. The skeletal remains, however, do not represent all areas or times, and about three-quarters of them are dated between 1500 BC and AD 500 (Middle Development Stage) and come from sites at Prince Rupert Harbour and the Strait of Georgia (Cybulski 1994). Full skeletal remains are not always available, narrowing the accuracy of differential diagnosis in such cases because assessment of lesion patterns is critical for discerning the likelihood that infectious diseases like tuberculosis or the treponematoses were present (Cybulski 1990:56).

Much of the writing about prehistoric coastal British Columbia emphasizes cultural continuity in the various regional sequences and depicts gradual social change over the 5,000 or so years that precede European contact. New research and interpretations suggest otherwise and emphasize the dynamic relationship between the various groups of people and their socio-ecological environment. Evidence from dental-abrasion facets caused by the use of labrets, coupled with diversity in head-shape modification practices over time and space suggests greater degrees of social change in the pre-contact period than has previously been suspected.

The social system encountered in the southern coastal area at contact, for instance, may have been 5,000 years old, while that known for the north appears to have been as recent as 1,300 years old. Changes in burial rituals may signify or be part of larger sociocultural transformations that might have occurred at that time. Below-ground burial of single individuals in shallow pits in shell middens, for example, was commonly practised until about AD 1000, in contrast to the above-ground burial practices typical of the historic period. The latter form of mortuary treatment may have begun 500 years before contact (Cybulski 1994).

Differences in the sex ratio of mortuary remains signal other forms of cultural diversity in the pre-contact period. The Prince Rupert Harbour remains, for example, contain almost twice as many males as females. Cybulski (1990:58) hypothesizes that since females periodically made up a large proportion of the slave population in consequence of intertribal warfare, their remains and those of other low-status individuals would have been interred elsewhere. He further speculates that the Prince Rupert Harbour people had a very different sociocultural context than the Strait of Georgia people, where there was little evidence for selective burial practices or warfare.

This is supported by differences in fracture frequencies at the two locales. At Prince Rupert Harbour almost 40 per cent of the individuals had limb and/or spinal fractures; the Strait of Georgia region shows much less, around 11 per cent. Interpersonal violence associated with tribal warfare at Prince Rupert Harbour likely accounts for most of the trauma. This is because almost 60 per cent of the traumatic injuries at the site consisted of depressed skull fractures from club blows, parry fractures, various defensive and disarming fractures of the hands and forearms, and cases of decapitation (Cybulski 1990:58).

The pre-contact maritime subsistence economy of the Northwest Coast is typically depicted as rich and plentiful. Intensive harvesting of almost the full range of marine resources, but with particular emphasis on salmon, provided the economic foundation for social organizational complexity, dense, sedentary village populations, and diverse forms of artistic expression (Suttles 1968). Cannon (1995) makes a case, however, for fluctuations in village prosperity in conjunction with periods of the failure of local marine resources, signalled by increased proportions of starvation foods (deer and ratfish) in archaeological assemblages. This interpretation is consistent with Suttles's (1968) observation that serious food shortages frequently occurred on the Northwest Coast in the wake of episodic maritime resource failures.

Attained adult stature is considered to be a good indirect measure of health and nutrition during childhood. Studies of growth and development in countries with developing economies support the contention that stunting and wasting in children, brought about through severe and prolonged nutritional and/or disease stress, can produce permanent reductions in achieved adult height (Stini 1975). In this regard, the apparent stability in stature among coastal peoples over a 3000- to 4000-year period is striking. Average heights of 162.4 cm estimated for skeletal remains for the Early Stage (3500 BC to 1500 BC) compare favourably to Boas's average measure of 164.2 cm for people living in the area in the late nineteenth century (Cybulski 1990:55 and 1994). The consistency of the stature estimates suggests that, periods of scarcity notwithstanding, the Northwest Coast people who survived to adulthood probably did not experience prolonged bouts of malnutrition or chronic and debilitating infectious disease during childhood growth. On the other hand, regional differences in the frequency of porotic hyperostosis have been detected, despite its coast-wide prevalence of 13 to 14 per cent (Cybulski 1977, 1990). This suggests that there was local variation in pathogen loads, the sources of which remain unexplained and which undoubtedly embrace a complex of sociodemographic factors (Stuart-Macadam 1992). It is evident, nonetheless, that coastal peoples were challenged by microorganisms to varying degrees, but not sufficiently to produce irreversible stunting of growth.

Dental health in the pre-contact period also seems to have been quite good, with dental caries affecting less than 1 per cent of all teeth[9] (Cybulski 1990:57). Caries are notably absent in Northwest Coast populations until the twentieth century, when the diet of fish, plant foods, and the meat of sea and land mammals began to be supplemented with foods rich in carbohydrates (Price 1934). Abscessed jaw sockets, which were undoubtedly quite painful, were common in the pre-contact period and affected upwards of 50 per cent of all adults. This marked tendency towards periapical abscesses probably resulted from a combination of dietary and cultural practices. Traditional food-preparation techniques introduced grit into the food which contributed to tooth wear. Trauma and wear to the anterior teeth sustained through use of the lower jaw as a tool by women, and associated with a high frequency of head and facial fractures among males, probably contributed to the prevalence of abscessed anterior teeth in the upper jaws of both sexes (Cybulski 1990:58).

Skeletal studies to date have failed to turn up any evidence for pre-contact tuberculosis or for malignant bone tumours, even though both of these diseases are present in historic Northwest Coast skeletal remains

(Cybulski 1990:57). While it is conceivable that they were unknown to pre-contact coastal people, their absence may equally reasonably be an artifact of poor bone preservation and age-related sampling (Cybulski 1994:17).

There is clear evidence, nonetheless, for treponemal infection well before AD 1492 from two Middle Development Stage sites (1500 BC to AD 500). Four out of ten skeletons from the Duke Point Site near Nanaimo (1490 BC +/− 125 years) show classic symptoms of treponematosis, and as many as six individuals, including a foetus, may have been affected. The widespread nature of the infection may be indicative of endemic non-venereal syphilis, at least in this sample. One female at the Boardwalk Site at Prince Rupert Harbour (325 BC +/− 90 years) shows clear signs of *caries sicca* (Cybulski 1990:57), the classic 'worm-eaten' cranial lesions considered to be 'the only reliable and pathognomonic lesion of syphilis' (C. Hackett 1983:113).

THE HALCYON AGE RECONSIDERED

The foregoing discussion should make it clear that the immune systems of pre-contact Americans were neither inexperienced nor pristine (see F.L. Black 1990), and that osteological analyses have demonstrated that there is no foundation for the perception that the Americas were disease-free prior to European contact (Larsen 1994:114). Infectious diseases were not 'filtered out' of people who crossed the Bering Strait from Asia to the Americas. Skeletal biological analysis from various regions in Canada provides substantial evidence for disease and nutritional compromise of varying degrees and kinds. Fungal, bacterial, and parasitic infections afflicted pre-contact peoples, depending on local socio-ecological conditions. Health patterns changed over time well before European contact, as illustrated by the prehistory of southern Ontario Iroquoia, and there was much diversity within and between regions, typified by the Arctic and Northwest Coast sequences. The concurrent infectious disease load supported by pre-contact Aboriginal groups, moreover, likely influenced the extent to which they were affected by introduced diseases (Herring 1992). We now consider the evidence for changes in health and disease in Aboriginal communities in Canada that were a consequence of contact with Europeans from the sixteenth to the nineteenth centuries.

3

Contact with Europeans and infectious diseases

One of the central pillars in the vision of the post-contact history of the Americas is the idea that European contact precipitated a catastrophic drop in the size of Aboriginal populations. The decimation and extinction of many indigenous peoples is a matter of historical fact, initiated by a cascade of interwoven sociopolitical, economic, and ecological changes. These include: ecological disruption resulting from the importation of new plants and animals, including pathogens (Crosby 1986); interference with and subversion of the social order by missionaries, traders, and government officials; the arrival of settlers to farm the lands of people already shattered by epidemics and the persecution of resisting survivors; and social fragmentation and reorganization as surviving groups coalesced on the margins of European settlement (Upton 1977:133).

The relative influence each of these processes, either alone or in combination, exerted on the size and demographic structure of Aboriginal populations varied from time to time and from place to place. Evaluating the nature and extent of depopulation, and the local, regional, and hemispheric factors that explain the phenomenon, continues to be one of the major thrusts of inquiry into the post-contact period. In recent years, particular weight has been accorded to the role played by pathogens introduced from Europe and Africa in this process.

As we have seen in the last chapter, the presence of new pathogens and the absence of immunity to them are insufficient as the sole explanation for epidemics in the Americas or elsewhere. Epidemics occur when the complex relationship between human populations and their social and physical environment is altered, disrupted, or conducive to the flourishing of micro-organisms. As Morse (1993:17) notes with respect to the contemporary problem of emerging viruses, 'Changing environmental

conditions are often responsible for viral traffic.' The problem then becomes one of teasing out the social histories of Aboriginal populations
and understanding how new opportunities were created for the transmission of infectious diseases through socio-ecological change resulting
from European contact. This includes determining the toll of lives taken
by individual or successive epidemics on specific populations and
regions, as well as evaluating how epidemics inhibited demographic
recovery and set in motion dramatic changes in the social order. It is a
difficult task, especially since the information available for addressing
these questions is sparse, spotty, and often of disappointingly poor quality.

   This chapter considers the main theories regarding the role of epidemics in the demographic transformation of Aboriginal populations in the
post-contact Americas and describes aspects of health and disease from
selected regions in Canada. We illustrate the complexity of social and
ecological changes that underlay population declines in Canada and emphasize that the new sociopolitical and ecological relationships that
emerged with European contact created the fundamental conditions that
allowed epidemics to flourish.

INTRODUCED DISEASES AND DEMOGRAPHIC DECLINE

Few researchers doubt that diseases of European origin figured prominently in the post-contact history of Aboriginal Americans. From the
seventeenth century onwards, smallpox, measles, influenza, dysentery,
diphtheria, typhus, yellow fever, whooping cough, tuberculosis, syphilis,
and various unidentifiable 'fevers' caused illness and death as they spread
from person to person and from village to village. Many of these are
believed to have been virgin soil epidemics. Virgin soil epidemics are
characterized by unusually high mortality in all age groups, rather than
the more usual high frequency of illness and death among the very young
and very old. This distinctive pattern of mortality occurs either because
the disease is new to the population, or because it has not been present
in it for such a long time that many individuals who had acquired antibodies to it have long since died. In either case, the population lacks
acquired immunity to the disease (Mausner and Bahn 1974:27).

   Although the presence of epidemics of European origin in the post-
contact period is well documented, an intense debate swirls around the
issue of the *extent* to which these epidemics shaped the post-contact de-

mography of the Americas (Trigger 1985:354). Indeed, the controversy about the depopulation of Aboriginal American societies has come to turn on this question. This has generated a large literature in which records of epidemics have been compiled; routes of disease spread plotted; and evaluations made of their social and biological impact on Aboriginal societies (cf Meister 1976; Helm 1980; Dobyns 1983; Hurlich 1983; Krech 1983a; Crosby 1986; Ramenofsky 1987; Decker 1988; Snow and Lanphear 1987; Dobyns 1989; Thornton, Miller, and Warren 1991; Ray 1976; Reff 1991; Verano and Ubelaker 1992; Herring 1993, 1994).

Some scholars accord extraordinary importance to the role of introduced diseases in post-contact disruption and population decrease (Borah 1976; Dobyns 1983, 1984; Cook 1973; Cook and Borah 1971). Russell Thornton contends, for example, that 'Without doubt, the single most important factor in American Indian population decline was an increased death rate due to diseases introduced from the Eastern hemisphere' (Thornton 1987:44). Alfred Crosby maintains, 'It was their germs, not these imperialists themselves, for all their brutality and callousness, that were chiefly responsible for sweeping aside the indigenes and opening the Neo-Europes to demographic takeover' (Crosby 1986:196). The fundamental problem is how to fill in the sketchy outlines of the picture with quantitative detail (Johansson 1982:139).

Scholars who embrace the idea that infectious diseases introduced from Europe were primarily responsible for the destruction of Aboriginal societies also often argue that infectious diseases reached many groups well before Europeans themselves did (Dobyns 1966, 1983). Accordingly, they contend that even the earliest population counts must be gross underestimates (cf Cook 1973; V. Miller 1976; Upton 1977) and therefore derive high initial population estimates through the application of depopulation ratios as high as 25:1 (Dobyns 1983) to the earliest recorded figures. This encourages the impression that even the most casual European contact resulted in immediate, catastrophic mortality, well before there were any written records to document it (Ramenofsky 1987:1).[1] Another related aspect of this point of view is the implication that Aboriginal population size declined continuously from the early sixteenth century onwards until a *nadir*, or minimum number, was reached, after which it rebounded, stabilized, or became extinct (Meister 1976:161).

An alternative interpretation of the history of the Americas takes the position that introduced infectious disease was not a significant agent of depopulation early in the post-contact period (cf Helm 1980). Severe population declines are thought to have occurred later in a slower and more insidious fashion (Johansson 1982:140) after sustained and intense European contact. This perspective conveys the impression that populations did not dwindle continuously from the time of contact, but declined later in concert with Aboriginal-European interaction that resulted in dramatic sociodemographic change. Scholars who espouse this point of view therefore tend to view early censuses of Aboriginal people as reasonable estimates, rather than depictions of relic populations already substantially depleted by epidemics (Mooney 1928; Kroeber 1934). Alfred Kroeber, for instance, was well aware that Indian populations had dwindled by the twentieth century, but attributed that decline to warfare, changes in subsistence patterns through intense European-Aboriginal interaction, and lack of political organization, rather than primarily to the effects of disease (Kroeber 1925, cited in Ramenofsky 1987:9). Helm (1980) explored the capacity of Dene hunting tribes in subarctic Canada to sustain their population size in the face of introduced disease. She concluded that selective female infanticide in the first half of the nineteenth century had a greater effect on mortality than introduced disease at that time.

In any event, the discourse on demographic change resulting from European contact is essentially couched in terms of these catastrophist or gradualist theories, with advocates of each arguing through the literature about the effects of disease on the population history of specific groups (cf Helm 1980 vs Krech 1983a; Snow and Lanphear 1987 vs Dobyns 1983, 1989). Since the late 1970s, the catastrophist view that introduced diseases were the primary agents of demographic change has come to dominate thinking about the post-contact history of the Americas (Johansson 1982:140–1). Recognition of the importance of epidemiological research was boosted by the coincidental publication of William McNeill's influential book *Plagues and Peoples* (1976), William Denevan's textbook *The Native Population of the Americas in 1492* (1976), and a special symposium on the topic at the 1976 meeting of the American Society for Ethnohistory (Dobyns 1976). Since then, it has become fashionable to question conservative estimates (Trigger 1985:234) and contact population estimates have spiralled. For central Mexico, for example, the numbers have soared from 2 million to 25 million during this period (Henige 1990:170). In less dramatic fashion, estimates of Huron numbers prior to the seventeenth-century epidemics have increased from 16,000–22,500 to 25,000–32,000 (Trigger 1985:233–5).

ESTIMATES OF POPULATION SIZE AT CONTACT

Given these very different visions and ways of interpreting the evidence, it is not surprising that an extraordinarily wide range of contact population estimates have been devised for North America (Ubelaker 1992:171). While most seem to hover between 1 to 2 million people, Dobyns's (1966) figure of 9.8 million, which he subsequently doubled to 18 million (Dobyns 1983), is substantially higher than the rest, as is Thornton's (1987:32) figure of 7 million.[2]

Over and above the differences in philosophical and theoretical orientation among researchers, Ubelaker (1992:170–2) notes that much of the variation in population estimates stems from disagreements about the geographical expanse of various regions in North America and from the disparate methodologies and sources of data used by the estimators. It bears recalling, however, that most historical demographic reconstructions stand or fall on the observations of a relatively small number of explorers, missionaries, physicians, traders, or government officials. A great deal of attention is therefore normally paid to evaluating the accuracy of recorded counts and to determining whether they are tainted by intentional or accidental bias (Ross 1977:1–3; Ubelaker 1988:289).

The amount of *reliable* information on population counts, birth rates, mortality rates, migration rates, and disease episodes varies from region to region and from time to time. During the late fifteenth and early sixteenth centuries, when fishermen and explorers plied the northeastern waters along the Atlantic coast of Canada, there is virtually no historical documentation of Aboriginal people, diseases, or epidemics. In fact, the series of outbreaks that swept through the Montagnais, Algonquins and Hurons of the St Lawrence and Ottawa Valleys between 1734 and 1741 are among the best documented early historic epidemics in the northeast (Trigger 1985:229–97). Unfortunately, the early explorers showed more interest in charting the coastline or recording and retrieving the available resources, including occasional human souvenirs to take back to Europe, than in commenting on Aboriginal life (Carlson et al. 1992:145–6). But this 100-year lacuna means that we can only speculate about the demographic results of Aboriginal-European interaction and the effects of virgin soil epidemics during this period.

Because of local and regional variability in the amount and quality of epidemiologic and demographic information, researchers look to increasingly complicated and sophisticated methods to circumvent the weaknesses in the primary source data. It is becoming more common to combine ethnohistoric and archaeological evidence, experiments with projective techniques, Monte Carlo simulations, mathematical models, and model life-table comparisons. The aim is to adjust as much as possible for errors in the initial observations and for distortions in the data due to sampling error, and to generate a range of possible demographic scenarios from as many sources as possible (cf Dobyns 1966, 1983; Helm 1980; Roth 1981; Joraleman 1982; Ramenofsky 1987; McGrath 1988; Thornton 1987; Thornton et al. 1991; Ubelaker 1988; Snow 1992; Storey 1992; Whitmore 1992).

Even the best methods, however, cannot compensate for the initial assumptions upon which they are built. Estimates of population sizes for the Americas are influenced, moreover, by the biases of scholars themselves (Borah 1976). The figures reflect the investigators' views on the density and complexity of pre-contact societies and the perception of the health of pre-contact indigenous North Americans. We have already seen, for example, that serious diseases with the capacity to erupt into epidemic form were present in the Americas prior to AD 1492. But because of the widespread assumption that infectious disease was not an important feature of pre-contact life, there have been few attempts to evaluate the extent to which extant infectious disease loads might have influenced the experience of introduced, post-contact disease (Herring 1992:154; see Molto, in press, for an exception).

It is tempting to ignore these theoretical and methodological hornets' nests or to dismiss them as academic trivia. Yet these issues have profound effects on the kinds of images projected in the literature about disease and the contact experience. Population estimates are important because they establish the baseline for all subsequent demographic estimates and for the construction of social histories (Johansson 1982:137). The larger the estimate of the initial population, the more devastating the impact of European contact is inferred to have been; the more conservative the estimate, the less demographically disruptive (Ramenofsky 1987:1). This helps to explain why the magnitude of the population estimates shifts with the political wind: conservative numbers typified the 1910s, liberal ones the 1920s, and so on (Ubelaker 1976). The most extravagant estimates date to the period between the 1960s and 1980s in concert with the shift in theoretical orientation towards appreciating and emphasizing the potential devastation of early contact epidemics (Ubelaker 1992:172).

Apparently, larger questions beyond the scope of the demographic data at hand are being discussed through the depopulation literature (Bruner

1986; Henige 1990), and estimates of Aboriginal population sizes and population dynamics remain incomplete, patchy (Ubelaker 1992:169), and speculative. This should caution researchers and students alike 'to establish what was, not what should have been' (Thornton 1987:36). The bleakest assessment waves all the estimates aside, claiming that the fundamental insufficiency of the evidence makes the endeavour no different from trying to guess the number of elves in J.R.R. Tolkien's Middle-earth (Henige 1990:169). At the very least, most estimates are influenced by political and cultural biases and deserve to be treated with caution (Johansson 1982:137). It is perhaps worth recalling Romaniuk and Piché's (1972) caution that *reliable* estimates of demographic rates for Canada's Aboriginal peoples begin in the 1960s (see also Piché and George 1973).

POST-CONTACT CHANGES IN POPULATION SIZE

The most recent reassessment of North American contact population figures was undertaken by Douglas Ubelaker (1988, 1992) of the Smithsonian Institution. To compensate for as many disparities as possible in the work of previous investigators, he based his study on forty-five articles for the Smithsonian's *Handbook of North American Indians* submitted in 1976 by scholars most familiar with the primary sources. The new estimates subsume ethnohistorical, archaeological, and ecological factors, as well as the possible impact of early epidemics. After independently assembling each tribal estimate, he calculated regional totals, population densities, and the per cent of reduction in population size, to correspond with the ten culture areas included in the *Handbook*. With the exception of the Southeast, by Ubelaker's account, all appear to have reached their nadirs in the twentieth century, with population depletions ranging from a low of 53 per cent in the Arctic to extraordinary highs of 89 per cent for the Northwest Coast and 95 per cent for California (Ubelaker 1988:293). Figure 3 shows the estimated population decline in the six culture areas in Canada.

Which of the two post-contact scenarios discussed earlier best explains this phenomenon? The problem in selecting *either* explanation is illustrated by Carl Meister's (1976) comparison of the demographic history of five groups of Indians from the western United States. His findings for the Pueblo, Maricopa, and California Indian/Ute appear to conform to the catastrophist model, suggesting that introduced diseases took a major toll of mortality early in their contact experiences. On the other hand, the

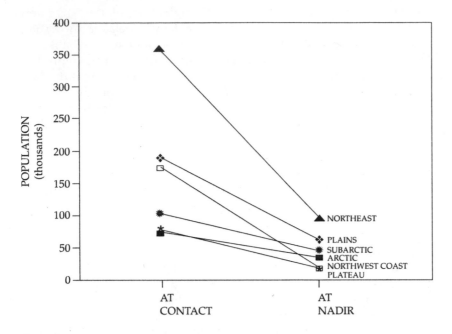

Figure 3
Estimated decline in Aboriginal population in selected culture areas in North America

SOURCE: Based on data from Ubelaker (1992)

Navajo and Gila River Pima histories do not fit the model at all. The Navajo experienced a brief, ten-year period of population reduction between 1860 and 1870, but at the end of that decline their population was still several times larger than it was at the time of initial contact. The Gila River Pima show yet another pattern, with two periods of population decline separated by periods of population growth, evidence that they were able to recover from epidemics well before the introduction of European medicine. Meister suggests that the increase in Pima mortality in the latter half of the nineteenth century was more likely the result of being driven from their land than to a lack of immunity to diseases of European derivation (Meister 1976:162–5).

Meister's study shows that no single pattern can be expected to apply to every Aboriginal group. Variation in the phenomenon of contact was so great that it is fundamentally meaningless to try to fit each Aboriginal social history into a rigid category of experience. Demographic change and encounters with new pathogens of European origin involved a complicated, multifactorial process located in the particular social histories and interaction networks of specific communities.

To illustrate the complexity intrinsic to the contact-disease problem in the Canadian context, we turn to the evidence for the extinction of the Beothuk of Newfoundland.

COMPLEXITY AND THE CONTACT-DISEASE PROBLEM: THE EXAMPLE OF THE BEOTHUK OF NEWFOUNDLAND

The Beothuk of Newfoundland were the first indigenous North Americans to encounter Mediterranean explorers and fishermen in the late fifteenth century (Upton, 1977:133).[3] In just over 300 years, by 1829, the last known Beothuk had perished. The uniqueness of their tragedy in Canadian history (Upton 1977; Pastore, 1987, 1989) and the complexity of its underlying causes exemplify the difficulties of evaluating the role that disease may have played in their demise and in the early contact period, as well as the diversity of social processes set in motion in the post-contact period.

Despite decades of archaeological and historical research, there are no firm and reliable estimates of Beothuk numbers at contact, which is generally defined as AD 1500. Archaeological reconstructions of the ecology of Newfoundland over the past 5,000 years show that while the island had the potential to support 'sizeable' human populations through its rich biome of marine and terrestrial resources,[1] many important food sources were available only on a seasonal basis and were subject to failures or periods of unavailability (Tuck and Pastore 1985:74). The fluctuating and precarious nature of the resource base meant that human populations were subject to recurrent booms and busts, as suggested by an archaeological record of at least three pre-Beothuk Aboriginal extinctions on the island[5] prior to the arrival of Europeans (ibid. 70–2).

Upton's (1977:134) review of the published best guesses of Beothuk contact population size reveals an extraordinary range of 500 to 20,000 people, an indication of the poor quality of the information on this question. This is in keeping with what is known about the early contact period, which essentially consisted of sporadic coastal encounters between Beothuk and transient European fishermen. Any trade conducted between them is judged to have been on a very minor scale and so marginal in nature that it may have taken the form of a silent trade, in which trade goods are left at a specific location and the trading parties do not meet (Pastore 1987:50).

As is the case elsewhere in the Americas (cf Henige 1990), some of the early population estimates for Newfoundland are entirely without foundation, while others have an air of crypto-science because they are derived from climatic considerations and from assessments of the capacity of northeastern forests and coastlines to support the Beothuk hunter-gatherer lifestyle[6] (cf Upton 1977:134, especially footnote 2). In fact, Beothuk contact population size will remain purely speculative except in the unlikely event of a systematic archaeological survey of the entire Newfoundland coast and much of the interior (Pastore 1989:55). Even so, it is extremely difficult to estimate Aboriginal population sizes from archaeological evidence (Trigger 1985:231).

Population estimates for the mid-eighteenth century to the early nineteenth century fare little better, for most were 'based on casual contacts with Beothucks and mostly on heresay [sic]' (Marshall 1977:234). This is largely the result of the Beothuk strategy of withdrawal to the island's interior by the early seventeenth century (Upton 1977:135) and apparent decision not to engage in trade with Europeans (Pastore 1987:59). Furthermore, the fishery-based economy of Newfoundland and unusual settlement circumstances meant an absence of the clergymen, traders, soldiers, or government agents (Upton 1977:153) who elsewhere recorded population estimates of indigenous peoples.

Whatever their numbers at contact, Marshall (1977:235) speculates that there could have been about 350 Beothuk in 1768, based on John Cartwright's map of their dwellings on the River Exploits, on the reckonings of planters in the area, and on accounts of Shanawdithit, the last surviving Beothuk. By 1811, there were only 72, and they had dwindled to 13 by 1823. With the death of Shanawdithit in 1829, the Beothuk vanished.

Without reliable population estimates, we cannot know how quickly their fate unfolded. On the other hand, the magnitude of decline and speed of the death of a people does not diminish in any way the fundamental tragedy of that loss.

Despite the scarcity of demographic data, there is a growing body of opinion that a constellation of events and processes contributed to the Beothuk extinction. Introduced diseases may have played a role, but there is so little evidence that it is impossible to do anything other than speculate about their impact. Smallpox was observed on the island from 1610 onwards, but no major outbreaks were recorded. Although measles and other epidemics were sporadically noted among European immigrants, Marshall (1981:73–5) considers that the isolation of the Beothuk made slim the chances of transmission of infectious diseases to them, except perhaps in the last 100 years or so when contact increased.

Tuberculosis is the *only* disease to have been documented among the Beothuk (Marshall 1981:75). Three women are said to have been suffering from pulmonary consumption when captured by furriers in 1823, 'which *they may have contracted prior to their capture*, and it must be *assumed* that this disease had taken its toll among the Beothucks' [italics ours] (Marshall 1977:236). Indeed, Marshall speculates that from 1730 onward 'this disease played a significant role in the eventual demise of the Beothuk group' (1981:76). Unfortunately, this quite plausible idea cannot be verified because there is no solid evidence with which to support or refute it. The argument is based on the single mention of tuberculosis in 1823, in conjunction with the estimated drop in Beothuk population from 350 in 1768 to 13 in 1823. It is also made with reference to the likelihood of increased contact between Beothuk bands as their territory shrank in the eighteenth century, and as their encounters with Europeans became more frequent; together, these social circumstances could have given rise to high tuberculosis mortality rates, such as have been recorded for Aboriginal groups elsewhere (ibid. 74–5).

Where Marshall's (1977, 1981) review of the literature suggests that introduced diseases became a more important determinant of Beothuk mortality after 1730, Upton (1977) focuses on their significance in the early contact period. Not only does he postulate that there was massive depopulation from the beginning of European contact, he also suggests that epidemics may have been the stimulus behind the Beothuk avoidance of contact with Europeans between AD 1612 and 1750 (Upton 1977:135). Following Cook's (1973) analysis of the decline of seventeenth-century Aboriginal groups in New England, he writes: 'Presumably the first phase of contact had the same results in Newfoundland as elsewhere in the northeastern coastal region. European diseases had been introduced there by casual trade and there is no reason why the Beothuks should be exempt' (Upton 1977:138). This is a remarkable proposition given that so many other features of Beothuk history stand in stark contrast to conditions elsewhere in the northeastern coastal region (Upton 1977:153) and the lack of supporting documentation (Marshall 1981).

Apart from the complete lack of evidence, there are other reasons for scepticism about massive initial depopulation of the Beothuk by introduced diseases. Marshall (1981) observes, for instance, that the sporadic encounters typical of the early contact period were not conducive to the transmission of acute community infections. Certainly the silent trade postulated by Pastore (1987:50) in the sixteenth and early seventeenth centuries would lend support to this inference. On the other hand, if Basque whalers plying the Strait of Belle Isle in the mid-sixteenth to early seventeenth centuries employed the Beothuk in shore-based activities, there would have been greater opportunities for the transmission of pathogens to them (Pastore 1989:70).

Having estimated an initial Beothuk population of about 2,000 for AD 1500, Upton (1977:152) assumes 'a rapid loss of population as a result of first contact diseases followed by a period of recovery and stabilisation.' This is a good example of the depopulation-to-nadir model. He then conjectures that if this assumed depopulation occurred on a similar scale as in New England, the Beothuk would have been reduced by disease to about 400 by the early seventeenth century (Upton 1977:137–8) and at an annual rate of 1.01 per cent from AD 1500 to 1811 (ibid. 152). Henige's observation is particularly apt here: 'It is all too easy to confuse the possible with the probable ... the notion that newly introduced diseases quick [sic] assumed epidemic (or "pandemic") proportions throughout the New World is, by its very nature, detached from any evidence' (Henige 1990:185). In the absence of documentation, it is tempting to begin with a story and locate the appropriate 'facts' within it (Bruner 1986:141–2).

Although it is not yet possible to resolve the extent of early cross-cultural contact or disease exchange, there is no doubt that the Beothuk opted for a pattern of avoidance of Europeans by the early seventeenth century, gradually withdrawing into the resource-poor interior of the island and disappearing from the written record until 1766 (Upton 1977:138). Whereas archaeological evidence indicates that the pre-contact Beothuk had a broad-based diet drawn from the seasonal exploitation of both marine and land resources, their displacement from the coastal regions by other ethnic groups meant that they were cut off from important foods, especially seal, and forced to rely on the relatively meagre resources of the interior. This strategy could not work in the long term, given the precarious nature and periodic failure of important staples like caribou and the lack of fallback foods such as porcupine, deer, and moose (Tuck and Pastore 1985:73–6). With a hostile settler population preventing access to coastal marine resources (Marshall 1977:3), the necessary conditions for a subsistence crisis were created. This exclusion from resource-rich areas was probably the major factor in the decline of the Beothuk (Tuck 1976:76). The Beothuk world appears to have gradually become more tightly circumscribed as Europeans moved inland along the Exploits River and its tributaries to hunt for furs (Upton 1977:139). With the loss of contact with Labrador, which could have provided a refuge and resources, the fate of the Beothuk was sealed (Pastore 1989:71).

The reasons for the Beothuk retreat inland remain unknown, but appear to have been closely associated with the growing exploitation of coastal resources by other ethnic groups and to increasingly hostile relations with them: 'Although the spread of permanent English settlement on the island may have been the most important factor denying the Beothuks access to vitally needed coastal resources, to that equation must now be added the Basque and Inuit presence in the Strait of Belle Isle, the Micmac use of the southern third of the island, and the French base at Placentia' (Pastore 1989:71). The Beothuk, moreover, never developed a full-blown fur trade with Europeans and, unlike the seventeenth-century settlers to Newfoundland, never became fur trappers (Pastore 1987:60); this gave rise to several important consequences. Because the Beothuk were interested in some European goods, a pattern of acquiring them through theft developed. This resulted in reprisals and killings of an unknown number of Beothuk by Europeans which, though clearly abhorrent, have been sensationalized by the popular press into 'the people who were killed for fun' (Horwood 1959, cited in Pastore 1989:56).

Another consequence of the lack of cross-cultural trade was the absence of cultural brokers in the form of European traders, whose own economic interests would have been served by intervening with the settler population on behalf of the Beothuk (Upton 1977:153): 'There was no missionary to plead for their souls, no trader anxious to barter for their furs, no soldier to arm and use them as auxiliaries in his wars, no government to restrain the settlers' (Upton 1977:153). It appears then that the Beothuk were not pushed to extinction by the effects of introduced diseases and epidemics. Rather, starvation from the loss of resource-rich territory and marginalization into the impoverished Newfoundland interior led to their demise. Evidently, post-contact economic and sociopolitical relationships were the ultimate sources of the Beothuk's crisis and tragic disappearance.

If the lack of cross-cultural trade in Newfoundland helped to buffer the Beothuk from disease (but not from starvation and marginalization), Aboriginal groups in other areas of Canada developed thriving cross-cultural trade networks. Ironically, this probably served to make them particularly vulnerable to epidemics.

TRADE CENTRES AND EPIDEMICS

Trade centres often became the nucleus for disease outbreaks and central points of diffusion of epidemics to the hinterland (Ray 1976; Dobyns 1983, 1992; Herring 1993). This is because they represented points of

convergence between Aboriginal people and Europeans and their pathogens, creating conditions conducive to the spread of infection from the
one to the other. Trade centres also attracted long-distance Aboriginal
trading partners who brought pathogens with them or acquired new ones
at the trade centre, which, in turn, they unwittingly took with them on
their return journey. Temporary and permanent settlers tended to cluster
around the fringes of trade centres, typically resulting in higher population densities than characterized the surrounding areas. The higher the
population density, the greater the chance that contagious diseases, either
introduced or local, would spread quickly from person to person.

This is well illustrated by the disease history of the central-Canadian
Subarctic. The establishment of Hudson's Bay and North West Company
fur-trade posts in mainland Canada not only stimulated significant relo-
cations of Aboriginal peoples and restructured intergroup exchange networks (Ray 1974), but also created novel patterns of Aboriginal-European
contact and brought together widely separated disease pools (Herring
1993). Exchange networks, centred on trading posts, created routes for
the spread of contagion, channelling the movement of micro-organisms
and patterning their dispersion across some regions, while bypassing
others (see Dobyns 1983:12–13; Reff 1991:119–24).

Clearly, the reorganization of trade relationships and the geographical
distribution of Aboriginal groups, along with alterations in intergroup
contact attendant upon the fur trade, were probably as significant for the
disease history of the Americas as the introduction of European diseases
per se. Examples from the post-1670 fur trade at York Factory and Norway
House, both in present-day Manitoba, illustrate how economic and social
circumstances associated with trading centres influenced the transmission of epidemic diseases between communities and over long distances.

York Factory, established in 1714 at the mouth of the Hayes River, was
one of the earliest posts on Hudson Bay and became the main port of
entry for trade goods for western Canada. As the most important source
of European cargo on the bay, York Factory housed a small European
population of young Hudson's Bay Company (HBC) officers and servants
and drew a far-flung network of Cree and Assiniboine from central and
southern Manitoba and Saskatchewan (Ray 1974:72). Post journal records and parish burial records from 1714 to 1801, show that Europeans
and Aboriginal people alike died from infectious diseases, including a
protracted epidemic of influenza in 1717 and a devastating smallpox
epidemic in 1782 (Ewart 1983).

By the nineteenth century, European physicians resided at the post,
and causes of death were identified with greater precision, allowing

Ewart (ibid. 573) to construct an unusually detailed profile of mortality (Figure 4). Tuberculosis, influenza, and dysentery were the leading infectious diseases, and the presence of poliomyelitis, typhoid fever, and puerperal fever indicate that sanitary conditions at York Factory were less than ideal during this period. The detail provided by this compilation underlines the danger of relying solely on accounts of epidemics as a means of fleshing out epidemiologic profiles. Not only does a focus on epidemics stress the unusual and catastrophic; it also fails to reveal the presence of many serious afflictions, such as bronchitis and meningitis, which Ewart was able to identify at York Factory.

Arthur Ray (1976) was one of the first scholars to try to go beyond the construction of disease inventories to examine the spatial dynamics of epidemic diseases of European derivation and to assess the cumulative effects of a *sequence* of epidemics on Aboriginal groups. His study focuses on the period between 1830 and 1850 in the western interior of Canada, a vast expanse of land that embraced present-day Saskatchewan, the Northwest Territories, Manitoba, and parts of northern Ontario. A series of major and minor epidemics of scarlet fever (1843), measles (1846–7), smallpox (1837), and influenza (1835, 1837, 1843, 1845, 1847, and 1850) affected the region during this time, with heavy tolls of mortality accompanying the 1835 influenza epidemic, the 1837 smallpox epidemic, and the 1846–7 measles outbreak. Because the post records do not contain precise information on the number of deaths or on the incidence of illness, the demographic consequences of these epidemics cannot be evaluated. However, Ray's analysis of the origins, patterns of diffusion, and processes that fuelled their spread reveals that York Factory and Norway House were central to the movement of pathogens through the region.

Boat, canoe, and cart brigades linked these two trade centres to a large network of HBC posts throughout the western interior. Most of the traffic moved through this widespread exchange network during the summer months when open water made transport easier. The summer season was also marked by large-scale population shifts. Assiniboine, Cree, and Ojibwa groups, for instance, spent the winters in the forested parts of the parkland, while summers were taken up with bison hunting and travel south to trade in the Missouri River valley. Any movement of people carries with it the potential concomitant movement of pathogens, with the result that summer eruptions were more likely to spread rapidly because of the larger encampments, increased visits to trading houses, and generally high volume of boat movement between districts that distinguished the season.

Nine of the outbreaks identified by Ray (1976) in the HBC post journals

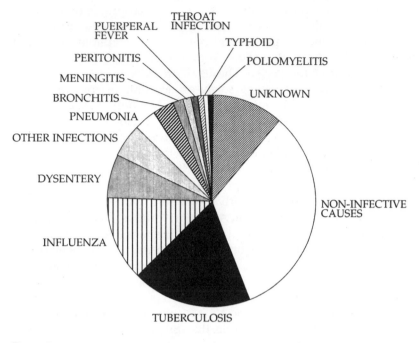

Figure 4
Distribution of deaths by cause at York Factory, 1801–1900

SOURCE: Redrawn from data in Ewart (1983)

struck two or more districts, spreading outward from trading centres. Both Norway House and York Factory experienced more epidemics than other, less central posts, and the Norway House District endured ten different epidemics, making it the most unhealthy of all. Since the HBC boat brigades were primarily responsible for the transmission of both cargo and disease from one district to another, the vulnerability of the Norway House District is not startling. In view of its key position in the fur-trade network and frequent contact with locations to the west, north-west, northeast, and south (Fort Garry), it was exposed to pathogens from a wide geographical area (Ray 1976:156–7). Even as recently as the 1918–19 influenza pandemic, Norway House continued to be a central source of infection and point of diffusion for infectious disease in the region (Herring 1993, 1994).

But boat brigades and trade routes were not the only means by which diseases spread. In the case of the 1780–2 smallpox epidemic, information gleaned from post journals and scrutinized from the perspective of epidemiologic principles led Decker (1988:18–24) to conclude that Indians, travelling overland or by river from their camps for the purpose of trade or to obtain aid, brought the dreaded 'red death' to York Factory and Cumberland House.

Building on Ray's work, Decker (1989) studied a series of epidemics that struck the northern Plains between 1774 and 1839, tracing the pattern of transmission and calculating mortality rates for each. How devastating was this series of smallpox, measles, influenza, and whooping-cough epidemics, and did they depopulate the people of the northern Plains?

Before addressing this question, it is important to recognize that all epidemics do not necessarily result in depopulation. *Epidemics* are outbreaks of disease which produce excessive morbidity or mortality compared to the norm for that population and are typically sporadic and short-term. They are generally followed by a return to pre-epidemic mortality levels and population age structure. Populations experiencing *depopulating epidemics* continue to be susceptible to the infectious disease and experience recurrent bouts of it, along with high mortality in selective age categories. Under these circumstances, the age structure of the population is fundamentally changed through the experience of recurrent epidemics, and this, in turn, may affect the population's ability to reproduce itself (Palkovich 1981:71).

Bearing this distinction in mind, it appears that of the four epidemics, only smallpox fulfilled the criteria for a depopulating epidemic in the northern Plains. Smallpox is also distinctive because of its enhanced capacity to spread, relative to other diseases. It could survive for long periods of time in a dried state on corpses and inanimate objects and had a long period of infectivity, lasting from the onset of its typical rash to the peeling of the last scars, allowing it to move explosively and inexorably over huge distances.

The smallpox epidemic of 1781–2 was the first severe epidemic recorded in subarctic Canada. Decker (1989:221) speculates that depopulation of the region observed between 1774 and 1839 resulted from depletion of the adults during the 1781–2 smallpox epidemic, reducing the number of marriages and births in the next generation. It appears, nonetheless, that all of the Plains groups recovered from the devastation and that a demographic turning point was reached around 1820.

Significantly, 'no group experienced a continual steady decline in population, despite the fact that nine major epidemics swept through the Plains within two generations' (Decker 1989:220). The demographic resurgence of the Plains Cree was aided in the 1830s by the absorption of entire extended families of Woodlands Cree, who migrated to the Plains in the wake of disease and resource depletion (ibid. 225). As McGrath (1991:418–19) emphasizes, social responses are instrumental in determining an epidemic's course and impact. Evidently, a complex configuration of social, ecological, and disease features were influencing the decline and subsequent recovery of northern Plains people at this time.

Hackett (1991), for instance, has linked the 1819–20 measles epidemic in the Canadian Northwest to the establishment of an endemic measles focus in the urban centres of Baltimore, Philadelphia, and New York in the northeastern United States. By 1818, the combined populations of these three cities had surpassed the critical size necessary to maintain a constant supply of new susceptibles (Black 1966), and measles was carried westward from the Atlantic coast by small groups travelling along major transportation routes, through the upper Great Lakes, along the north shore of Lake Superior, and on into the Northwest. As Dobyns (1983) emphasizes, previously isolated Aboriginal groups were nevertheless affected by outbreaks in distant locations, even in the absence of direct contact.

It appears that the first quarter of the nineteenth century constitutes a watershed in the disease history of the Northwest, after which epidemics other than smallpox began to strike Aboriginal peoples with greater frequency (Decker 1989:145; Hackett 1991:136). This widening of the infectious-disease spectrum was closely connected to the westward expansion of the American frontier and to improvements in transportation efficiency. Together, these two developments opened up the Northwest to diseases such as measles, influenza, and scarlet fever that are characterized by shorter periods of infectivity and a lower diffusion potential than smallpox (Hackett 1991:140). At the same time, large and small game alike were being depleted in the Northwest, and declining fur harvests prompted the HBC to close many trading posts.

The important relationship between diet and disease is well known. Malnutrition and undernutrition can occur for many reasons, but whatever the cause, they increase susceptibility to infectious disease.[7] Places like Norway House were basically 'trapped out' by the mid-nineteenth century, with the result that it was necessary to travel long distances to hunt furs – sometimes as far as 300 miles. Reports of scarcity and hunger in the HBC post journals are quite frequent during this period, but it is difficult to interpret their meaning or connect them specifically to outbreaks of disease because 'starvation' has connotations beyond its literal definition (Black-Rogers 1986). In any event, the combined effects of the depletion of local resources, periodic hunger, and the introduction of more exogenous acute community infections, at greater frequency, must have reduced the resistance to disease and exacted a high toll of morbidity, if not mortality.

TUBERCULOSIS EPIDEMICS AND RESERVES

While smallpox was the scourge of the sixteenth to the eighteenth centuries (see Stern and Stern 1945), tuberculosis overtook it thereafter to become a genuine plague of enormous proportions. It remains a serious health problem in many Aboriginal communities today (see chapter 4). The disease has a long history in the Americas and has been identified in skeletal remains from Canada well before the arrival of Europeans, as discussed in chapter 2. While there is no need to treat tuberculosis as a newly introduced disease, it is critical to examine the social circumstances that allowed it to flourish and permitted its resurgence in the post-contact period.

There are scattered reports of scrofula, consumption, and phthisis during the early contact period that suggest that the disease was quite common (Graham-Cumming 1967). Scrofula, or glandular tuberculosis, is among the first diseases noted by Jesuits in 1633–4, and tuberculosis appears to have been quite widespread among the Montagnais by 1637 (Thorpe 1989:61). Other accounts suggest that Indians along the Hudson Bay and James Bay coasts were exposed to English and French rife with tuberculosis some 200 years earlier than their counterparts in the interior (Hurlich 1983). Graham-Cumming (1967:130) suggests that eastern Indians had been exposed to tuberculosis for so long that by the last quarter of the nineteenth century the disease had become endemic and probably no more prevalent among them than among non-Indians in comparable living conditions.

By the twentieth century, however, tuberculosis was a major health problem both as a specific cause of death and as an underlying condition that reduced resistance to other infectious diseases (Stone 1925:79). The soaring tuberculosis problem resulted in a tuberculosis death rate among Indians in the western provinces ten to twenty times higher than that for non-Aboriginal people (Stewart 1936:675). The prevalence of acute forms of the disease, the wide range of expressions of it, and the extraordinarily

high rates relative to other groups (Figure 5) led some observers to conclude that North American Indians had a special susceptibility to tuberculosis because they lacked 'racial immunity' (McCarthy 1912:207). Some
feared the complete extinction of Aboriginal North Americans (Hrdlicka
1908).

Others noted that the idea of unusual genetic susceptibility was simply
an assumption rather than an established scientific fact (Wherrett 1965).
It is now generally accepted that ethnic differences in susceptibility to
tuberculosis can be fully explained in terms of how long and under what
circumstances the population has experienced the epidemic, and the extent to which herd immunity has been acquired through experience with
it (Bates 1982).

A community's experience of a tuberculosis epidemic is intimately tied
to local conditions. A deterioration in living conditions or the development of an environment conducive to the spread of tubercle bacilli can
propel low, endemic rates into a full-blown epidemic. Ferguson's (1928)
work in the Qu'Appelle Valley of Saskatchewan from the 1880s onward
emphasized the importance of radical social, spiritual, and ecological
disruptions which underlay the rising tuberculosis mortality rates there.
He asserts (1955:6) that tuberculosis became a serious problem among
western Aboriginal populations only after they were settled on reserves.
This was linked, moreover, to other dramatic changes to the social and
physical landscape at the time, such as the construction of the Canadian
Pacific Railway, which facilitated the spread of people and pathogens to
the west, and the inflow of European immigrants, many of whom likely
harboured the tubercle bacillus.

Most important, the relocation of Aboriginal people to reserves with
minimal resources, where people lived in crowded houses, and where
children were concentrated in boarding schools, essentially guaranteed
their complete and rapid tuberculinization. As Walker noted in 1909
(cited in Bryce 1909:282), increasing tuberculosis mortality on Canadian
reserves in the early twentieth century represented 'the whole story of
the passing of the Indian from the nomadic to the settled habits of life.'

CONCLUSIONS

Infectious diseases, especially acute community infections introduced
from Europe, struck Aboriginal communities in Canada from the time of
contact, adding to the infectious-disease load already present before contact. The opportunities for the transmission of diseases of European der-

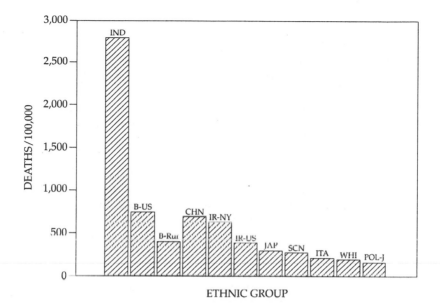

Figure 5
Estimates of tuberculosis mortality rates by ethnic group, United States, late nineteenth and early twentieth century

Key
IND   Indians (9 reservations)
B-US   Blacks (U.S. Census, 1900)
B-Rur   Blacks (Rural United States)
CHN   Chinese (Cities)
IR-NY   Irish (New York City, 1890)
IR-US   Irish (Total United States, 1900)
JAP   Japanese
SCN   Scandinavians
ITA   Italians
WHI   American Whites
POL-J   Polish Jews

SOURCE: Based on data from McCarthy (1912)

ivation varied extensively, however, as did the effects they had on each community. Over and above the distinctive features of the pathogens themselves (which include the severity of symptoms, ease of transmission, and capacity to induce immunity), the *social circumstances* surrounding the encounter with pathogens are of paramount importance. No single depopulation model can explain all cases; the social history of each Aboriginal community must be evaluated to determine the extent to which infectious disease debilitated and depleted it.

It is likely, however, that Aboriginal communities in closer and more intense contact with European settlements were at greater risk of contracting introduced diseases than more isolated communities, or than those that chose not to become entangled in social and economic relationships with European groups. The Beothuk case shows, however, that strategies of avoidance brought their own survival risks, especially when there was no viable hinterland to which to escape.

As the larger sociodemographic fabric of the North American continent changed during the post-contact period, the capacity for diseases to afflict Aboriginal communities was enhanced. Given the poor quality of most early population estimates in Canada, it is difficult to evaluate the demographic consequences of this unfolding epidemiologic transformation. Ewers's (1973:104) observation twenty years ago that 'the long range effects of successive epidemics on the populations of particular tribes have not been sufficiently studied' remains as true today as it was then. And it is unlikely that scholars will ever be able to determine with any degree of precision or certainty the extent to which Aboriginal populations in Canada (or elsewhere) declined, or to specify the impact made by infectious diseases on this process, in isolation from the social and economic circumstances that allowed the diseases to thrive.

The inescapable conclusion, however, is that across the continent, regional and local developments all contributed to the increasing ease of spread of infectious diseases, indigenous and introduced, to Aboriginal communities in Canada. The growth of North American cities in the nineteenth century through immigration and natural increase created population densities necessary to support acute community infections in endemic form. Increasingly extensive and numerous trade and transportation routes opened up previously isolated parts of the country to the movement of pathogens, old and new. The escalating speed of travel made possible by the invention of the steam engine allowed infectious diseases with short incubation periods, such as influenza, to diffuse more widely along waterways, and later via road and railway routes. Poor living conditions on reserves ensured that chronic infections, like tuberculosis, took firm root in Aboriginal communities.

By the twentieth century, the infectious-disease load in many Aboriginal communities was high. It is against this backdrop of persistently high infection rates that yet another epidemiological profile began to emerge.

4

New epidemics in the twentieth century

In the last two chapters we have had a glimpse of the likely state of health of Aboriginal peoples in Canada from before the arrival of Europeans. While an idealized, disease-free paradise was unlikely ever to have existed, there is sufficient documentary evidence to suggest that a series of epidemics and famines of varying extent, severity, and duration affected different regions at different times subsequent to contact. We have also seen that the latest of the major epidemic diseases – tuberculosis – still remained largely out of control by the middle of the twentieth century.

In this chapter, we review the pattern of health and disease of Aboriginal peoples from the end of the Second World War to the early 1990s. During this period, most infectious diseases were increasingly brought under control, although they have by no means been eradicated. Many infectious diseases remain at a persistently higher level than for the rest of the Canadian population, pockets of high endemicity remain across the country, and fresh epidemic outbreaks, albeit of short duration and geographically localized, continue to occur. Concurrently there has been a shift to diseases such as heart disease, diabetes, hypertension, and obesity, which previously were insignificant causes of mortality and morbidity. An even more alarming trend is the new epidemic of injuries – both intentional and unintentional – which have overtaken all other causes of ill health.

In addition to reviewing statistical data on contemporary health status, this chapter pays special attention to the methods of obtaining such data. The complexities of data sources for Aboriginal peoples need to be recognized before the results of contemporary epidemiological studies can be interpreted and evaluated.

MEASURING ABORIGINAL HEALTH

Even from the 1950s onwards, when the delivery of health care to Aboriginal peoples was greatly expanded and the collection of health statistics much improved, the reconstruction of a 'health history' of Aboriginal peoples remains a difficult task. Furthermore, not all groups of Aboriginal people are equally well represented in surveys and studies. In general, registered Indians, particularly those residing on reserves, and Inuit in the Northwest Territories are best documented. The least is known about non-status Indians and Métis, particularly those residing in urban areas. Wigmore and McCue of the Native Council of Canada, the national organization of non-status Indians, are critical of the lack of health data relating to this group of Aboriginal people, a lack which has rendered invisible their serious health problems, particularly among those residing off-reserve and in urban areas. They see a clear link between the lack of health information and the lack of policy and cultural sensitivity on the part of governments (Wigmore and McCue 1991).

Health researchers have long attempted to summarize the overall health status of a population by using a single measure. In Canada, Connop (1983) proposed a composite health index for Indians in northwestern Ontario by combining traditional mortality and hospitalization data, weighted by values of health priorities assigned by community members in a survey. A convenient summary measure often used in international comparisons is life expectancy, which is based entirely on the mortality experience of the population. Substantial gains in this area by Aboriginal peoples in Canada have been recorded. The life expectancy at birth of the Inuit in the Northwest Territories more than doubled between 1941-50 and 1978-82, when it reached sixty-six years (Robitaille and Choinière 1985). Registered Indian men gained 4.3 years between 1960-4 and 1982-5 while women gained 9.3 years, although there is still a gap of nine years in men and seven years in women compared to the national average (Norris 1990). The major contribution to the reduced life expectancy at birth among Aboriginal peoples has been their higher rate of infant mortality. While substantial gains have also been made in the post-Second World War years (Figure 6), the registered Indian rate in the early 1990s was still about twice as high as the national rate. The decline has been the steepest among Northwest Territories Inuit, although it still remains higher than the registered Indian rate.

Internationally, Canadian registered Indian and Inuit infant mortality rates are comparable to those of some countries of southern and eastern

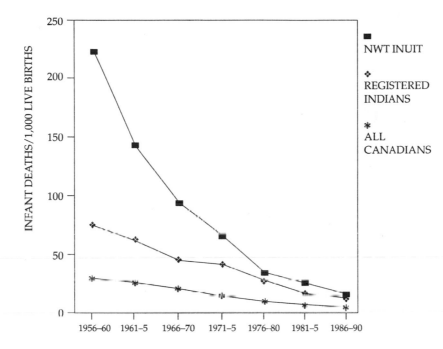

Figure 6
Infant mortality rate among Canadian registered Indians, Northwest Territories Inuit, and all Canadians

SOURCE: Data from Medical Services Branch, Health Canada; Northwest Territories Department of Health; and Statistics Canada

Europe and several of the newly industrialized countries of East Asia and Latin America. While the epithet 'Canada's Third World' is often used to depict the sorry state of health of Aboriginal peoples, the rate of infant mortality among Canadian Aboriginal peoples has in the past two decades been greatly reduced to levels much lower than those rates commonly found in the so-called least developed countries, for example, in sub-Saharan Africa. Figure 7 shows how registered Indians and Inuit rank in relation to all the countries in the world. Figure 8 compares life expectancy between the Aboriginal and national populations in several industrialized countries with large Aboriginal populations – Canada, Australia, New Zealand, and the United States – based on data compiled by Kunitz (1990).

There have been many studies on the causes of mortality and morbidity.

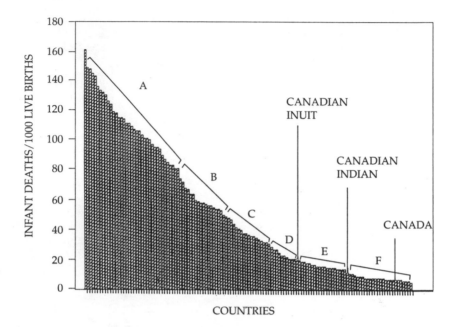

Figure 7
International comparison of infant mortality rates

Note: Data are collected by UNICEF from 130 countries and generally refer to the late 1980s.

Examples of countries:
A: most sub-Saharan African countries, Afghanistan, Bangladesh, Haiti
B: some North African countries, India, central America, Brazil
C: Venezuela, Argentina, China, some Asian and Middle-Eastern countries
D: Korea, Malaysia, Chile, Panama, Uruguay, Romania, USSR
E: Costa Rica, Cuba, Jamaica, Greece, Portugal, Eastern Europe
F: Western Europe, North America, Australiasia, Israel, Japan, Hong Kong

Many are regional in scope: for example, studies in Alberta (Millar 1982), northwestern Ontario (T.K. Young 1983), Labrador (Wotton 1985), and Nouveau Québec (Robinson 1988). Attempts have been made to survey mortality on Indian reserves nationally (Mao et al. 1986, 1992; Morrison et al. 1986), based on the Canadian Mortality Database (CMD). In general, Aboriginal peoples suffer from an excess of injuries and infectious, respiratory, and endocrine diseases, while the risk of cancer and circulatory diseases is lower, although the gap for some of these conditions has also

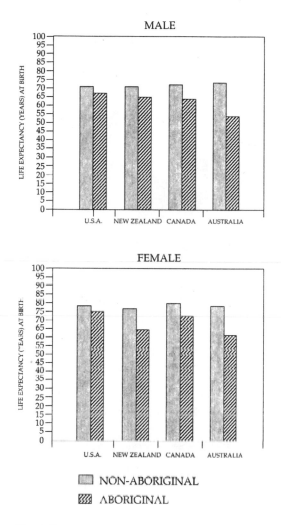

Figure 8

Comparison of life expectancy between Aboriginal and non-Aboriginal populations of
Australia, Canada, New Zealand, and the United States

SOURCE: Based on data from the 1980s reported in Kunitz (1990)

narrowed in recent years. The time trend in mortality for selected causes
is shown in Figure 9.

While, in general, mortality is the most easily obtainable of the health

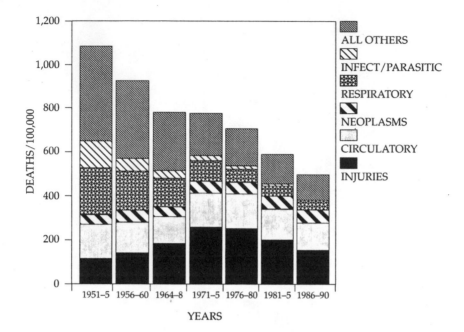

Figure 9
Change in the crude mortality rate by selected causes among Canadian registered Indians, 1951–1986

Note: Inuit are included in 1971–5 data; Ontario Indians are excluded in 1964–8 data; B.C. Indians are excluded after 1985; and Northwest Territories data are excluded after 1987.

SOURCE: 1955–60, 1971–5 data from annual reports of Medical Services Branch, relevant years; 1964–8 data from Latulippe-Sakamoto (1971); other years from Canada, DNHW (1988, 1991)

indicators, there is no convenient single source of mortality data for Aboriginal Canadians nationally. The Medical Services Branch (MSB) of the Department of National Health and Welfare (DNHW) routinely collects vital statistics from its administrative regions. In addition to its annual reports, periodic monographs have been produced which present an overview of the health status (predominantly mortality) of its client population (see, for example, Canada, DNHW 1988, 1991). However, MSB serves only about 75 per cent of the on-reserve registered Indian population in Canada.

An important source of data is the Canadian Mortality Database

(CMD), which has been collecting detailed cause-of-death information on all deaths in Canada since 1950. It does not, however, contain information on ethnic origin, at least not since the early 1970s. Since deaths are coded by the usual place of residence, it is possible to identify deaths among residents of Indian reserves. Although such deaths may theoretically include non-Indians, in reality the probability is low, since most non-Indians who reside on Indian reserves are for the most part transient government workers. On the other hand, such deaths would include a substantial number of non-status Indians who reside in many reserves in Canada. Mao and colleagues (1992) at the Laboratory Centre for Disease Control in Ottawa have analysed data from the CMD for six provinces during the period 1979–88. The mortality rates for selected causes of death among residents of Indian reserves under age sixty-five and their risk of death relative to all Canadians are presented graphically in Figure 10.

It should be noted that not all provinces, and neither of the two territories, have separate residence codes for Indian reserves. Aboriginal peoples who do not reside on reserves are, of course, not even included. Data on the Métis are practically non-existent. Thus, a national picture of Aboriginal mortality still remains elusive.

Central to all epidemiologic analyses is the need for population data from which rates of health events can be computed. For registered Indians, there are two sources of population data: the Indian Register operated by the Department of Indian Affairs and Northern Development (DIAND) and the census conducted by Statistics Canada. Since the census is based on self-report of ethnic origin, it is the only source of information on non-status Indians, Métis, and Inuit. There are problems associated with both sources. Late reporting of births and deaths to the Indian Register has been documented. Non-cooperation of a large number of Indian bands with Statistics Canada during recent censuses has resulted in incomplete enumeration. In 1981, 6 bands were not enumerated. In 1986, 136 bands with an estimated 45,000 residents were incompletely enumerated. In 1991, the number of bands not participating in the census declined to 78, which means that approximately 38,000 Aboriginal persons were not counted. Viewed nationally, this number accounted for less than 5 per cent of the total Aboriginal population. However, for specific regions or cultural and linguistic groups, the proportion of the undercount would be considerably higher.

Because the census's determination of ethnic status is based on self-identification, it can be influenced by the respondents' social experience

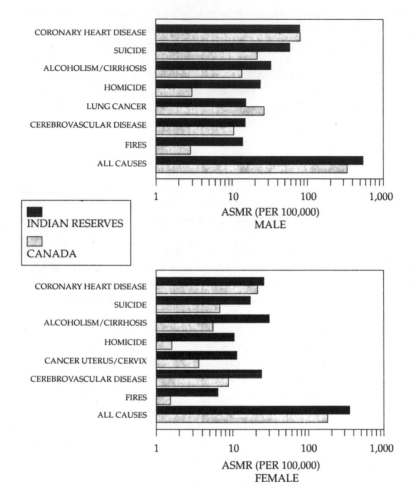

Figure 10
Age-standardized mortality rate (ASMR) by selected causes among residents of Indian reserves in six provinces, 1979–1988, compared to Canada

SOURCE: Based on data reported in Mao et al. (1992)

and cultural ties. The failure of individuals to identify with any Aboriginal
categories, particularly for non-status Indians and Métis, will significantly
affect the population count of those with Aboriginal ancestry. On the
other hand, heightened cultural pride and perceived benefits (such as

entitlements to government services, or land-claims settlements) may increase the number of self-identified Aboriginal Canadians.

Data-collection and -processing procedures may not be comparable from census to census; for example, those relating to the number and labelling of Aboriginal categories, the reporting of multiple origins / mixed heritage, the inclusion of reserve residence and legal status in the definition of Indian status, and differences between information obtained by self-enumeration (since 1971) and by enumerators. (For a historical review of data about ethnic origin in Canadian censuses from 1871 to 1986, see Kralt [1990].)

In most studies, the DIAND Register annual population counts of the on-reserve registered Indian population have been used to provide the denominator for mortality rates. The passage of Bill C-31, an *Act to Amend the Indian Act*, in 1985, which restores Indian status and band membership rights to a large number of Indians (particularly women), has had a significant impact on the registered Indian population. By 1990, the registered Indian population was estimated to have increased by 19 per cent over and above the rate of natural increase (Canada, DIAND 1990).

The pattern of mortality provides only a partial picture of the health status of a population. Most sicknesses, after all, do not result in death. The existence of universal health insurance plans in all Canadian provinces and territories, all of which maintain databases of all utilization of hospital and physician care, can potentially provide a source of data on morbidity. However, ethnic identification is not available, although special identifiers of registered Indians are provided in some Western provinces. Where such data are available, registered Indians have been found to have higher rates of hospital admission than the total provincial population, and the morbidity pattern for different disease categories parallels the pattern for mortality (Canada, DNHW 1988, 1991). In the James Bay region of Quebec, the age-standardized hospitalization rate among the Cree was 1.4 times the provincial rate for all diagnostic categories combined. The ratio was as high as 4 times for skin conditions. On the other hand the rate for cancer was only about half that of Quebec in general (Robinson 1988). It should be cautioned that data on the utilization of health services do not reflect entirely the burden of illness in a population. Many other factors, particularly those relating to access to health care facilities and the practice styles of health care providers may account for differential use.

The only way to capture information on health conditions that do not result in any kind of formal contact with the health care system is to ask people directly about them. Health surveys also provide an opportunity to gather data on health behaviours, practices, attitudes, and beliefs – more positive measures of health beyond those of death, disease, and disability. While there have been many large national health surveys since the 1970s, most have the irritating habit of specifically excluding the northern territories and Indian reserves. A rare exception is the Nutrition Canada Survey (Canada, DNHW 1975b), conducted during 1970–2, which had a separate Indian sample selected from twenty-nine bands across the country (n=1,808) and an Inuit sample from four communities in the Northwest Territories (n=346). This survey provides a wealth of health and nutritional data collected by interviews, physical measurements, and laboratory tests. The Health and Activity Limitation Surveys of 1986 (Statistics Canada 1990), which provides a national perspective on the prevalence of disabilities, did sample the Territories and Indian reserves.

The Aboriginal Peoples Survey (APS) conducted in 1991 has rectified some of the deficiencies in survey data on a national scale. The APS is the most comprehensive national survey of Aboriginal peoples with a significant health and social component. It included not only Indians on- and off-reserve, and Inuit, but also, for the first time, Métis.

For many specific diseases and health conditions, many special disease registers and surveys, usually covering a particular community or region, have been conducted over the years. In the rest of the chapter, some of these studies will be reviewed. In view of their contribution to the overall burden of mortality and morbidity, three groups of diseases will be discussed: infectious diseases, chronic diseases, and injuries. Within each group, an assessment of the extent and magnitude of the problem, the factors which predispose or determine its occurrence, and intervention programs which have been tried to control it will be made. Because most health problems tend to be studied only once in one location, a historical narrative is rarely possible. It should be noted that 'infectious' is used here to refer to a disease caused by micro-organisms such as bacteria or viruses. Not all infectious diseases are 'contagious' in the non-technical sense of the word, meaning easily passed from person to person. Chronic diseases represent a mixed group of diseases usually characterized by slow, insidious onset and are not caused by micro-organisms. The term 'injuries' has by and large replaced 'accidents' in the prevention literature to highlight the health impact on the person and the existence of preventable factors in their causation.

The disease-based discussion that follows is chosen out of convenience, primarily because of the disease orientation of the biomedical literature in which most of the studies on Canadian Aboriginal health can be found. A useful alternative, illustrated in Table 1, is one based on life-cycle phases – infancy, early childhood, adolescence, early and late adulthood, and old age – which would convey a sense of changing health risks over the life span. Such an approach would also facilitate targeting special intervention strategies for specific age groups. Yet another alternative would be one based on causal factors, particularly preventable ones, such as personal lifestyle (smoking, physical inactivity, inappropriate diet, etc.), socio-economic conditions (poverty, unemployment, overcrowding), 'stress,' and so on. It should be noted that among many practitioners and commentators in the public health community, it is almost an article of faith that 'health promotion' is preferred over 'disease prevention,' as if the two are in conflict. It would be a major achievement for any health care system if the level of major causes of mortality and morbidity – diseases and injuries – were reduced, even though the more intangible goal of improving health is still to be accomplished.

INFECTIOUS DISEASES

The success of immunization programs has reduced the epidemiological significance of diseases such as measles, rubella, mumps, poliomyelitis, tetanus, and diphtheria in Aboriginal communities. As late as the 1950s, virgin soil epidemics of these diseases still occurred in some areas in the Arctic, for example in Yukon during the construction of the Alaska Highway by the U.S. military during the Second World War (Marchand 1943). In Chesterfield Inlet, Northwest Territories, 8 per cent of the Inuit population contracted polio from non-Aboriginal workers stationed in Churchill, Manitoba, and 2 per cent of the population died (Adamson et al. 1949). In 1952, a measles epidemic swept through Baffin Island, Northwest Territories, and the Ungava Peninsula in northern Quebec, afflicting 99 per cent of the population, between 2 per cent and 7 per cent of whom died. This epidemic was traced to Inuit visitors to the Armed Forces base at Goose Bay, Labrador (Peart and Nagler 1954).

The availability of effective anti-tuberculosis therapy and the large-scale control efforts of the 1950s resulted in a steep decline in tuberculosis mortality. Despite such improvements, the disparity between Aboriginal and non-Aboriginal Canadians remains great, with the former having an incidence as much as ten times higher. The rates were lowest in eastern

TABLE 1
Age-specific health risks for Aboriginal peoples

	Infants (<1)	Children (1-14)	Adolescents/Young Adults (15-24)	Adults (25-64)	Elderly Adults (65+)
Infectious Diseases	* Acute respiratory infections * Meningitis * Gastro-enteritis	* Acute respiratory infections * Meningitis * Gastro-enteritis	* Sexually transmitted diseases	* Tuberculosis	* Pneumonia/influenza
Chronic Diseases			* Diabetes	* Diabetes * Gallbladder diseases * Cirrhosis	* Diabetes * Cancers * Heart disease * Stroke
Injuries	* Accidents	* Accidents * Child abuse	* Suicide * Violence	* Accidents * Violence	
Other Causes	* Immaturity * Birth-associated * Congenital defects * Sudden Infant Death Syndrome	* Congenital defects			

Note: 'Risks' refer to health problems where the risks of mortality and/or morbidity among Aboriginal peoples are higher than among other Canadians. Some conditions are also included for their importance to the Aboriginal population, even though their risks relative to other Canadians may not be substantially different.

Canada but highest in the prairie provinces and the northern territories (Enarson and Grzybowski 1986). Figure 11 shows the decline in incidence among Canadian Indians, Inuit, and the national population from 1961–5 to 1986–90. It can be seen that by the late 1970s the Inuit rate had declined to a level below that of Indians, among whom the rate had remained stable at a relatively high level.

Regional studies, for example those among the Cree-Ojibwa in north-western Ontario (T.K. Young and Casson 1988), support the national trend of a levelling off in the decline. Sporadic outbreaks of tuberculosis still occurred in Aboriginal communities throughout the 1980s and 1990s (for example, among the Lubicon Cree in Alberta). The recrudescence of tuberculosis is indicative of deteriorating socio-economic conditions and the inability of existing health and social services to prevent and cope with the outbreak.

Several strategies are available in the prevention and control of tuber-culosis: vaccination with Bacille-Calmette-Guérin (BCG), prophylaxis or preventive treatment with isoniazid (INH), mass screening with tuber-culin skin tests and/or chest x-rays, and definitive treatment of active cases. All or some of these methods are used by different jurisdictions around the world, to some extent dictated by the financial and human resources available to the health care system.

Tuberculosis is potentially a completely treatable disease, and a variety of efficacious drugs are available. The emergence of strains of *Mycobacteria* that are resistant to currently available anti-tuberculosis drugs in some populations, particularly transient 'skid-row' patients, is cause for con-cern. However, in a review of anti-tuberculosis drug resistance in Mani-toba, only 7 per cent of all cases during 1980–9 were drug resistant, and the risk of resistance among status Indians was not different from that of other Manitobans (Long et al. 1993). The former practice of prolonged hospital treatment, often at centres far removed from the home commu-nity, which imposed severe personal hardship and family disruption among Aboriginal patients, has been generally superseded by shorter courses of intermittent and supervised therapy since the 1970s. Poor compliance with treatment regimes has often been cited as being respon-sible for treatment failures among Aboriginal patients. A key informant survey in thirty-one Indian reserves in British Columbia revealed a wide-spread belief that tuberculosis was a disease of the past and little knowl-edge about recent improvements in treatment. There was also substantial resentment towards and mistrust of non-Aboriginal health professionals (Jenkins 1977). Successful therapy requires not only individual respon-

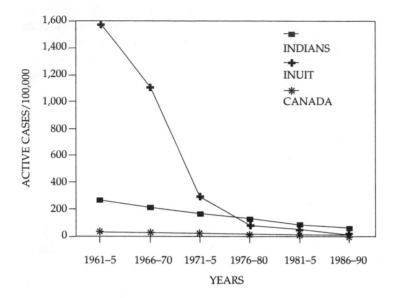

Figure 11
Trend in incidence of tuberculosis among Canadian Inuit, Canadian Indians, and all Canadians

SOURCE: Based on data from Medical Services Branch and Statistics Canada

sibility, but also the existence of a continuing source of care, as well as commitment and sensitivity among the health care staff providing the treatment.

In terms of prevention, Aboriginal people are one of the few groups in Canada which receive the BCG vaccine at birth. One of the early field trials of this vaccine, conducted among Indian infants in Saskatchewan during the 1930s, found it to be highly protective, in the 80 per cent range (R.G. Ferguson and Sime 1949). In the 1980s, studies conducted among Indians in Manitoba (T.K. Young and Hershfield 1986) and Alberta (Houston et al. 1990) still showed a protective effect of at least 60 per cent. Mass prophylaxis with the drug isoniazid or INH was also tested among the Inuit in various circumpolar regions, including Frobisher Bay, Northwest Territories (Dorken et al. 1984). These studies are examples of situations where the high burden of illness among Aboriginal communities has led to their being selected as sites for intervention trials. The results of such studies have broader national and international implications and applications beyond the individual communities where they originally took place.

Another infectious disease which strikes particularly hard at Aboriginal communities is meningitis, an infection of the linings of the brain which can have serious, often fatal, consequences. A study of infant mortality on Indian reserves in five provinces during 1976–83 showed that the risk of death from meningitis was 4 times that of all Canadians during the post-neonatal period (Morrison et al. 1986). In Manitoba, the Indian rate was 1.4 times the non-Indian rate among children under five and 1.8 times among infants under one. For Inuit in the Keewatin region of the Northwest Territories, the excess was 20 times among the under-fives and 33 times among infants (Hammond et al. 1988).

Although diarrhoeal disease or gastro-enteritis is less severe in Aboriginal communities than in many developing countries, isolated outbreaks continue to be reported – for example, from the James Bay coast of northern Quebec (Robinson and Moffatt 1985). In 1991 a large outbreak of gastro-enteritis occurred in the Keewatin region of the Northwest Territories. It was traced to food contaminated by the toxin-producing micro-organism called *Escherichia coli* 0157:H7. It was reputedly the largest such outbreak ever reported, with 521 cases during the six-month course of the epidemic, 22 of whom developed, and 2 of whom died from, the serious complication called hemolytic uremic syndrome, which may lead to kidney failure (Keewatin Regional Health Board 1992). Far more epidemics have occurred than are reported in the literature. Even in non-epidemic situations, Aboriginal children suffer from diarrhoea far more frequently than non-Natives. In southwestern Ontario, Evers and Rand (1982) reported 573 episodes of gastro-enteritis and 73 hospitalizations per 1,000 infants during their first year of life, respectively 3 and 24 times more often than non-Natives in the same area.

While in the long term the improvement of community infrastructure such as water supply and sanitation will reduce or eliminate the health impact of diarrhoeal diseases, individual-based efforts directed at encouraging breast-feeding can be effective. The protective effect of breast-feeding against diarrhoeal disease has been demonstrated among Indian infants in northern Manitoba (Ellestad-Sayed et al. 1979).

Botulism is a disease caused by the consumption of food contaminated by the toxin-producing bacterium *Clostridium botulinum*. In Canada, between 1971 and 1984, 61 outbreaks involving 122 cases and 21 deaths were reported, almost exclusively from among Inuit in northern Quebec and the Northwest Territories, and Indians from British Columbia. The sources of botulism in the Aboriginal population are contaminated traditionally prepared foods: raw, parboiled, or fermented sea mammal meat among the Inuit and fermented salmon eggs or fish among Indians in British Columbia (Hauschild and Gauvreau 1985).

Pneumonia and infections of the respiratory tract can cause serious illness among the very young and the very old. In rural southwestern Ontario, 46 per cent of Indian infants, compared to 18 per cent of non-Indians, experienced lower-respiratory disease during their first year of life. Indian infants were also more likely to have multiple episodes of illness (Evers et al. 1985). The high risk of hospital admission for lower-respiratory infection continued during the second year of life (Evers and Rand 1983). A study of hospitalization data of children under five years of age living in seventeen Indian communities in British Columbia estimated that rates for upper- and lower-respiratory infections were 5 and 8 times the rates for non-Aboriginal children (Thomson and Philion 1991). Various housing surveys and successive censuses have documented the high proportion of Aboriginal dwellings characterized by overcrowding, inadequate heating, and poor ventilation (Clatworthy and Stevens 1987), factors which contribute to the high risk of respiratory infections.

Although solid statistical data on a provincial or national basis are lacking, sexually transmitted diseases such as gonorrhoea and chlamydia are important health problems in Aboriginal communities. In urban areas, the situation is likely to be far more serious, because of the social circumstances associated with city living, including prostitution and drug abuse. The new epidemic of acquired immune deficiency syndrome (AIDS) has by the end of 1993 resulted in about 9,000 cases in Canada, fewer than 1 per cent of whom are of Aboriginal origin, according to data available from Health Canada's Laboratory Centre for Disease Control. Despite the relatively small number of Aboriginal AIDS victims, the potentially explosive situation has been recognized by Aboriginal political leaders, health care professionals, and the federal government. The number of Aboriginal cases may indeed be misleadingly low, as reporting of ethnic identity is available for only about 60 per cent of AIDS cases. Furthermore, the situation has deteriorated: the number of Aboriginal cases during the three years from 1991 to 1993 was double the total number of cases in the previous six years. Also, the proportion of women was 11 per cent among Aboriginal cases, compared to 6 per cent among all cases. The proportion of the Aboriginal population infected by the AIDS virus (called human immunodeficiency virus, or HIV), demonstrable in a blood test (HIV positive) but without the signs and symptoms of the disease, is simply not known. In some localities, anonymous testing of banked blood specimens collected for other purposes in the course of medical care is under way. Such testing will give some indication of the extent of HIV infection in the population, but individuals who test positive will not, and cannot, be identified.

A study of Aboriginal knowledge, attitudes, and practices related to AIDS in eleven Indian reserves across Ontario provided some data on the extent of at-risk behaviour. While two out of five men and one out of five women reported having multiple sexual partners, only 1 per cent reported intravenous drug use. However, some 80 per cent of respondents reported unprotected sexual intercourse at least some of the time (Myers et al. 1993). It should be emphasized that local attitudes and practices can be expected to vary widely, resulting in differences in the probability of disease transmission, case-finding, reporting, and treatment.

A Joint National Committee on Aboriginal AIDS Education and Prevention, consisting of all key 'stakeholders,' was established in 1989 and embarked on a public education program across the country (Canada, DNHW 1990a, 1990b). This committee established several guiding principles. Any education and prevention strategy should: be holistic, rooted in Aboriginal culture and traditions, and positive; empower communities and individuals; provide equity of access to services; be sensitive to different views of sexuality; and be tolerant of those who are infected. An important stumbling block is the reluctance of communities to admit the existence of the problem or the prevalence of risk factors related to sexual practices and intravenous drug abuse. There have also been cases of communities resorting to ostracism, expulsion of infected individuals, and the banning of sex education in schools. On the other hand there are also courageous Aboriginal persons with AIDS who travel across the country to increase awareness, promote safe sex, and plead for tolerance.

While diseases such as AIDS are new to Aboriginal communities, there are also 'old' infectious diseases which are disappearing because of changing ecological factors and cultural practices. Parasitic infections are one group of diseases which are very sensitive to changes in methods of food gathering and preparation, and the relationships between humans and domesticated animals. Sporadic cases of the roundworm infection trichinosis, which can be contracted by eating infected game meat such as bears and foxes, have been reported from northern Quebec and Labrador. In the 1950s the fish tapeworm diphyllobothriasis was widely distributed across northern Canada (Wolfgang 1954). Stool surveys in various parts of the Arctic and Subarctic during the 1950s and 1960s showed relatively high prevalence, as high as 80 per cent in some localities, but more recent surveys showed a much reduced prevalence (Watson et al. 1979; Sole and Croll 1980; Brassard et al. 1985).

Hydatid disease, a cystic disease of the lungs and liver, is caused by various species of the tapeworm *Echinococcus* which infect animals. In northern Canada its life cycle involves deer and moose (intermediate hosts), which are preyed upon by wolves (the definitive host). Domestic dogs become infected when they are fed internal organs of infected animals killed by hunters. In many Aboriginal communities, where dogs live in close proximity to human beings, the latter can become infected from accidentally ingesting eggs released in the faeces of dogs. A large number of cases have been reported from northwestern Canada, characterized by mild clinical illness (Meltzer et al. 1956). With the decline of the dogsled in transportation, this disease has declined substantially. A recent survey of blood samples in northern Quebec found only 1 per cent of Inuit and 3 per cent of Indians to have levels of antibodies suggestive of past infection (Tanner et al. 1987).

Infection with the protozoans *Entamoeba histolytica* and *Giardia lamblia* can result in diarrhoeal diseases, which in the case of amoebiasis can be severe and fatal and manifested clinically as amoebic dysentery. During the 1960s, frequent outbreaks of amoebiasis occurred in Aboriginal communities in northern Saskatchewan (Eaton 1968). A stool survey in 1964 found that 70 per cent of those sampled had some intestinal protozoa, 31 per cent had *E. histolytica*, and 12 per cent *G. lamblia* (Meerovitch and Eaton 1965). Elsewhere in the country, more recent surveys indicated that the prevalence was much lower (Watson et al. 1979; Brassard et al. 1985).

CHRONIC, NON-COMMUNICABLE DISEASES

Over the past several decades the predominant role of infectious diseases as causes of mortality and morbidity affecting Aboriginal peoples has been taken over by the chronic, non-communicable diseases and by accidents and violence. The division of diseases into 'infectious' and 'chronic' is entirely arbitrary. Indeed it is only certain chronic diseases, particularly those labelled by some researchers as 'diseases of modernization' or 'Western diseases' (see, for example, Trowell and Burkitt 1981) that are of interest because of their ability to serve as an 'indicator' of lifestyle and social change. We shall look in more detail at such chronic diseases as cancer, heart disease, stroke, hypertension, and diabetes.

Most studies of cancer mortality and incidence indicate that among Aboriginal peoples as a group, cancer is still less of a problem than it is among Canadians nationally, with the exception of certain specific types. A rise in incidence over the period 1967–86, however, has been documented among both registered Indians and northerners in Saskatchewan (Gillis et al. 1991).

A survey of all Indian Health Service facilities during 1948–52 found an overall lower risk of cancer among Indians, with the exception of cancer of the cervix, compared to Canadians (O.H. Warwick and Phillips 1954). In the 1970s, data from British Columbia, northwestern Ontario, and Manitoba (Gallagher and Elwood 1979; T.K. Young and Frank 1983; T.K. Young and Choi 1985) all showed a lower incidence among Indians when all cancer sites were combined. The few sites for which an increased risk has been found among Indians include gallbladder, cervix, and kid- neys. Although cancer is less likely to occur among Indians, those who suffer from the disease tend not to survive as long as non-Aboriginal patients. In Saskatchewan, an overall lower survival among Indians com- pared to the province as a whole has been observed (Gillis et al. 1991). The reasons for the lower survival are unclear, but may be related to differences in the stage of disease at diagnosis and access to and utilization of available health services.

The Inuit cancer pattern has generally been different from that of In- dians. Of particular interest is the extremely high risk of several cancers which are relatively rare in other populations: nasopharyngeal, salivary gland, and esophageal cancer (Gaudette et al. 1993). These have been called 'traditional' Inuit cancers. According to Schaefer and Hildes (Schae- fer et al. 1975; Hildes and Schaefer 1984), between 1950–66 and 1974–80 in the central and western Arctic, there has been a decline in the incidence of these 'traditional' cancers, corresponding to a rise in those cancers more commonly found in most industrial societies (lung, cervix, colon, and breast).

While the incidence of and mortality from cancer of the cervix have been steadily declining for Canadians since 1970, the opposite trend is observed among some groups of Aboriginal women. In Saskatchewan, the age-standardized mortality rate among Indians rose by 52 per cent between the two periods 1967–71 and 1982–6, while in the province overall there had been a 43 per cent decline. From twice the provincial rate, the Indian rate has increased to 6 times in the second period (Irvine et al. 1991).

While many consider cancer to be a 'mystery' disease, many risk factors – preventable by either individual or societal means – have been known for some time. One of the most important of such risk factors is cigarette smoking, responsible for lung and a host of other cancers, not to mention other diseases of the heart and respiratory tract, and deleterious effects on the foetus. The high prevalence of smoking among Aboriginal peoples in Canada is evident to the casual observer and confirmed in regional surveys in southern Manitoba (Longclaws et al. 1980), northwestern Ontario (McIntyre and Shah 1986), and the Northwest Territories (Imrie and Warren 1988). The Northwest Territories Health Promotion Survey found that 64 per cent of Indians and 78 per cent of Inuit were cigarette smokers, compared to only 39 per cent among non-Natives in the Northwest Territories and 34 per cent among Canadians nationally (ibid. 1988). What is of particular concern is the even higher rate of smoking among adolescents: in a 1987 survey of school students in the Northwest Territories, 71 per cent of Inuit and 63 per cent of Indians, compared to 43 per cent of non-Aboriginals, were regular smokers by the age of nineteen (Millar 1990).

Cancer may be prevented by reducing the prevalence of risk factors (primary) and by early detection (secondary). In terms of primary prevention, educational efforts directed at behavioural changes in smoking, alcohol consumption, delaying the onset of sexual activity, limiting promiscuity, and increasing protection against sexually transmitted diseases, and also at changes in diet (reducing the percentage of energy derived from fats, increasing the intake of fibre, fresh fruits, and green vegetables, and maintaining an ideal body weight) could bring about a reduced incidence of disease, although data from community preventive field trials in support of such conclusions are lacking. However, from a policy perspective, such educational efforts could not do much harm, and there may even be beneficial effects for other non-cancer diseases as well.

Many strategies for the early detection or secondary prevention of cancer exist, but the effectiveness of all of them has not been demonstrated. Pap smear for cervical cancer, and manual examination and mammography for breast cancer are two of the few for which the evidence is strong. In British Columbia, where a computerized cervical cytology screening registry exists, Hislop and others (1992) found that only 52 per cent of Indian women aged thirteen to fifty-nine belonging to twenty-eight bands had had one Pap smear during the past three years, about a third lower than the overall provincial coverage rate. Improving access to and participation in an effective screening program should help reduce the burden of cervical cancer, one of the few cancers for which Aboriginal women are currently at higher risk than the rest of the Canadian population.

Diseases of the heart, particularly 'heart attacks' (ischaemic or coronary heart disease), have often been considered to be rare among non-industrialized societies. With rapid social and cultural change, these diseases tend to increase. Among male residents of Indian reserves under sixty-five, the risk of dying from ischaemic heart disease during 1984–8 was not significantly different from that among Canadians nationally; among females, the Indian rate was 1.6 times higher. For stroke, the Indian female rate was twice as high as the Canadian rate, while that of Indian men was 1.4 times higher (Mao et al. 1992). The low incidence of cardiovascular diseases among the Inuit has been recognized for some time. Autopsies of Canadian Inuit (Lederman et al. 1962) during the 1950s indicate that cases of atherosclerosis, while not an important cause of death, were by no means absent. The age-standardized mortality rate for ischaemic heart disease in the Northwest Territories has remained consistently lower than the national rate, although that of Indian women approached that of all Canadians and exceeded that among the Inuit and non-Aboriginal people (T.K. Young et al. 1993).

A considerable literature has been accumulated on social and cultural influences in cardiovascular diseases, conducted in a variety of ethnic groups around the world (see the review by Dressler 1984). Little research has been conducted among Aboriginal peoples beyond establishing the presence of a differential in disease burden or, at most, explaining the differential in terms of the prevalence of classical risk factors such as elevated levels of blood pressure and cholesterol.

In Canada, a survey among the Ojibwa and Cree in the 1980s showed higher mean diastolic blood pressure in all age-sex groups compared to Canadians nationally, while for systolic blood pressure, the Indians' level was lower above the age of forty-five (T.K. Young 1991). Much interest has been shown in whether blood pressure rises with age among the Inuit, a phenomenon not demonstrated by some non-industrial populations around the world. In Igloolik, Northwest Territories, a survey of 400 subjects in 1969–70 showed a low mean blood pressure but no rise with age (Hildes and Schaefer 1973). Later surveys showed an age-dependent increase in blood pressure in both sexes in Inuvik, a large town, but not among males in remote Arctic Bay (Schaefer, Timmermans, et al. 1980).

For cholesterol, national data are available from the Nutrition Canada Survey conducted during the early 1970s, which showed generally low levels of serum cholesterol among Canadian Indians and Inuit (Canada, DNHW 1975a, 1975b). Health surveys in two Arctic communities revealed higher serum cholesterol levels in the more 'acculturated' group (Schaefer, Timmermans, et al. 1980).

From work done among the Inuit in Greenland, it has been hypothesized that long-chain omega-3 fatty acids found in a diet based on sea mammals and fish may be protective against ischaemic heart disease (Dyerberg 1989). Chemical analyses of adipose tissues in various Inuit foods have been done in the Northwest Territories (Innis and Kuhnlein 1987). High levels of eicosapentaenoic (EPA) and docosahexaenoic (DHA) acids, two of such fatty acids, have also been found in the salmon-based traditional diet of Tsimshian Indians on Vancouver Island (Bates et al. 1985). Abandoning a traditional diet for one which is likely to be high in fats, particularly saturated fatty acids, can be expected to have a detrimental impact on the risk of heart disease.

Most public health authorities advocate primary prevention to reduce the prevalence of multiple risk factors. While smoking cessation, cholesterol reduction, control of hypertension, maintenance of ideal body weight, and regular exercise all appear to reduce the risk of heart disease substantially, the effectiveness of currently available strategies to modify personal risk behaviour and lifestyle is variable. While there are scattered efforts by health professionals in individual communities to influence lifestyle, to date no large-scale, systematic primary prevention trial has been attempted and evaluated in an Aboriginal population.

To be effective, strategies for behavioural change must be directed both at individuals through education and at social factors through protecting traditional subsistence activities, ensuring the availability of foods at affordable prices, and promoting the marketing of appropriate foods.

Health professionals within the western biomedical tradition generally lack an understanding of or interest in Aboriginal concepts of disease causation, manifestation, and treatment. Working among the Ojibwa in southern Manitoba, Garro (1988a, 1988b) found that the cultural model of hypertension can be at odds with the prevalent biomedical view on the chronicity of the illness and the importance of 'compliance' with treatment. Hypertension is conceived by the Ojibwa as episodic in nature, accompanied by perceptible symptoms, and treatment is needed only when symptoms are present. Thus, hypertension control is considerably more complex than recalling patients for blood-pressure checks and pill counts.

The high prevalence of obesity has been documented in many Aboriginal groups in North America (McIntyre and Shah 1986; T.K. Young and Sevenhuysen 1989; Broussard et al. 1991). Yet only a few decades ago, many remote communities were still hovering on the brink of starvation, with deficient energy and nutrient intakes (Vivian et al. 1948; P.E. Moore et al. 1946). Among the Inuit, data on skinfold thickness collected by

Schaefer (1977) in various parts of the central and eastern Arctic during the 1960s revealed a generally lean population. According to Rode and Shephard (1992), who have monitored residents of Igloolik over two decades, substantial increase in subcutaneous fat has occurred since 1970, accompanied by a decline in physical fitness and muscular strength.

Of all the chronic diseases, diabetes – more specifically non–insulin-dependent (NIDDM) or type II diabetes – has achieved particular prominence because of its high prevalence among most Aboriginal groups studied, such as the Cree-Ojibwa (T.K. Young et al. 1985), Mohawk (Montour et al. 1989), Oneida (Evers et al. 1987), and Algonquin (Delisle and Ekoé 1993). Some groups, such as the Inuit and Athapaskan Indians, appear to be at lower risk for the disease (T.K. Young et al. 1992; Szathmary and Holt 1983). In Manitoba, a trend towards earlier onset of NIDDM during the young teen years has been observed (Dean et al. 1992).

The extent of geographical variation in the prevalence of diabetes among Aboriginal Canadians was demonstrated in a national review of diagnosed cases undertaken in 1987 (T.K. Young, Szathmary, Evers, and Wheatley 1990). The lowest rates were observed in the Northwest Territories, while the highest were found in the Atlantic region. In comparison to Canadians nationally, the prevalence of diabetes in Aboriginal peoples was higher in all regions except British Columbia, Yukon, and the Northwest Territories. In other regions, Aboriginal rates were 2 to 5 times higher than in all other Canadians.

The prevalence of diabetes also varied according to language family and culture area, and was lower in more northern latitudes, western longitudes, and geographically remote regions, findings that suggest an interaction between genetic susceptibility and environmental factors in accounting for the observed spatial distribution of diabetes. Language affiliation can be used as a proxy measure of genetic relationship among groups, since genetic distances (summary statistical measures based on a variety of genetic markers) between language families are larger than genetic distances within language families. Culture area reflects the subsistence pattern before European contact and is useful in some regions as an indicator of the baseline from which sociocultural changes proceeded after contact. Longitude and latitude, within certain regional groups, provide a rough measure of the intensity and duration of non-Aboriginal influences. Such differences are also reflected in the degree of geographical isolation and proximity to urban areas.

Diabetes is an example of a chronic disease with a multifactorial etiology. To date, epidemiological evidence of varying consistency has implicated heredity, obesity, physical activity, diet, and metabolic factors as potential risk factors. Among the Cree-Ojibwa, several factors have been found to be associated with diabetic status or high plasma glucose levels, including age, the level of serum triglycerides, measures of obesity and central fat patterning, and education (T.K. Young, Sevenhuysen, Ling, and Moffatt 1990). The independent role of fat distribution, particularly 'central' or 'centripetal' fat, in predicting diabetes or glucose intolerance has also been demonstrated in the Dogrib Indians in the Northwest Territories and the Oneida in southwestern Ontario (Szathmary and Holt 1983; Evers et al. 1989).

Diabetes is of public health importance primarily because of its association with various acute and chronic long-term complications such as coronary and peripheral vascular disease, retinopathy, nephropathy, and peripheral neuropathy (Macaulay, Montour, and Adelson 1988). In a study of mortality on Indian reserves in seven provinces during 1977–82, the risk of death from diabetes was 2.2 and 4.1 times higher among Aboriginal men and women respectively than in the national population (Mao et al. 1986).

In a national survey of chronic renal failure (or end-stage renal disease [ESRD]) the overall risk of ESRD from all causes among Aboriginal Canadians was 2.5 to 4 times higher, and the risk of ESRD due to diabetes specifically was at least 3 times higher than among non-Aboriginals (T.K. Young, Kaufert, McKenzie, et al. 1989). Similar excesses have also been observed regionally, such as among the Cree on the west coast of James Bay (Wilson et al. 1992) and in Saskatchewan (Dyck and Tan 1994).

As diabetes is considered to be a 'new' disease which has rapidly increased in magnitude and extent, Aboriginal peoples have little previous collective experience of it and the cultural response is still evolving (R. Hagey 1984; Garro and Lang 1994). Health professionals who serve Aboriginal peoples are confronted with the need to adapt their treatment regimen and education programs to the culture and the social environment of their patients. Innovative education programs can be found in scattered localities in Canada (Macaulay and Hanusaik 1988), designed to help patients manage their illness better and prevent the development of complications.

ACCIDENTS AND VIOLENCE

Among the most serious health problems affecting Aboriginal peoples in the decades since the end of the Second World War, particularly the younger age groups, are injuries sustained as a result of accidents and violence. The excessive risk begins from infancy onwards. Compared to Canadians nationally, Indian infants from five provinces during the period 1976–83 were 6 and 4 times more likely to die from some injuries in the neonatal and post-neonatal period respectively (H.J. Morrison et al. 1986).

The high level of mortality from injuries has often been attributed, on the general level, to the prevailing economic conditions and social stress that Aboriginal peoples experience. Alcohol abuse is often found to play a major role in many violent and accidental deaths when detailed investigations into the circumstances surrounding such deaths are undertaken (Trott et al. 1981; Jarvis and Boldt 1982).

In many remote Aboriginal communities (in British Columbia and northwestern Ontario, for example), where roads and motor vehicles are few, the risk of mortality from motor-vehicle accidents may be lower than that of the national population. On the other hand, the risk of death from accidents involving other types of transport (such as railways and boats), where these are the chief means of transportation, is extremely high (T.K. Young 1983; Hislop et al. 1987).

On Indian reserves, the number of fires have been increasing linearly throughout the 1970s and 1980s: the mean annual number of fires increased 70 per cent between 1970–9 and 1980–9. On the other hand, mortality from fires has been declining steadily by about 5 per cent per year during these two decades. The causes of these fires were attributed to heating equipment (18 per cent), arson (14 per cent), electrical installation (19 per cent), child-related accidents (11 per cent), smoking (7 per cent), and burning grass and trash (6 per cent) (Canada, DIAND 1989).

Many factors are responsible for the high number of residential fires in Aboriginal communities. Factors relating to the person directly involved include personal behaviours such as smoking, drinking, leaving children unattended, and having suicidal intent. The agents responsible for the fires may be candles, oil burners, woodstoves, electrical appliances, and faulty wiring in the dwelling. The presence in the physical environment of unsecured combustible materials, buildings with blocked exits, nonfunctional fire extinguishers, inflammable clothing and mattresses, and the lack of piped water in the homes contribute to injuries from fires. Contributing factors from the social environment are largely attributable to poverty, which lead to disconnected electricity due to non-payment of bills, alcoholism, lack of fire protection service in the community, nonadherence to building codes, and lack of child care and mental health programs (Friesen 1985).

Acts of violence are intimately related to the mental health of individuals and the social health of the community. Such violent acts may be self-inflicted or directed at others, and often result in suicide and homicide. Epidemiological data on Aboriginal suicides and homicides are very variable in quality. Nationally, the much higher risk of suicide and homicide among Aboriginal peoples is evident from data from the Canadian Mortality Database. Between 1984 and 1988 the age-standardized suicide rates among male residents of Indian reserves were 3 times and female residents 2 times that of all Canadians nationally. For homicide, the rates were 6 times higher in men and 4 times higher in women (Mao et al. 1992). Within the Aboriginal population, considerable regional variation also exists. In Manitoba between 1973 and 1982, the suicide rate was 2.6 times higher in southern Indian reserves than in the remote, northern ones (Garro 1988d). The higher suicide rate in the south is also demonstrated in Saskatchewan, where the Fort Qu'Appelle Zone had more than twice the rate of more northerly Prince Albert and North Battleford Zones (Federation of Saskatchewan Indian Nations 1986). The direction of the north-south gradient, however, was reversed in Alberta, where the rate in northern reserves was 2.3 times that in southern ones. In addition to varying by region, the suicide rate was also positively correlated with a lower per-capita income and greater distance from an urban centre (Bagley et al. 1990).

Aboriginal homicide victims are distributed evenly in all age groups, whereas for suicide, the highest risk is among young adult males, with few cases beyond age forty-five (Figure 12). One characteristic of adolescent suicides is their tendency to occur in epidemics, or clusters (Ward and Fox 1977; C.A. Ross and Davis 1986). Such epidemics continue to occur in scattered locations across the country, as in the Ojibwa community of Pikangikum in northwestern Ontario in 1994. Suicide mortality represents only the tip of the epidemiological 'iceberg.' For every successful suicide, there are many more suicide attempts (also called parasuicide). These may or may not result in any contact with the health and social service systems, and their true magnitude is thus difficult to estimate.

One particular form of violence which has received increasing attention in recent years is the abuse and neglect of children. Accurate data are extremely difficult to obtain, and media reports of flagrant cases do not necessarily reflect the true scope of the problem. In 1981 the proportion of Indian children living on reserves who were 'in care' was more than 5 per cent. This slowly declined to 3 per cent by 1987, still 3 times the national average (N.J. Hagey et al. 1989). Although children are taken

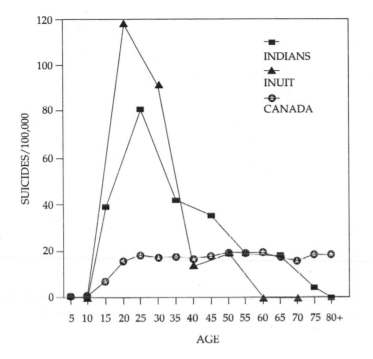

Figure 12
Age-specific suicide rate, registered Indians and Northwest Territories Inuit, mid-1980s

SOURCE: Medical Services Branch and Statistics Canada

away from their homes by social welfare agencies for a variety of reasons, a violent and abusive family environment is a major cause of this extreme action. Many Aboriginal leaders are convinced that physical, sexual, and psychological abuse of children in residential schools, an increasing number of cases of which are brought to public attention, may have produced a generation of adults who in turn inflict violence on their own children.

A study conducted among inmates incarcerated for criminal homicide in British Columbia in the mid-1970s involved extensive record reviews and standardized psychiatric interviews of twenty-two Aboriginal inmates and a group of Euro-Canadians matched on the basis of sentence, age at first homicide, and IQ (Jilek and Roy 1976). While Aboriginal peoples were overrepresented in the prison system, manslaughter charges far exceeded capital murders. The typical homicide committed by an Aboriginal person was directed against another Aboriginal, usually female and a relative of the offender. The non-Aboriginal victim of a homicidal Aboriginal, on the other hand, tended to be male and a stranger. The Aboriginal homicide offenders generally had only limited education, were occupationally unskilled, and had a past history of alcohol abuse, but were less likely than the non-Aboriginal offender to show evidence of psychiatric illness or sexual deviance. In terms of personality development, a lack of exposure to traditional Indian culture was associated with the early onset of antisocial behaviour. Those who showed a positive identification with their Aboriginal heritage, however, were more likely to benefit from education and therapy provided in the institutions (ibid.).

There are very few formal evaluations of the many suicide-prevention programs in Aboriginal communities. A study on Manitoulin Island, Ontario, five years after a suicide outbreak in the mid-1970s, attributed an apparent decline in suicide, parasuicide, and violent deaths to a multidimensional program consisting of residential alcoholism treatment, family counselling, community feasts, job creation for youths, and self-esteem enhancement in the schools. Aboriginal mental health workers were employed to provide crisis intervention as well as liaison with the non-Aboriginal professional health and social service sectors (Fox et al. 1984).

Many Aboriginal people recognize that the interrelated problems of self-inflicted and interpersonal violence (including child and spouse abuse) can be resolved only through a healing process undertaken by the communities themselves. The re-establishment of individual and community self-esteem requires overcoming the denial of embarrassing and/ or painful community problems on the one hand, and emphasizing and enhancing positive traditional values and customs on the other. In British Columbia, spiritual leaders involved their young people in the revived Spirit Dance ceremony where they found a renewed Aboriginal identity and cultural pride (Jilek 1982b). In northern Saskatchewan, one project aimed to empower abused Aboriginal women by developing mutual support networks (Dickson 1989). Various resource guides and training manuals to assist communities have been developed by the Nechi Institute of Alberta (Martens et al. 1988) and Les Femmes Autochtones du Québec (Lamoureux 1991). A landmark conference entitled 'Healing Our Spirit Worldwide' brought together in Edmonton in 1992 Aboriginal groups from around the world who shared their experiences in healing the wounds of violence and substance abuse.

Alcohol and substance abuse have been found to be contributing factors in a high proportion of violent acts. Among the types of substance abuse, gasoline sniffing is particularly prevalent among Aboriginal children and adolescents in some areas, with results ranging from acute intoxication to long-term neurological disorders, even death. In some communities in northern Manitoba in the 1970s, between 50 and 100 per cent of children and adolescents were believed to be current and recent sniffers (Boeckx et al. 1977). On one Indian reserve in northwestern Ontario, 25 per cent of children five to fifteen years of age, or 10 per cent of the total population, were identified as sniffers (Remington and Hoffman 1984). Early in 1993, a group of Innu children in Davis Inlet, Labrador, were recorded on amateur video sniffing gasoline in an unheated shack. The film was broadcast on national television, and substantial media attention and public outcry ensued. Entire families were airlifted across the country to undergo treatment and rehabilitation at Poundmaker's Lodge in Alberta, an Aboriginally operated centre. After six months, the children returned with their counsellors, accompanied again by much media fanfare. Unfortunately, the causes of the substance abuse, which are rooted in the poverty and despair of the community, remained unchanged – within months, most of the children reverted to their gasoline sniffing.

In a survey of residents over the age of five in an Ojibwa community in eastern Manitoba, it was found that adults and school pupils who participated in hobbies were less likely to use alcohol. Young people who reported good family relationships were also less likely to use alcohol and marijuana (Longclaws et al. 1980).

Barnes's review of solvent abuse in a variety of populations concluded that parental alcohol abuse was the most significant determinant of gasoline sniffing. He proposed a causal model which listed four environmental risk factors – low social assets, acculturative stress, parental drug use, and peer/sibling influence – mediated through a filter of 'psychological vulnerability' consisting of learned helplessness and alienation (Barnes 1979).

The approach to alcohol and drug abuse in most health jurisdictions is one of the treatment and rehabilitation – whether residential, out-patient, or 'community-based' – of those who have demonstrated a problem. Many programs are operated by Aboriginal agencies, a notable example being Poundmaker's Lodge in Alberta, mentioned above. Both in terms of professional manpower and facilities, the demand for Aboriginally controlled and culturally sensitive programs far exceeds the supply. There are instances also of successful transformations of non-Aboriginal solutions such as Alcoholics Anonymous into Aboriginal revival movements (Jilek-Aall 1981).

Nationally, the Medical Services Branch of National Health and Welfare developed the National Native Alcohol and Drug Abuse Program (NNADAP) as a pilot project in 1975; it became a permanent program in 1982. Contributions are given to communities for prevention programs, in-patient and out-patient treatment services, construction of facilities, training, and research. Expenditure on the program – $16 million in 1982–3 – had tripled by 1986–7 (Canada, Auditor General 1987: Section 12.68).

Prohibition as a systemic approach to alcohol abuse has a long tradition in many societies. In Canada, various amendments to the *Indian Act* prohibited the possession and use of alcohol by Indians until 1963 (J.A. Price 1975). According to Price, prohibition created a new class of legal offences, stimulated conflict with the police, led to financial exploitation by middlemen and 'bootleggers,' reinforced the pattern of binge drinking, and prevented the development of internal social controls. Yet beneficial effects of prohibition have also been observed. In an Inuit community, O'Neil (1985) observed over a four-year period that alcohol prohibition had contributed to an increase in family integrity and respect among generations, an increase in youthful interest in traditional values and lifestyles, and a decrease in aggressive behaviours and abuse of other substances. Enforcement of the by-law was through local social pressure without resort to the externally imposed law enforcement and justice systems. To be sure, clandestine drinking occurred, but it was tolerated as long as it remained private and did not result in disruptive behaviours in public. The difficulty of supply meant that even habitual heavy drinkers had to reduce their consumption level substantially (ibid.).

Physical training has been identified as a potential means of enhancing Aboriginal adolescents' self-image and reducing drug and alcohol abuse. In an Algonquin community in northwestern Quebec, Scott and Myers (1988) studied the impact of assigning students aged twelve to eighteen to a twenty-four-week fitness program designed to enhance aerobic capacity, flexibility, and strength. Alcohol and drug use remained stable in the intervention group but increased among controls. Scores of self-esteem and body image did not change in either group, while physical 'self-efficacy' (perceived physical ability and self-confidence) did increase over time in the intervention group (ibid.).

Whether alcohol abuse or alcoholism has any genetic basis has been the subject of much controversy, particularly in relation to its policy implications among Aboriginal peoples. Reed (1985) enumerated nine categories of alcohol response where ethnic differences have been shown to occur: consumption rate, absorption rate from the digestive tract, metabolism rate, prevalence of variants of the enzymes alcohol dehydrogenase (ADH) and acetaldehyde dehydrogenase (ALDH), alcohol sensitivity, cardiovascular changes, psychological changes, and alcohol abuse. Of these, he concluded that enzyme differences were very probably due to single genes, while rates of absorption and metabolism were likely under the control of many genes.

The speed with which alcohol is absorbed from the stomach can be measured by the time it takes to reach peak blood-alcohol concentration (BAC) after a test drink. Once absorbed into the blood stream, alcohol is metabolized in the liver first to acetaldehyde (catalysed by the enzyme ADH), and ultimately to acetate (catalysed by the enzyme ALDH).

A study in Alberta (Fenna et al. 1971) compared Euro-Canadian volunteers with Inuit and Indian hospital patients and found that with alcohol administered intravenously, both Aboriginal groups had slower rates of disappearance of blood alcohol. This differential response persisted even after stratifying for the history of usual alcohol consumption (categorized as light, moderate, and heavy drinkers). This study lent credence to the impression that Aboriginal drinkers took a longer time to 'sober up.' The Alberta study, however, was not corroborated by subsequent studies in other Aboriginal groups, some of which actually showed the opposite trend. In their comparative study of Euro-Canadians, Chinese, and Ojibwa Indians, Reed and colleagues (1976) showed that, in tandem with the fastest decline in blood-ethanol concentration among the three groups, at various times after the ingestion of ethanol the Indians also showed the highest levels of acetaldehyde, the metabolic by-product of alcohol believed to be responsible for such symptoms of intolerance as facial flushing.

Sensitivity to alcohol and its metabolic by-products would appear to be a 'protective' mechanism in populations with deficient or abnormal enzymes. Even if this were the case with Aboriginal peoples, and the evidence is by no means consistent, it would appear that socio-economic and cultural factors could overcome this physiologically based aversion to alcohol such that some members of this group appear to experience significant social and health problems related to alcohol abuse. Even if there are substantial genetic differences in alcohol metabolism among ethnic groups, it remains to be seen if such differences are in reality translated into differences in social response, the frequency of abuse, and the potential for successful interventions. On the other hand, the demonstration of metabolic differences does not mean that the problem of alcohol abuse is immutable and that broader strategies addressing social and economic determinants are necessarily futile.

CONCLUSIONS

This chapter has described some of the most important health issues and considered many of the difficulties associated with gathering information on the demographic composition, nutrition, and patterns of illness and disease in Aboriginal populations today. Taken together with the previous chapters, the evidence reveals a pattern of rising rates of infectious disease in the nineteenth and twentieth centuries linked to the transformation of the North American continent in conjunction with accelerated European migration and settlement. Recent trends since the Second World War show a lowering of mortality caused by such infectious diseases as tuberculosis, but also demonstrate a concomitant increase in morbidity and mortality from certain new infectious diseases (such as AIDS), chronic diseases (cancer, cardiovascular disease, and NIDDM), as well as from accidents, violence, and substance abuse.

Of course, in the pre-contact period, Aboriginal peoples had their own complex medical systems to deal with ill health. These systems continued to exist and adapt to the changes in health and disease associated with European colonization. The next chapter begins our discussion of this important area.

5

Medical traditions in Aboriginal cultures

The previous three chapters have described in some detail the state of Aboriginal health prior to contact and in the post-contact years up to contemporary times. Like all peoples, Aboriginal North Americans had complex and diverse medical and healing traditions to deal with the health problems which affected them. These traditions not only predated European contact, they also developed and adapted to the environmental, economic, and political changes wrought by Europeans. The intent of the present chapter is to survey elements of these traditions, including theories of disease and illness, treatment approaches, and the range of healers. It is not possible to be comprehensive in this examination;' rather, the emphasis will be on describing some elements of selected healing traditions of the past that have relevance today. A subsequent chapter will examine the context of traditional medicine in the contemporary world.

HISTORICAL IMAGES OF ABORIGINAL HEALING

Most of the data on the medical traditions of the past are derived from accounts by European and Euro-Canadian traders, missionaries, physicians, and government personnel, as well as scholars such as anthropologists. Two points need to be made about this. First, there was a time when many details of healing were freely provided to inquisitive outsiders, to the point where some were allowed to witness and document various healing activities. By the end of the first quarter of the twentieth century, there appears to have been a shift in this attitude of Aboriginal healers, and a period commenced in which the traditions went underground, shielded from the watchful eye of government administrators and others. Only since the 1980s has a degree of cautious openness emerged regarding healing. Second, it can be said that most early observers of Aboriginal healing retained an obvious bias in their writing. Aboriginal healing traditions were often seen as primitive, fraudulent, and even harmful; the healers as charlatans; and the patients as superstitious and ignorant. Healers were often labelled 'conjurers,' 'jugglers,' or 'magicians,' and their healing activities were often described as 'performances.' Yet, close examination of these texts often also reveals a grudging acknowledgment that many elements of Aboriginal healing did, indeed, work.

Writing in 1795, explorer Samuel Hearne described Dene-speaking healers as 'conjurers' who 'pretend to perform great cures' using techniques that involved 'laughing, spitting, and ... uttering a heap of unintelligible jargon.' Yet Hearne was also moved to write, 'I have often admired the great pains these jugglers take to deceive their credulous countrymen, while at the same time they are indefatigably industrious and persevering in their efforts to relieve them' (Glover 1958:123–4). Like many European observers, Hearne was hard-pressed to explain, in his own rational way, some of the 'tricks' the healers used. In one instance, he watched a healer swallow a bayonet as part of a healing ceremony, and when queried by the Indians admitted he was not close enough to detect the 'deception.' He did note, however, that the patient subsequently recovered (ibid. 125–6). Similarly, trader Andrew Graham wrote that 'Their conjurors pretend to great skill in the medieval way; and by an abstemious regime accompanied with superstitious rites, effect such an alteration in the habit of body and mind of the patient that sometimes is of real service' (G. Williams 1969:230).

George Nelson was a trader with the Hudson's Bay Company in northern Saskatchewan in 1823. A devout Christian, he took an avid interest in the religious and healing traditions of the Cree, and his journal represents one of the best published sources on Aboriginal healing' (Brown and Brightman 1988). Amazingly, Nelson actually seemed to be converted after observing many so-called 'performances' by 'conjurers.' For instance, in describing a ceremony known as the 'shaking tent' (to be described in detail later in this chapter), he wrote, 'I have almost entirely converted myself from these foolish ideas of Ghosts and hobgoblins, but I assure you in truth that I more than once felt very uneasy' (ibid. 104). At the conclusion of the shaking tent ceremony, Nelson was humbled: 'I am fully convinced, as much so as that I am in existence, that Spirits of some kind did really and virtually enter [the shaking tent], some truly terrific, but others again quite of a different character. I cannot enter into a detail by comparisons from ancient and more modern history, but I found the consonance, analogy, resemblance, affinity, or whatever it may be termed so great, so conspicuous that I verily believe I shall never forget the impressions of that evening' (Brown and Brightman 1988:106–7).

The unmistakable air of superiority which Europeans felt when commenting on Aboriginal medicine is clear even from the following passage written in 1886, despite the author's attempts to be sympathetic: 'The false and mistaken notions as to the principles and practice of medicine which prevailed among our forefathers are recalled by some of those in vogue among the red-man; and while, in the light of our own superior knowledge, we may be disposed to laugh at their primitive ideas, we are reminded that many – perhaps the majority – of the doctrines once taught among our own people were absurd enough' (Bell 1886:456–7).

Unflattering statements about Aboriginal medicine continued on through the twentieth century (and indeed are not uncommon today). A medical doctor writing in 1923 described his frustration with the 'interference from medicine men who chanted weird songs over the sick, removed imaginary fishbones from various parts of their bodies, pocketed evil spirits, and in other ways negated the work of the physician and made them despise the white man's medicine' (Shaw 1923:659). In his 1934 history of medicine in Canada, Bull (1934: 19) began by describing the 'conjurer' or 'witch doctor' and 'his bag of tricks,' but was brought to admit nevertheless that 'these horrific-looking medicine men were not entirely without practical knowledge.' Likewise, P.E. Moore (1946:141) stated that, 'The medicine men undoubtedly played on the superstitions of the natives, but they also possessed some knowledge of the use of herbs and native medicine.' American ethnologist Francis Densmore in 1929 described a Chippewa (Ojibwa) healer's actions as follows: 'he startled, amazed, terrified, and stimulated the sick person, and it is not impossible that in some cases the excited nervous condition produced an apparent or even real improvement in his condition' (1929:45). Even Canada's foremost anthropologist and academic 'expert' on Aboriginal peoples, Diamond Jenness (1972:387), sceptically referred to the 'medicine-men' and 'their supposed powers.'

There is no need to prolong this discussion. It is clear that Europeans have often viewed Aboriginal medical traditions through biased eyes, and even where forced to admit that success in treating patients was not uncommon, were nonetheless unable to see traditional medicine for what it really was: sets of coherent beliefs and practices which were well integrated within Aboriginal societies and which served important social and religious as well as medical functions.

DISEASE THEORY

Aboriginal medical systems, like all such systems throughout the world, are built upon coherent, rational understandings of the universe and people's place within it. 'Rationality' must be understood to be a culture-specific notion; one culture's rational thought is not necessarily the same as another's. Indeed, the rational thought that underlies scientific inquiry and biomedical practice is but one type of thought. Inherent in any group's medical system are ideas about how disease is caused, and what types of treatment are called for.

In general, Aboriginal peoples in Canada saw disease as the product of either natural or supernatural occurrences.[2] It is not the case, as some authors (such as Beardsley 1941:486; Balikci 1963:384; McKennan 1965:79; Grinnell 1972:281; Hultkrantz 1992:1) have suggested, that disease was thought to be caused only by supernatural intervention; Aboriginal peoples believed in disease causation which was devoid of any spiritual or supernatural significance. For instance, while not likely having knowledge of the existence of bacteria, they were cognizant of the need and means to reduce infection in wounds. Much of the use of plant and herbal medicines was based on a disease theory of natural causation.

Certainly the greatest attention throughout the literature has been on the understanding of and types of treatment for disease caused by or otherwise related to supernatural forces. In order to understand this, it is essential first to realize that Aboriginal terms which have been subsequently translated into English as 'medicine' actually refer to a much broader phenomenon than drugs or the practice of healing. Generally, these Aboriginal terms referred to a kind of 'power' in a spiritual sense, something that was influential on the lives of people, which was difficult to know fully or understand, and which therefore required certain preventive, propitiating, and/or prophylactic activities to occur. Hence, 'medicine' was partly within the realm of what we would call the religious, and many healers were also involved in religious activities. It is not possible to separate much of Aboriginal 'medicine' from 'religion' as Euro-Canadians would understand these terms.

One of the most comprehensive examinations of the role of disease in the world-view of an Aboriginal people is that in Hallowell's (1963) study of the Ojibwa of the Berens River area of Manitoba. According to Hallowell, the terms 'natural' and 'supernatural' are not even appropriate for describing the components of their world-view; instead of such a dichotomy, he suggests that there existed 'a basic metaphysical unity in the ground of being' (ibid. 267). Their world consisted of human beings ('anishanabek' in Hallowell's lexicon), and 'other-than-human beings.' One class among these latter beings were the 'pawaganak,' or 'dream visitors,' a term synonymous with 'grandfathers.' The pawaganak were willing to share some 'power' and knowledge with human beings if the humans behaved in a socially prescribed manner, and in so doing served to protect individuals and bring them good fortune. Both the ability to heal and the ability to protect oneself from disease or illness were predicated upon the assistance of these other-than-human beings. However, those individuals with stronger than normal power could actually use that power to cause illness. Most Aboriginal healing traditions recognized that the power to heal also entailed the power to cause harm, illness, and misfortune to befall a particular victim (this is often referred to today as 'bad medicine'). Such activity was not, however, socially acceptable, and represented a heightened example of disreputable and amoral behaviour which was invariably punished.

Within this world-view, minor illnesses such as colds, headaches, and digestive disorders were not likely to arouse anxiety, and were treated with herbal remedies. Serious illness, in contrast, was viewed as a penalty for a prior transgression of the moral order, and therefore required the assistance of a specialized healer. Such transgressions could involve only human beings, or they could involve a breach in the relationship between human beings and the other-than-human beings. The cause of illness was sought within the web of interpersonal relations involving both sets of beings; hence both the occurrence of disease and its treatment served to reinforce the social and moral order of Ojibwa society, an important function in a society where informal mechanisms of maintaining the moral order were the norm. Indeed, confession by individuals, detailing breaches of the order that they had committed in the past, was an essential ingredient of treatment.

In general, then, the Ojibwa case underscores a principle common to Aboriginal healing systems: the world is seen as a place in which harmony and balance exist between and among human beings and spiritual or 'other-than-human' entities, and serious illness is indicative of a disruption in this balance. Furthermore, it is apparent that these healing traditions encompassed a holistic view of manifestations of illness in the individual; there is little evidence of a clear distinction between what science would call somatic disorders and disorders of the psyche. Notions of 'sanity' and 'insanity,' and of personality disorders were not strictly defined, as in the case of the biomedical tradition. The mind, body, and spirit were seen as an integrated whole. Part of the problem Euro-Canadians have had with understanding these elements of Aboriginal healing traditions can be found in both the cognitive and linguistic realms. For instance, Trimble and colleagues (1984:201) have suggested that in the Lakota language, 'mental health' translates as *being* in a state of well-being, and not a *state* of well-being.

It is possible to identify a small number of generally applicable theories of disease causation. In addition to natural causations, these would include spirit intrusion, object intrusion, soul loss, and sorcery or 'bad medicine.'

Spirit intrusion refers to the possibility that malevolent spirits or ghosts are inhabiting the body. Object intrusion is similar, in that some object has entered the body and is causing illness. The object may not be something intrinsically pathogenic; upon extraction it is frequently demonstrated to have been a piece of hair, bone, wood, or some other benign substance (Ritzenthaler 1963:316). Soul loss involves the loss of one's soul or spirit from the body, which must then be recaptured (McKennan 1965:79). Soul loss was fairly common among the Indians of the Northwest Coast (Trimble et al. 1984:206). 'Bad medicine,' as noted above, involved the practice of sorcery or witchcraft, in which a malevolent healer, usually at the request of another individual, undertook to cause illness or bad luck to befall an unaware victim. Soul loss could occur with bad medicine when, for instance, a malevolent shaman abducted a victim's soul at night (Hallowell 1942:61). The symptomatology for each of these problems varied somewhat from group to group, and included both somatic and psychological changes. Lethargy, anorexia, changes in emotional status or behaviour, and overt physical conditions such as tremors or palsy-like symptoms were common. Non-physical complaints might include the inability to attract a lover, or poor luck in hunting. In some cases, the symptoms of whatever type could actually be experienced by someone other than the individual who had caused the problem by breaching the moral order. So, for instance, since children were usually not viewed as being fully socialized into the normative order, serious illness among them was viewed as the product of a transgression by an adult.

As one can see, each of these types of disease causation implies a fairly direct intervention of spiritual or supernatural agents; these are not diseases as biomedicine would recognize them, although in recent years the psychological dimension of these problems has been recognized. Unlike biomedical approaches, however, Aboriginal medical systems were probably more concerned with delineating the etiology of the problem, since in so doing the type of treatment required became obvious. And since the cause often involved a breach of the normative order, repairs to the moral fabric of society became central to healing activities. Indeed, the communal nature of Aboriginal healing is in marked contrast to the more circumspect practices of biomedicine.

HEALERS AND HEALING PRACTICES

There were a great many types of healers among the Aboriginal peoples of Canada. While there has been a general acceptance of the appellation 'medicine man/woman' in recent years to describe these individuals, such a term is somewhat meaningless in that it glosses over very important distinctions among the types of healers, their knowledge and skills, and how they acquired the status to heal.

It is first essential to emphasize that there existed among Aboriginal peoples a 'popular' sector of medicine (see Kleinman 1980), wherein certain knowledge regarding the maintenance of health and the treatment of illness or trauma was extant. As in any society, what we might call home management of illness was common. Individuals tended to possess a generic knowledge of medicinal plants and what amounts to first-aid techniques, and applied this knowledge when necessary. The ability to do this did not represent the product of specialized training, which separates treatment within the popular sector from that of the 'folk' sector, where we find non-professional medical specialists of varying types.

Hultkrantz (1992:17–18) has suggested that there are basically three types of healers: herbalists, 'medicine men,' and shamans. The difference between them, it would seem from Hultkrantz, is the degree to which spiritual assistance is required in the healing. The herbalists employ various botanical substances, often in combination, with which they treat a wide variety of disorders, including dressing wounds. Their knowledge is gained largely through experience and tradition handed down to them by older herbalists. The term 'medicine man' denotes a healer 'who has supernatural sanction to make a person well and who follows supernatural dictates in his curing activities' (ibid. 18). The 'shaman,' according to Hultkrantz, is an individual with the ability to fall into a deep trance or 'ecstasy' and undertake spirit flight or summon spirits to counsel him.

The distinction by Hultkrantz is somewhat arbitrary, for he notes that 'The ordinary medicine man may certainly heal the sick while in a light trance, but he does not sink down into the deep trance that is necessary for making contact with the supernatural world' (ibid. 19). In reality, the situation may be much more complex than Hultkrantz suggests.

Andrew Graham (G. Williams 1969), in his observations along Hudson Bay in the late eighteenth century, distinguished between the 'conjurers' or 'jugglers,' who were directly involved with spiritual powers, and the 'tuckathin, or doctors' among the Cree who were highly knowledgeable herbalists. He also described 'itinerant druggists' who came up from the south every year to barter roots and herbs. The literature suggests that some Aboriginal groups had greater knowledge of plant medicines than others, and that borrowing (or bartering) often took place. For instance, D. Smith (1973:21) states that the Chipewyan 'have freely borrowed root medicines from the Cree ... and are quick to give the Cree credit as the "inventors." ' Jenness (1938:73) suggests that the Plains Indians in general had a 'scanty' knowledge of herbal remedies, and groups such as the Sarcee borrowed from the Cree, 'who seemed to know the mysterious virtues of every plant and shrub.' It would not be correct to suggest that herbalists always lacked spiritual assistance in their work, or that other healers were excluded from the use of herbs, for neither is true. Herbalists and other healers could even obtain knowledge of particular combinations through spiritual assistance.

It is virtually impossible to present a coherent and comprehensive discussion of the many botanical medicines which are known to have been used by Aboriginal peoples. There are many sources on this topic, of which the most useful are Hutchens (1973), Hellson (1974), Arnason and colleagues (1981), Ford (1981), Leighton (1985), and Moerman (1986). There have been relatively few pharmacological studies of these plants, and hence much of their value may well have been lost to time. Nevertheless, the testament to their efficacy can be found in two basic facts. First, the earliest fur traders, missionaries, and settlers often turned to the Aboriginal herbalists for treatment, and second, more than 170 drugs which have been or still are listed in the *Pharmacopoeia of the United States of America* owe their origin to Aboriginal usage (Vogel 1970:111–23, 267). Various Aboriginal groups were able to prevent scurvy by brewing tea from spruce bark (rich in vitamin C); they were able to reduce pain by using willow extract, which contains salicin (similar to the product 'aspirin'); they had various kinds of anaesthetics, emetics, diuretics, and medicines that could induce labour or numb labour pains. Plant extracts also acted as antibiotics when applied to wounds. There is no doubt that the Aboriginal herbalists had a different understanding of how and why such plants worked in comparison to biomedicine; but clearly, through thousands of years of adaptation to their environments, and through experimentation, they had developed an impressive array of botanical medicines and preparation techniques. Perhaps only a minority of these have been made readily available to non-Aboriginal peoples, and many formulations have no doubt been lost as a result of the colonization of the Americas.

Beyond the herbalists is a variety of healers who, while they may still use botanical medicines in their healing, tend to rely more on spiritual activity. In this regard, the ability to contact spiritual entities to assist in diagnosis and treatment is essential, and the degree to which an individual can do this is a measure of the person's standing within his or her society. As in all medical traditions, some practitioners were better than others, and their techniques included a number of inspirational, spiritually directed approaches, plus pragmatic and learned techniques which no doubt required practice.

In the late eighteenth century, Andrew Graham described these shamans thus:

Jugglers or conjurers are very numerous amongst them [Cree]. They are generally men who are good hunters, and have a family; some of them are very clever at it. They are supposed to have intelligence with the Evil Spirit [actually 'the Creator'], and by that means can procure anything to be done for the good or injury of others, foretell events, pacify the malignant spirit when he plagues them with misfortunes, and recover the sick. They have also several tricks of sleight hand; such as swallowing a string with a musket ball hanging to it; taking it directly out at the fundament; pretending to blow one another down; swallowing bears' claws, and vomiting them up; extracting them from wounds, or the breast, mouth etc. of a sick person; firing off a gun and ball to remain behind; and a thousand other pranks which make them be held in great esteem by the rest. (G. Williams 1969:161)

The notion that such healers played tricks on their patients is rife in the historic literature. Techniques known today as 'sleight-of-hand' were particularly noted, including swallowing objects, making objects disappear, and undertaking 'surgery' in which objects were removed from the body of the patient without any subsequent wound, suture, or scar. There is no question that such techniques were a part of healing, and some healers

have, on occasion, even disclosed such practices. For instance, anthropologist David Mandelbaum (1979:162–3) relates that one of his inform-
ants, Fine-Day, a Plains Cree, was once shown how to take hot coals into
his mouth by a healer, but could not bring himself to do it. Mandelbaum
notes, 'Officially, however, all these feats were performed in accordance
with directions imparted in a vision' (ibid. 163). Bell (1886:461) noted
that some shamans who had become Christians had subsequently 'con-
fessed that their former course had been all imposture.' Insofar as we are
in a position to posit that some degree of deception was employed in
treating patients, a number of logical reasons for this activity are evident.
First, the ability to undertake apparently impossible feats no doubt served
to impress upon the patient the degree of skill and spiritual power of the
healer; it served as a kind of measure of competence. Second, there is also
the likelihood that a placebo effect occurred as a result of such feats, in
which some individuals subsequently recovered without the intervention
of a pharmacological agent or surgical procedure. Samuel Hearne, writing
in 1771, perfectly described the placebo effect among the northern Dene-
speaking peoples: 'Though the ordinary trick of these conjurers may be
easily detected, and justly exploded, being no more than the tricks of
common jugglers, yet the apparent good effect of their labours on the sick
and diseased is not so easily accounted for. Perhaps the implicit confidence placed in them by the sick may, at times, leave the mind so perfectly
at rest, as to cause the disorder to take a favourable turn; and a few
successful cases are quite sufficient to establish the doctor's character and
reputation' (Glover 1958:142).

As Moerman (1983) has indicated, the placebo effect is an essential
ingredient of all medical traditions, including biomedicine with its highly
visible system of healer validation (degrees on the wall, white lab coats,
and stethoscopes, for instance) and the inclination for doctors to prescribe
inappropriate medicines to help the patient feel that something is being
done (prescribing antibiotics for viral infections is a good example).
Clearly, Aboriginal healing traditions had developed a similar view towards the need to validate the healer's abilities and to empower the
patient to heal himself or herself. Such is an integral, and essential, element of healing, no matter what the culture.[3]

A common shamanistic method of healing has been referred to as
'sucking' or 'cupping,' and its practitioners are often referred to as 'sucking doctors.' This technique is called for particularly when it is believed
that an object has entered the body and is causing a problem, or where
an internal poison or body tissue is implicated. Most accounts suggest

that a sucking horn or tube of some sort is used, although the healer may place his or her lips directly onto the flesh. By sucking and blowing, the object is ultimately removed, and usually shown to the patient and the others attending. The ceremony involves prayer and singing, sometimes blowing on a whistle, all designed to summon the supernatural assistance required to locate and extract the object. Alexander Henry (1976:120–1) described an incident of sucking in 1763, likely among the Chippewa:

After singing for some time, the physician took one of the bones out of the bison: the bone was hollow; and one end being applied to the breast of the patient, he put the other into his mouth, in order to remove the disorder by suction. Having persevered in this as long as he thought proper, he suddenly seemed to force the bone into his mouth, and swallow it. He now acted the part of one suffering severe pain; but, presently finding relief, he made a long speech, and after this, returned to singing, and to the accompaniment of his rattle. With the latter, during his song, he struck his head, breast, sides and back; at the same time straining, as if to vomit forth the bone. Relinquishing this attempt, he applied himself to suction a second time, and with the second of the three bones; and this also he soon seemed to swallow. Upon its disappearance, he began to distort himself in the most frightful manner, using every gesture which could convey the idea of pain: at length, he succeeded, or pretended to succeed, in throwing up one of the bones. This was handed to the spectators, and strictly examined; but nothing remarkable could be discovered. Upon this, he went back to his song and rattle; and after some time threw up the second of the two bones. In the groove of this, the physician, upon examination, found, displayed to all present, a small white sub-stance, resembling a piece of the quill of a feather. It was passed round the company, from one to the other; and declared, by the physician, to be the thing causing the disorder of his patient.

Mandelbaum's informant, Fine-Day, described a number of cases of sucking among the Plains Cree, and the similarities with Henry's account are striking. For instance, in the 1930s Fine-Day related the following incident:

All at once he drops his rattle and sucks at the sick man's temple. The thing was lodged in the back of the neck but he sucked it out through the temple. As soon as he got it he clapped his hand to his mouth and starts to reel backwards. His wife grabs the moccasins and hits him on the back with them. He straightens up and grabs the thing from off his tongue and holds it between his cupped palms. He shakes it and then gives it to me. I take it. It feels as though it is burning me. I shake all over. I feel it move between my fingers. I blow on it and soon it cools. I give it to my cousin. It burns him and he blows just as I did. We look at it later. It has a dragon fly's head with the wings folded back over the body. (Mandelbaum 1936)

Fine-Day also described Plains Cree sucking in a more general way: 'Some doctors pass their hands over the sick person and hold him for a while. They lay their hands on him and feel where the sickness is and point it out. When they locate the spot, they take a buffalo horn, put some sweet-grass in it, put an ember on and clap it over the place. It sucks out the matter and has to be taken off sideways. You can see a yellow stuff in the horn after it is taken off.'

Another important and widespread healing ceremony has been re-ferred to in the literature as the 'shaking tent' or the 'conjuring lodge.' Similar to the sucking procedure discussed above, the shaking tent seems to have had a very broad geographical range in Canada, although most of the literature pertains to Subarctic and Plains hunting peoples. It has been identified among Montagnais (Flannery 1939), northern Cree (Pres-ton 1975), Ojibwa and Saulteaux (Hallowell 1942), Plains Cree (Mandel-baum 1979), Blackfoot (Cooper 1944; Schaeffer 1969), Assiniboine (Coo-per 1944), and no doubt many more. There are remarkable similarities in the description of the shaking tent rite. The best eyewitness accounts of this are those of trader George Nelson, writing of the Cree in northern Saskatchewan in 1823 (Brown and Brightman 1988), and anthropologist Richard Preston (1975), writing of the James Bay Cree in the 1960s. Their descriptions are far too lengthy and detailed to recount here; however some of the most common elements of the shaking tent can be presented.

The shaking tent ceremony had a variety of functions. Communion with the spiritual world was integral to all ceremonies, and through such contact the shaman, among other things, was able to predict the future (such as the weather, where game might be found, or that a sickness would soon arrive), locate lost objects, and diagnose the cause of illness. Characteristically, the shaking tent itself was a small, often conical lodge made of branches and skin covering, in which the shaman was seated or knelt. Frequently the shaman was bound hand and foot by his assistants before being placed in the lodge; sometimes he was gagged as well. Shortly after the commencement of the ceremony, with assistants and community members seated around the outside, the ropes that bound the shaman would be thrown out the door or the top of the tent. Then the shaman would sing and invite his spirit helpers, and indeed any spirits, to enter the lodge. When they did so, the lodge would often shake violently back and forth. The people outside would then hear a succession of voices of the spirits as they entered and communicated with the shaman. These were not in the voice of the shaman, however, and sometimes were in a language unintelligible to those on the outside (often considered an ancient language). Some of the discussion in the tent was jovial, with the spirits and the shaman exchanging jokes, but the spirits also provided important information at the shaman's request. On occasion, an outside participant, such as the sick person, would be invited to enter the tent to see the spirits. Nelson (Brown and Brightman 1988:106) was provided such an opportunity and saw a variety of small lights. The existence of the spirits in the form of small lights has been reported by others who have witnessed the ceremony (for example, Hallowell 1942),[4] although it is suggested that among other groups they appeared as hominoid [sic] figures or birds (Brown and Brightman 1988:159).

One of the functions of the shaking tent was to provide news of distant relatives and events. Hallowell (1942:47) provided one example of this, in which an outside participant queried the spirits: 'The other Indian, who had left a brother sick with double pneumonia at the mouth of the river a few days previously and for whom there seemed no hope of recovery, wanted to know how the sick man was. The answer in this case was that he would recover. When we arrived at the mouth of the river he was up and walking about. And when I [Hallowell] arrived home at the end of the summer I found mikinak's [the spirit's] report concerning my father's health was not only judiciously phrased but quite true. He was no worse. Neither had he improved in health.'

As noted earlier, among the Ojibwa and many other Aboriginal groups, serious illness was often seen as the product of a transgression of the moral order of the society. Hallowell (1942:55–6) has described an incident in which the shaking tent was used to diagnose why a man was having problems passing urine. Ultimately, the spirits examined the issue by first questioning why the medicines offered by a previous healer for this complaint had not worked, adding 'Perhaps some of the old people did something wrong.' Subsequently, an older woman spoke up, admitting that many years earlier, she and a group of youngsters had forced a sewing thimble onto a smaller boy's penis and then told him to go urinate. The boy responded that he couldn't, and that it hurt, and he began to cry. When the confession was over, the conjurer said, 'I thought there was something that stopped the medicine from working.'

While the shaking tent was a common feature of many Aboriginal healing traditions, even more common was the sweat lodge. Indeed, as Lopatin (1960) has demonstrated, a form of sweat bathing is common to many societies throughout the world, including those in other Nordic areas such as Russia and Scandinavia. The function of the sweat lodge for North American Aboriginal peoples was multifaceted: it was used for purposes of prayer, to maintain health, and to address particular health problems or social concerns. It was also used as a precursor to other religious and healing ceremonies. Among the specific health problems for which the sweat lodge was used, we find 'febrile symptoms, chronic rheumatism, headache, fast pulse, catarrh, and sore muscles' (Beardsley 1941:489), as well as more general colds and fevers (Ritzenthaler 1963:327); in general it was used as a panacea for most types of health problems (Vogel 1970:256). Although the structure of the lodge varied from group to group, as did the actual ceremony, Grinnell's (1972:282–3) description of the Blackfoot sweat lodge in the late 1800s is typical:

The sweat lodge is built in the shape of a rough hemisphere, three or four feet high and six or eight in diameter. The frame is usually of willow branches, and is covered with cowskins and robes. In the centre of the floor, a small hole is dug out, in which are to be placed red hot stones. Everything being ready, those who are to take the sweat remove their clothing and crowd into the lodge. The hot rocks are then handed in from the fire outside, and the cowskins pulled down to the ground to exclude any cold air. If a medicine pipe man is not at hand, the oldest person present begins to pray to the Sun, and at the same time sprinkles water on the hot rocks, and a dense steam rises, making the perspiration fairly drip from the body. Occasionally, if the heat becomes too intense, the covering is raised for a few minutes to admit a little air. The sweat bath lasts for a long time, often an hour or more, during which many prayers are offered, religious songs chanted, and several pipes smoked to the Sun.

The effect of the sweat lodge ceremony is to encompass the individuals in complete darkness; sometimes only the soft glow of the heated rocks is noticeable. Some sweat lodge leaders will use a variety of herbs, either mixed into the water or sprinkled directly onto the rocks. On the prairies today, it is common to have four rounds, with the lodge being opened between each round for a brief period. And, unlike Grinnell's description, prayers today tend to be offered to the 'Creator' instead of the 'Sun.'

The therapeutic benefits of the sweat lodge have obviously been recognized widely, as evidenced by its global presence. Some of the early settlers to North America also participated in sweats with Indians. For instance, LeClercq wrote, 'The sweat-house ... is the great remedy of the Gaspesians; and it can be stated as a fact that a number of the French have also found therein a cure for chronic inflammations and sufferings which seem incurable in France'; and Denys wrote, 'Our Frenchmen make themselves sweat like them, and throw themselves into the water similarly, and are never incommoded thereby' (cited in Bailey 1969:121).

Setting aside the religious significance of the sweat lodge, a variety of explanations have been posited to explain its apparent therapeutic benefits. First, of course, is that the sweat acts as a placebo, empowering the mind to begin the healing process and opening the individual to subsequent treatment. The appeal to intervention by spiritual forces, based on the faith of the participants, is an integral part of this effect (Swartz 1988). This may well be a lesser effect, however. It is quite likely that the combination of sensory deprivation in some areas (lack of sight) combined with heightened sensory stimulation in others (the heat on the skin; the smell of herbs) induces an 'altered state of consciousness' which, among other things, facilitates the body's release of endorphins. Aboriginal sweat lodge participants have suggested to one of the authors (Waldram) that one must participate a few times before the mind is able to concentrate on prayer and ignore the intense heat and discomfort. Adair and colleagues (1969) have suggested that the sweat has a sedative effect, and Achterberg (1985) has suggested that the high temperature of the body in a sweat mimics that of the body during a fever, which may stimulate the body's natural reactions to toxins (and the high temperature may kill heat-sensitive bacteria and viruses). D.E. Young, Swartz, Ingram, and Morse (1988:84) have postulated that the steam releases salicylic acid from the willow branches of the lodge frame, a compound which is used today in various antiseptics and anti-neuralgic compounds, among other things.

THE MIDEWIWIN

The Midewiwin is a religious and healing movement believed by many historians to have arisen first among the Ojibwa in the 1800s, possibly as a reaction to the intrusion of and disruption caused by the arrival of Europeans. Subsequently, it spread to neighbouring Woodlands and Plains Indian groups, such as the Saulteaux, Plains Cree, and Dakota (as well as other groups on the American side of the border), where it was adopted in various forms. The Midewiwin is important because it represents an indigenous, hierarchical, religious and medical system with a

well-defined structure. It contrasts with the less structured, individual-
istic approach of much Aboriginal healing in Canada.

The Midewiwin, sometimes referred to as the 'Grand Medicine Society'
in the literature, was a society of individuals who, periodically, came
together to perform various religious and healing ceremonies, and to
induct new members into the group (Vecsey 1983:179). It was built upon
the foundations of traditional Ojibwa religion, as detailed earlier in this
chapter. One of the major concerns of the Midewiwin was the maintenance of health, and the instruction of novices involved teaching them to
identify and prepare botanical medicines. Other instruction involved
ways to commune with the spiritual world to enhance individual power
to heal; in a more general sense, the Midewiwin taught general principles
of health maintenance, particularly as they pertained to the need for the
individual to maintain harmony with the world and to refrain from breaking social norms or offending the pawaganak.

Members of the Midewiwin are often referred to as 'priests' in the
literature, although this term fails to do justice to the broad role of these
individuals within Ojibwa society. Individuals were initiated into the
society, whereupon they were exposed to the knowledge of its members.
A person could have a dream that he should enter the society, or he could
fall ill and require the services of a Mide healer, which would result in
his being initiated. There were at least four 'degrees' or levels of knowledge within the Midewiwin, with each higher level requiring the master-
ing of more complex knowledge and being rewarded with unique designations, such as furs and coloured scarves specific to the rank. Since
illness was one means of entering the society, most community members
attained at least the lowest rank. Rising further required one to apprentice
with a teacher who acted as a sponsor or mentor, and the higher the rank
aspired to, the greater the cost to the initiate (Ritzenthaler 1963:317–19).

The Midewiwin served to maintain social order as well as health. According to Densmore (1929:87), 'The ethics of the Midewiwin are simple
but sound. They teach that rectitude of conduct produces length of life,
and that evil inevitably reacts on the offender. Membership in the Midewiwin does not exempt a man from the consequences of his sins. Respect
toward the Midewiwin is emphasized, and respect toward women is
enjoined upon the men. Lying, stealing, and the use of liquor are strictly
forbidden. The Mide is not without its means of punishing offenders.
Those holding high degrees in the Midewiwin are familiar with the use
of subtle poisons which may be used if necessary.'

Howard (1977:134) in his report on the Plains Ojibwa, has hypothesized that the Midewiwin was a response to the general anxiety created among the Ojibwa as a result of the presence of so many shamans capable of causing illness and misfortune. In effect, through membership in the Midewiwin, these individuals were co-opted, and since almost everyone in the community was a member, the possibility of 'bad medicine' was greatly reduced.

It was once believed that the Midewiwin was on the verge of extinction, and that it had ceased to function by the middle part of the twentieth century. However, like many other aspects of Aboriginal religion and healing, the pronouncements of its demise were incorrect. Quite likely, the Midewiwin went underground for many years; by the 1980s it had begun to resurface, particularly among the Saulteaux of Manitoba. Midewiwin ceremonies are currently held on an annual basis.

ANATOMICAL KNOWLEDGE AND SURGICAL PRACTICES

Virtually all the Aboriginal societies in what would become Canada were hunting peoples of some sort, and hence it is logical that some degree of anatomical knowledge would have been attained. The processing of meat and skins would afford ample opportunity to develop an understanding of the basic body organs and their functions. In some instances, deliberate autopsies of animals may have been carried out, as in the case of the Inuit in the western Arctic (Lucier et al. 1971:253). However, the extent to which pre-contact Aboriginal peoples understood human anatomy is, unfortunately, unknown. And, despite claims by authors such as Bell (1886:534) that, 'They never attempt any grave operation, although their general knowledge of anatomy is not to be despised,' there is little historical record of how that anatomical knowledge may actually have translated into surgical procedures.

For the most part, the surgical procedures that have been documented tended to be relatively minor.[5] The treatment of wounds and trauma was certainly important, as both the palaeopathological and the historical records demonstrate. The Earl of Southesk (Southesk 1875:329), for instance, recorded two cases of gunshot wounds, one Indian and the other European, that were successfully treated by an Indian healer using herbal medicines. The frequent application of various botanical medicines on wounds indicates an understanding of the need to prevent infections; the use of tourniquets and bandages is also noteworthy.

Bloodletting, of various forms, was common. Morice (1900–1) described a number of different approaches used among the Dene to treat such ailments as headaches and general pains. His description of surgery on the temporal artery records a procedure that was likely fairly common: 'This is slightly cut with as sharp an instrument as can be procured, and the blood is allowed to escape until a rich red colour has succeeded the dark hue of the first flow which is supposed to be the cause of the ailment. The wound is then compressed by the application of a piece of skin or of a green leaf, according to the season. The head is afterwards bandaged so as to ensure the speedy healing of the wound.' In general, only a little blood was ever allowed to escape.

Bone setting was also important, and some Aboriginal groups had individuals with special skills in this area. Stone (1935:82–3) has written that 'their skill in the care of wounds, fractures and dislocations equalled and in some respects exceeded that of their white contemporary.' Typically, fractures and bones were set and splinted with wood, or tightly wrapped with reeds or other firm but flexible materials. The palaeopathological record demonstrates that many times these wounds healed effectively, although the record also suggests that limping or impaired function, combined with some degree of pain, likely plagued some individuals subsequent to injury.

Scarification was practised by many groups. Morice (1900–1) reports that the Dene would sometimes treat rheumatism, local aches, and sprains by scratching numerous lines on the affected limb with a sharp instrument, then applying herbs which acted as antibiotics. Vogel (1970:192) suggests that this was one of the commonest surgical practices among Aboriginal North Americans. Amputation was also known, in instances where limbs were crushed or where irreversible infections such as gangrene had set in.

The degree of sophistication of Aboriginal surgical practices is difficult to ascertain. However, two examples demonstrate that at least some surgeons operated with great skill. Morice (1900–1) has described the manner in which Dene surgeons removed cataracts by carefully scraping the surface of the eyeball with a sharp instrument. He reports that they were usually quite successful at this. Kidd (1946) has described cases of trepanation of skulls, as found in some British Columbia Indian remains. In these cases, surgical openings were made in the skull using some type of instrument, for reasons which still remain somewhat unclear. Kidd postulates that patients may have sought the release of 'demons' enclosed within the skull, and it is likely that the theory behind the operation was not unlike that for bloodletting: some malignant influence contained within the body was causing problems and needed to be released. At any rate, Kidd notes that the surgeons would have required great skill in carrying out the operation without killing the patient, and that the pain of the operation would have been so great that some kind of local anaesthetic would have been required, in addition to the ability to dress wounds.

In order to undertake surgery of various kinds, well-refined instruments would have been required. The archaeological record demonstrates that many stone and bone implements were fashioned for this purpose. For instance, bone was particularly useful for piercing and suturing (with animal sinew as stitching), and cutting instruments and awls were common. Certainly the technology that facilitated the manufacturing of weapons and tools in general would have been applied to the creation of surgical implements, and much skill and practice would have been required to execute the surgery successfully (Fortuine 1985:36–41). Skilled surgeons might also be shamans, and highly skilled individuals no doubt gained renown as a result.

GENDER AND THE HEALING TRADITIONS

There exists a widespread belief, among both analysts and some Aboriginal peoples, that the healing roles were primarily occupied by males. The ubiquitous term 'medicine man' is now part of the vocabulary of many people, both Aboriginal and non-Aboriginal. Part of the problem no doubt stems from a historical record which is based almost exclusively upon the observations of male traders, explorers, and missionaries. Not only were these observers largely unconcerned with female roles in Aboriginal societies, but also, by virtue of their gender, they were no doubt excluded from observing many female activities and talking to females. Although a close examination of the literature demonstrates that females did, indeed, occupy healing roles, the poor state of the literature on this topic makes it impossible to determine whether healing roles were equally available to, or filled by, both men and women (Osgood 1931, 1936; Cruikshank 1979; Hultkrantz 1992).

A good example of the male bias in historical accounts is that of the Earl of Southesk (Southesk 1875: 329), who wrote in 1859 of the Saulteaux and other northern Indians that certain herbs were 'known only to the medicine-men, – who are a sort of masonic brotherhood, consisting of women as well as men ...' The contradictions of a brotherhood with female members was clearly lost on the Earl.

Mandelbaum, in the fieldnotes for his published study on *The Plains*

Cree (1979), recorded an incident in which his informant's uncle was unable to 'doctor' an ill young man:

They got an old woman to do it. I peeked in through a hole in the tipi. She was naked save for a breech clout. Her arms and legs were painted with horizontal lines. She made a big fire in the tipi. I watched her pick out of the fire something that looked like a section of gun barrel. It was red hot. All of a sudden it disappeared. She kept on rattling and soon reached around to her back and she had it again. One side was cool and she dropped it into a cup of water. The water steamed. She picked up a gun screw from the fire and did just the same thing, dropping it into another cup of water. Her husband was beating the drum. She blew all over the young man. She took the two pieces of metal out. They disappeared. Then she stood away from the sick man and sucked. The young man had to be held down so powerful was her sucking.

This account demonstrates that this medicine woman was fully versed in the techniques of sucking and sleight-of-hand. McLean (1889:27), in a late-nineteenth-century account, suggested that in some Aboriginal groups, medicine women were particularly feared because of their power.

Among the Inuit, evidence suggests that both males and female occupied shamanistic roles as '*angakkuq*.' A survey of the literature has led Oosten (1986) to conclude that, as for Indians, ambiguity also exists with respect to the existence of specialized gender roles among the Inuit. Oosten (1986:128) concludes: 'The angakkuq has to cross the ideological boundaries between life and death, men and spirits, human beings and game to maintain or restore the religious order. From this point of view it may be that it is essential that his being a man or a woman is indifferent. When his soul leaves his body to explore the world of the dead or to recapture a lost soul his gender is no longer of importance. The soul itself is neither male nor female.'

There is no concrete evidence in the literature that there were gender limitations on most of the healing roles. Common knowledge today would suggest that women were more likely to be herbalists and midwives, and men shamans, but there is no solid evidence to support this. Hence, we could speculate that most healing roles were not gender specific.

THE ASSAULT ON ABORIGINAL HEALING TRADITIONS

The traditional medical systems of Canada's Aboriginal peoples were subjected to a variety of oppressive measures, particularly between 1880 and the mid-twentieth century. Undertaken by government and the churches (the latter with government support), for the most part these measures were not aimed at medical practices *per se* but rather at elements of Aboriginal spiritual and social life which were deemed by these agents to be barriers to assimilation. However, as noted previously in this chapter, Aboriginal medical systems were intertwined with other aspects of religion and culture, and hence an attack on the latter constituted an attack on the former. In this section, we will briefly detail the assault on two prominent Aboriginal traditions: the potlatch and the Sun Dance.

The potlatch was an integral part of the cultures of most Northwest Coast Indian societies. These societies were based on complex systems of status and rank, with 'chiefs and nobles' holding titles to large tracts of land in the name of their lineages or 'houses.' The potlatch was a ceremonial which was undertaken to signify ascension to a title by an individual, or any other change in the status quo which required witnesses (such as high-status marriage, the raising of a carved pole). Potlatching was a means of validating individual status and responsibility. A key aspect of the potlatch was the distribution of wealth gathered by the potlatch sponsor and his supporters. Blankets and food items were popular 'give-aways' during the late nineteenth century. The ceremony served to redistribute wealth, and a family which appeared to impoverish itself at its potlatch would benefit by being guests at others. Another important aspect of the potlatch was that it enabled individuals and families to recount their histories and reaffirm their hereditary rights; hence, the potlatch served as an important institution reaffirming the oral tradition and history of the people (McMillan 1988:187–9).

There was no specific medical function to the potlatch, but the attack on it by government and missionaries had a diffuse effect on various aspects of Northwest Coast healing. The potlatch came to be viewed by the government as a 'foolish, wasteful and demoralizing custom' as early as the 1870s (cited in Fisher 1977:206). Part of its objection was to the fact that some Northwest Coast groups had escalated potlatching to the point of destroying, rather than giving away, the various goods in a form of competition. This was due, in part, to the deadly effects of epidemic diseases which had decimated the villages and blurred lines of ascension. The government was also prodded by the missionaries, who viewed the potlatch as heathen and an obstacle to the Christianization of the Indians. The views of the Rev. Cornelius Brant (Methodist), writing in the 1880s, were likely typical: 'The Church and school cannot flourish where the "Potlatching" holds sway ... Thus all the objects or advantages to be secured by good government are frustrated by this very demoralizing custom; and as the wards of the Government the native tribes should be prevented by judicious counsel and governmental interference, that is by some kind of paternal restraint from indulging in their Potlatching feasts' (cited in LaViolette 1973:42). Brant then added, somewhat prophetically, 'Of course my knowledge of the Indian character suggests the danger of attempting coercive measures.'

In 1883, Prime Minister John A. Macdonald issued a 'proclamation' stating that the potlatch was 'the parent of numerous vices which eat out the heart of the people. It produces indigence, thriftlessness, and habits of roaming about which prevent home association and is inconsistent with all progress' (cited in ibid. 38). The proclamation called upon the lieutenant-governor of British Columbia to 'use his best efforts for the suppression' of the potlatch. This was followed in 1884 by an amendment of the *Indian Act* of 1880, representative of the first attempt to outlaw an Indian ceremonial. Section 3 of the amendment stated: 'Every Indian or other person who engages in or assists in celebrating the Indian festival known as the "Potlach" [*sic*] or in the Indian dance known as the "Tamanawas" [*sic*] is guilty of a misdemeanour and shall be liable to imprisonment for a term of not more than six or not less than two months in any gaol or other place of confinement; and any Indian or other person who encourages, either directly or indirectly, an Indian or Indians to get up such a festival or dance, or to celebrate the same, or who shall assist in the celebration of same is guilty of a like offense, and shall be liable to the same punishment' (*Statutes of Canada* 1884, 47 Vic., c.27).

Unlike the potlatch, the 'tamananawas' had more direct relevance to Aboriginal medicine. The term 'tamananawas' referred to shamanistic acts, including healing, and ritual cannibalism (Cole and Chaikin 1990:12). It was ritual cannibalism (involving dogs, corpses, and living individuals), including ritual biting,[6] which was offensive to some non-Aboriginal people. Both the Indian agents and the missionaries sought to have this ceremony eliminated.

The 'Potlatch Law' proved to be difficult to enforce, with the federal and British Columbia governments somewhat confused over jurisdiction. Efforts to repeal the law began as early as 1887, when the Indians of the Cowichin agency sent a petition to the government (LaViolette 1973:57). In 1886, the relevant section was repealed and substituted with a new section making it an indictable offence to participate in or encourage 'any Indian festival, dance or other celebration of which the giving away or paying or giving back of money, goods or articles of any sort forms a part, or is a feature' (*Revised Statutes of Canada* 1886, c.43, S.114). This new section broadened the prohibition, however, by outlawing 'any celebration or dance of which the wounding or mutilation of the dead or living body of any human being or animal forms a part or is a feature.' This new clause was directed at both the tamananawas of the Northwest Coast Indians and the Sun Dance of the Plains Indians. The law in some form or another remained on the statutes until the 1951 revision of the *Indian Act*.

According to Jilek (1982b:14), the potlatch law was used to suppress the Coast Salish healing ceremonial known as 'Spirit Dancing,' and some older people recalled the prosecutions which ensued. The result was a decline in Spirit Dancing to the point where dancers from neighbouring groups (especially from the United States) had to be brought in to assist in its revival in the late 1960s.

The Sun Dance of the Plains Indians was also subjected to both legislative action and formal discouragement by government and the churches (Pettipas 1994). This dance (also known as the 'Thirst Dance') was a multi-day ceremony held in the summer to honour the sun and other spirits. Critics were offended by a number of aspects of the dance and its related activities. For one thing, the dance took as many as four days to perform, and related activities took many more days before and after. Indeed, the Sun Dance was an important social occasion, and Indians from many different tribes and regions often attended. Furthermore, government agents held the view that dancing was not compatible with a settled, agricultural way of life (E. Titley 1986:165). Second, the dance was considered to be repulsive by some non-Aboriginal people because of the practice of piercing the flesh on the chest of some dancers as a means of offering more suffering to the Great Spirit. Leather thongs were tied to skewers pushed through the skin, and tied at the other end to the central Sun Dance lodge pole. The dancers then attempted to pull the skewers out by straining against the rope.

At first, the government was uncertain as to how to proceed to terminate the Sun Dance. One approach was to implement the 'pass system,' wherein individuals wishing to leave the reserve for any reason were required to obtain the written permission of the Indian agent. This system was conceived in 1885, in part as a reaction to the 'rebellion' in the Northwest, but was never formally or legally adopted by the government. As Barron (1988) has noted, it could not be legally enforced, and while the North-West Mounted Police and the Indian agents worked together to enforce the system as a way of reducing the Indians' mobility on the western prairies, they were not very successful. Sun Dances continued to be held, sometimes in open defiance of the pass system, and sometimes more covertly in remote areas.

The 1886 amendment to the *Indian Act* described above, was a clear legislative attempt to ban some elements of the Sun Dance. And, as with the potlatch, Indian agents were advised to proceed cautiously. Dancing *per se* was not illegal, but piercing and extensive giveaways were. There were some arrests. The number is unknown, but use of summary conviction facilitated the legal process.[7] Threats of fines and jail sentences were commonplace. Some individuals requested permission to hold the dances, with variable success. For instance, in 1918 the Onion Lake (Saskatchewan) Band wrote to Duncan Campbell Scott for such permission, suggesting that the dance was in reaction to the Spanish influenza epidemic which had been wreaking havoc on the band. They were refused, but attempted to hold the dance anyway, only to be thwarted at the last moment by the police. In contrast, a dance on the Blackfoot reserve in 1921 was allowed to proceed, without the piercing and with a police officer in attendance (Lux 1992).

A further amendment to the *Indian Act*, in 1906, made it illegal for Indians to leave the reserve to participate in any 'Indian' dances or to participate in exhibitions without permission (*Revised Statutes of Canada* 1906, c.81, S.8). In the years following, a new problem arose for the government: it believed that the large dance camps were also being used for political purposes, as Indians began to organize politically (E. Titley 1986:177). Police patrols and intervention increased at dances after 1921. In effect, the participants were subjected to harassment, as suggested in the following circular issued by Duncan Campbell Scott in 1921:

Sir – It is observed with alarm that the holding of dances by the Indians on their reserves is on the increase, and that these practices tend to disorganize the efforts which the Department is putting forth to make them self-supporting. I have, therefore, to direct you to use your utmost endeavours to dissuade the Indians from excessive indulgence in the practice of dancing. You should suppress any dances which cause waste of time, interfere with the occupations of the Indians, unsettle them for serious work, injure their health or encourage them in sloth and idleness. You should also dissuade, and, if possible, prevent them from leaving their reserves for the purpose of attending fairs, exhibitions, etc., when their absence would result in their own farming and other interests being neglected. It is realized that reasonable amusement and recreation should be enjoyed by Indians, but they should not be allowed to dissipate their energies and abandon themselves to demoralizing amusements. By the use of tact and firmness you can obtain control and keep it, and this obstacle to continued progress will then disappear.

To the consternation of the government, Indians began to seek legal advice on the question of holding dances, and they were advised that dances could be held without breaking the law. And many continued to ignore the laws prohibiting the dances and their absences from reserves (E. Titley 1986:178–9). Like the Potlatch Law, the regulations affecting the Sun Dance and other dancing and religious activities were finally eliminated in the 1951 *Indian Act.*

The legacy of these repressive measures is still with us today. While there was a time when Aboriginal medicine was open to non-Aboriginal people, more recently the notion that healing and other spiritual activities are 'secret' has become pervasive. Clearly, this is a reaction to very real fears in the past that individuals would be prosecuted if they undertook certain ceremonials; it is also likely that the specific laws against the potlatch and the Sun Dance were perceived as laws against many other Aboriginal traditions as well. Indeed, there are many stories in the west of sweat lodges being prevented or disrupted by government agents. In recent years, some healers have begun to discuss their medicine more publicly, but this represents a radical departure from the norm, and such individuals are often chastized by other Aboriginal people for doing so.

CONCLUSIONS

Aboriginal healing traditions, like the cultures themselves, were very complex at the time of first contact with Europeans. It has been possible to examine only a few aspects of these traditions, and we warn against overgeneralization. However, we do know that despite government repression, Aboriginal healing traditions continued in spite of the development of early European medical services in the New World, a topic to which we now turn.

6

Traders, whalers, missionaries, and medical aid

The strong healing traditions of the Aboriginal peoples were not easily pushed aside with the arrival of Europeans and their own medicine in North America. This tenacity was due, in part, to the relative lack of sophistication of European medicine (especially in the colonial context), as well as the fact that the delivery of biomedical services was hardly organized in the first century or two after contact. Indeed, the delivery of health services to Aboriginal peoples prior to Confederation was primarily on an ad-hoc basis by traders and missionaries. As noted in a previous chapter, from the time of contact the Indians and Inuit in what would become Canada suffered from various epidemic diseases, such as smallpox, influenza, and measles. Much of the rudimentary medical care they received from Europeans had as its intent the rescue of as many disease victims as possible. Although much aid was provided for humanitarian reasons, not all of the motives of both missionaries and traders were altruistic. Diseased (and dead) Aboriginal people were a burden on local accounts, and were not economically or spiritually productive: they could neither hunt nor trap, and although their souls could be 'saved' on death's doorstep, they certainly could not be truly converted. Furthermore, after the formation of Canada in 1867, the federal government slowly came to see the obvious advantages of allowing the traders and missionaries to continue to deliver medical services.

THE FUR TRADERS

Even though most European expeditions to the northern New World included a physician, it is evident that the skills of these individuals were questionable. While it is evident that traders and whalers often had possession of basic medical kits or 'chests' from which they could dispense medicines to their employees or charges, very few had any actual medical training. Brett (1969:521) concludes that such individuals likely had little time to treat Aboriginal patients anyway, being overburdened with the demands of treating the ship's crew. Indeed, many crew members suffered extensively from nutritional deficiency diseases such as scurvy, as well as from the effects of the cold weather, including frostbite and exposure. As a result, 'instead of the European bringing medical attention to the Eskimo, the latter ministered to the explorer in matters of health by instructing him in the principles of Arctic survival and in preventing scurvy by the simple expedient of eating fresh raw meat or, in the more southerly latitudes, consuming a distillate of the bark of the spruce tree' (ibid. 522).

The story of Hudson's Bay Company (HBC) trader and doctor William Todd provides an excellent example of the ad-hoc care provided by the company to northern Indians. As well documented by Ray (1984), Todd's career spanned thirty-five years, from 1816 to 1851, during which time he served as both a trader and a medical doctor, becoming 'the most famous surgeon in the western interior of Canada before 1850' (ibid. 13).

In addition to his medical work for company personnel, including HBC Governor George Simpson, Todd played an important role in reducing the effect of disease among the Indian population in western Canada. When in 1837 it became known that smallpox was afflicting some Indian groups along the Missouri River, Todd commenced a vaccination program using a relatively new cowpox vaccine that had been sent to Canada by the HBC in London; this represents the first use of this type of vaccine in western Canada. Todd trained an Indian to administer the vaccine to his family and the others in his camp. Todd's initiative proved highly successful, and many Indians avoided the dreaded disease. Todd's use of the vaccine was somewhat controversial; not only did he initiate vaccination before confirmation that the disease was, in fact, smallpox, but medical science at the time was not completely convinced of the efficacy of the cowpox vaccine that Todd used. Western medical science in the early 1800s when Todd entered the service of the HBC was still rudimentary, with the causes of many diseases and the process of immunization not well understood (Ray 1975:12).[1] Nevertheless, Todd's actions contributed to the development of an 1838 policy directive by HBC Governor George Simpson in London, which suggested the basic motives behind treating the Indians: 'We have long endeavoured to impress on the [traders] the importance of introducing vaccination ... both as a measure of humanity ... and with a view to the welfare of the Business ... but we fear that sufficient attention has not been paid ... and that consequences may be very calamitous. We now forward to each of the Factories Packets of vaccine matter, and we desire that it be distributed throughout the Country, and that the Gentlemen in charge of Posts exert their utmost influence ... to induce [the Natives] to submit to inoculation' (cited in T.K. Young 1988:36).

While his medical endeavours may have been appreciated, Todd was considered by the company to be only an average trader, and hence unworthy of promotion. Indeed, when in 1849 he requested a promotion and remuneration for services rendered as a medical doctor, he was denied on the grounds that 'every medical man in the service is bound to give his professional aid to the Company's Servants and Indians when there is occasion for such aid, although there may be no stipulation to that effect either in his contract when he enters the Service, or in the Deed which he signs on receiving a Commission' (Ray 1984:23). Despite the fact that Todd's medical skills were significant in attracting a loyal Indian following for the company trade, and that only healthy Indians could effectively hunt and trap, his efforts were obviously considered secondary to the ultimate aims of the company as a business.

In general, the medical services which the traders for companies such as the HBC made available to Indians concentrated on groups near the posts themselves, or Indians arriving at the posts from inland. The 'Home-guard Indians' in particular benefited from their proximity to the posts. These northern Indians, usually Cree, Ojibwa, or Chipewyan, congregated around the posts and, over time, became more or less full-time residents. They worked for the traders as hunters and provisioners, and labourers. When illness struck these people they were unable to fulfil their roles in the fur trade; furthermore, their suffering was plainly evident to the traders. Indeed, a 1683 directive from the London Committee of the HBC directed Governor Henry Sergeant at the Albany post that the policy of the company was to 'treat the Indians with Justice and humanity ...' (cited in Van Kirk 1980:14). At most coastal posts, listed among the 'officer' class could usually be found a 'surgeon,' whose services were made available to company personnel and Indians alike (Brown 1980: 28). As the trade moved inland in subsequent years, only the largest posts were likely to have physicians or apothecaries, although all posts had a dispensary of medicines (T.K. Young 1988:100).

The availability of medical services (however crude) at the posts, as well as food supplies, was important for the Homeguard Indians, who, according to Van Kirk (1980:16), 'came to look upon the [HBC] Company posts as welfare stations which would provide succour, especially for the crippled, sick or starving' (cf Brown 1980:19; Thistle 1986:65). Food supplies, such as flour and oatmeal, were routinely provided to the local Indians by the traders (Brown 1980:19; Krech 1983b:132). Indeed, in the late 1700s trader Andrew Graham described in self-laudatory terms the provision of such services: 'The hungry are fed, the naked clothed, and the sick furnished with medicines, and attended by the factory surgeon; all this gratis ... I appeal to any gentleman of probity and justice, whether a method so humane, kind, and benevolent, was ever adopted by any people connected with Indians' (G. Williams 1969:327).

In contrast, Francis and Morantz (1983:93) have suggested that the provision of food supplies to the Indians of eastern James Bay during times of scarcity 'was not an act of charity.' They continue: 'For one thing, it was in the traders' interest to keep the hunters alive and healthy and able to continue gathering furs. But more importantly, it may have been an act of compensation, since starvation among the homeguard was exacerbated by the company itself in its desire to have them present at the spring goose hunt.' Furthermore, these authors present evidence in one instance of an HBC official in 1842 who felt compelled to feed starving Indians because 'I imagine I would be censured did I permit them to Starve under the immediate eye of our Pastor' (ibid.163).

As we saw in chapter 5, many of the early traders and explorers had little of a positive nature to say about the Indian medical skills and knowledge. The Earl of Southesk, writing of his travels throughout the west in 1859–60, wrote of the Saulteaux of the Fort Pelly area: 'The Indians are not so healthy a race as is sometimes imagined, stomach and chest complaints frequently occurring, and the women being subject to various female ailments that are common in Europe. As physicians their own "medicine-men" appear to be useless. When an Indian is ill he generally applies at the nearest Fort, where he obtains good medicine, and medical advice if the Company's officer-in-charge has studied the subject, as he often has. Food and shelter too are sometimes given him until health is restored' (Southesk 1875:329). Unclear from this passage, of course, is the extent to which Indians may have been selectively using the traders' medical assistance, perhaps for certain conditions or diseases, or after unsuccessful treatments by their own healers. Alexander Mackenzie, for one, noted that the Cree often sought European medicines as trade items (G. Williams 1969:327), and these no doubt formed part of the Indians' intertribal trading networks.

Fur traders also made efforts to assist Indians afflicted by the various epidemic diseases, but their efforts met with mixed and marginal success. Thistle (1986:62) has documented the intrusion of smallpox into the Cumberland House area in the early 1780s, noting that many Indians came to the post for medical assistance but that there was little the traders could do. However, two subsequent epidemics, in 1824 and 1838, were less virulent due to HBC efforts to vaccinate Indians, and their training of Indians and Métis in the methods of vaccination to ensure as wide coverage as possible (ibid. 62). Attempts were also made at isolating non-infected new arrivals at the posts. The effects of the epidemics on the company were great, however, and Thistle (ibid. 62) cites one trader who lamented in 1782 that 'Indeed it is hard labour to keep the House in fuel and bury the dead.' Nevertheless, traders did often collect debts from deceased Indians (through their families), and some even took furs left as sacrifices to 'the good Spirit' by Cree Indians (ibid. 63).

With respect to smallpox, some Indians apparently believed the disease to be so deadly that little hope for recovery was held out for those who contracted it. William Walker, writing in 1781, stated, 'They think when they are once taken bad they need not look for any recovery. So the person that's bad turns [so] feeble that he cannot walk, they leave them behind when they're pitching away, and so the poor Soul perishes' (Rich 1951–2: 265). Undernourishment of the sick clearly contributed to their demise, according to Ray (1974:106), as did the practice of jumping in cold lakes and rivers when feverish.

It is clear that the HBC's hiring of Indians led to the development of the Homeguard Indians, with the result that areas around the posts became more heavily populated, at least on a seasonal basis, leading to periodic famine and, of course, the spread of disease. However, it would be wrong to suggest that the company was simply looking after its own economic interests in providing food and medical assistance. As Brown (1980) and Van Kirk (1980) have documented, there were many stable relationships formed between traders and Indians, and hence assistance given to Indians and mixed-bloods often involved assisting kinsfolk and loved ones. Indeed, Van Kirk (ibid. 76–7) has suggested that Indian women were particularly likely to receive assistance from the HBC and North West Company (NWC) traders, and she describes one case of a Carrier woman nursed back to health by NWC traders after being beaten by her husband. When she regained her health, she was allowed to remain at the post, as it became evident that her family no longer wanted her. In another documented case, Van Kirk (ibid. 17) details the story of an Indian woman left at Albany in 1769 who was 'exceeding ill.' She was nursed back to health by the HBC traders, and her children cared for, until the following spring when all four were able to rejoin her husband. While the traders' attitudes towards the women may have been more favourable than towards the men, due to their 'bourgeois European notions of how women should be treated' (ibid. 17), the fact remains that individual traders' motives extended beyond simply ensuring a profitable business.

Alexander Mackenzie, a Scottish trader who worked for the North West Company, embarked on a journey to the Arctic in 1789. His journals of explorations in 1789, and again in 1793, demonstrate a willingness to treat sick Indians he encountered. In July of 1793, he described one encounter on the west coast (perhaps with a Bella Coola Indian); his description of Indian medicine is ill-informed and unflattering:

At an early hour this morning I was again visited by the chief, in company with his son. The former complained of a pain in his breast; to relieve his suffering, I gave him a few drops of Turlington's Balsam° on a piece of sugar; and I was rather surprised to see him take it without the least hesitation. When he had taken my medicine, he requested me to follow him, and conducted me to a shed, where several people were assembled round a sick man, who was another of his sons. They immediately uncovered him, and showed me a violent ulcer in the small of his back, in the foulest state that can be imagined. One of his knees was also afflicted in the same manner. This unhappy man was reduced to a skeleton, and, from his appearance, was drawing near to an end of his pains. They requested that I would touch him, and his father was very urgent with me to administer medicine; but he was in such a dangerous state, that I thought it prudent to yield no further to the importunities than to give the sick person a few drops of Turlington's Balsam in some water. (Mackenzie 1971:331–2)

Undaunted, the 'native physicians' took up the challenge of healing the ulcer victim. After 'they blew on him, and then whistled,' 'they also put their fore fingers doubled into his mouth, and spouted water from their own with great violence into his face.' Then, according to Mackenzie, 'they laid him upon a clear spot, and kindled a fire against his back, when the physician began to scarify the ulcer with a very blunt instrument, the cruel pain of which operation the patient bore with incredible resolution' (ibid. 332–3). This represents an early example of the simultaneous utilization of both European and traditional Indian medicine.

The provision of medical services was not entirely unidirectional. In a variety of ways, Indians assisted the traders in medical matters. Scurvy was a particularly pervasive problem. One of the earliest known examples occurred during the winter of 1535 when Jacques Cartier's men experienced a severe bout of scurvy, ameliorated when Iroquoians taught them to concoct a vitamin C-rich drink from white cedar (cited in Trigger 1985:131–2). James Isham, an HBC employee at York Factory in the 1740s, referred to the use of a plant by Indians and traders alike to treat scurvy and a variety of other disorders (Rich 1949:216–17). Decker (1989:45) cites an 1843 case at York Factory in which the Indian women and children gathered cranberries, gooseberries, and currants to help the HBC traders stave off scurvy. Indeed, many deaths from smallpox during the 1780s reduced the number of hunters for the HBC to such an extent that scurvy outbreaks occurred. Other services were provided as well. For instance, Zimmerly (1975:77) notes that in Labrador in the late 1800s, the death of an Inuit woman was particularly mourned by many of the Euro-Canadians because of her active role as a midwife to them. Additional aids, especially various herbal preparations and the treatment of wounds and injuries, were also provided.

The role of traders in the delivery of medical services continued after Confederation, particularly in remote northern areas. Writing of the early twentieth century, Felton (1959:36) described these services in glowing, uncritical terms: 'Good medicine chests and surgical implements supplied by the [HBC] Company – and the character of the men they employed – took care of all emergencies and anyone who needed treatment received it.' Noting that nursing stations had begun to supplant the traders' medical role, Felton (ibid. 37) suggested that the latter were relieved to have the 'burden' lifted, having 'shouldered it willingly but often with misgivings.' When influenza broke out at an Arctic post in 1928, a company ship organized a 'soup kitchen' and provided blankets to sick Indians; under the supervision of the HBC physician, HBC staff (and some members of the Revillon Frères missionary society) 'tended the sick day and night for two weeks' (ibid. 37). An outbreak of cerebrospinal meningitis at Cape Dorset in 1943 was met by the delivery of an inadequate supply of sulpha drugs, all that was available at an HBC post some twenty miles away. While awaiting a renewed supply of the drug (which took a month to arrive), the post manager quarantined some Inuit and, travelling by dogsled with an Inuk trapper, did what he could to help. Overall, fifty cases were diagnosed, out of which there were twenty deaths. Of course, many of the traders themselves lacked medical training, and if there were no company physicians available, they were forced to resort to what could be referred to as lay-persons' knowledge. Hence, Felton (ibid. 38) describes the case of a trader at Bathurst Inlet who, unable to diagnose a problem with an Inuit girl, gave her Oxo (beef bouillon) and rum; she died after two weeks. As Felton (ibid.) notes, these traders received a 'Post Manager's Medical Guide' describing common ailments and treatments, and a first-aid course; otherwise, they received no specialized medical training.

The interest of the Hudson's Bay Company in the health of Aboriginal people remained throughout the first half of the twentieth century, despite the fact that the Canadian government had taken on the responsibility for Indians under the *British North America Act*. In 1925, the company formed a 'Development Department,' including as one of its responsibilities the welfare of Aboriginal people (Ray 1990:218–19). One project entailed the development of cottage industries. Indeed, Col. E.L. Stone, medical superintendent in the Department of Indian Affairs, 'gave his entire approval to this and stated that his Department was really in need of the Company's help, and in fact had only the Company to turn to' (cited in Ray 1990:219). With respect to the company's plan to distribute cod-liver oil and meal to the Indians, Stone 'stated his desire of joining us in this and obtaining the product from the company for distribution amongst those Indians with whom the Company was not in contact' (cited in Ray 1990:220).

The head of the HBC's Development Department, Charles Townsend, convened a meeting in 1927 with Dr Frederick Banting (co-discoverer of insulin) to discuss Aboriginal health issues. Banting agreed with Townsend's view that malnutrition was the key reason for high infection rates with diseases such as tuberculosis and influenza. Banting informed Townsend of a similar program of improving the health of farm labourers in Central America which had the effect of reducing production costs to the companies involved. Reports authored in 1925 and 1926 by Drs Stone and Wall, respectively, of the Department of Indian Affairs strongly advocated reform to the trapping industry as a measure to improve the health of northern Indians; copies of these reports were submitted to Townsend, for whom they were of obvious interest (Stone 1925; Wall 1926). Ray (1990:220) notes that, by 1928, the HBC was distributing vitamin supplements, powdered milk, and antiseptic to Indians. However, for a variety of economic reasons, by the end of the 1930s the HBC was no longer realizing returns on its labours in the areas of medical services to Indians, and it began to curtail its activities. Nevertheless, as Ray (ibid. 221) suggests, the HBC's role in providing medical services and food to Indians laid 'the groundwork for the modern state welfare system so prevalent in the north today.'

While the HBC had provided medical services and relief to Indians prior to Confederation as a means of retaining a productive and loyal coterie of trappers and hunters, after Confederation the company attempted to convince the federal government to take over these responsibilities; the loyalty of Aboriginal trappers was no longer assured, and many were trading with rival companies and individuals. However, Ray (ibid. 227) notes that the government responded by channelling services through other trading companies as well as missionary societies, further undermining the HBC's tenuous hold on the trappers. As a result, some post managers were reluctant to surrender their relief role. The federal government, in general, was apprehensive about taking on the responsibility of providing relief to the Indians, in part out of fear of the cost, but also out of concern that Indians would become dependent wards. Hence, the Indians became something of a ping-pong ball between the company and the federal government (a position they would subsequently occupy with the federal and provincial governments). The HBC had little choice but to assist the Indians, through its Development Department, even knowing that such efforts were unlikely to buy Indian loyalty. Ray (ibid. 227) states unequivocally that 'the northern natives were better off with the company than with government bureaucrats.' But, by the end of the Second World War, the federal government's involvement in Indian relief and medical care would begin to dominate.

THE WHALERS

Along the northern coasts, contact between Aboriginal inhabitants and Europeans frequently occurred in conjunction with whaling activities. The effects of the introduction of diseases for these Aboriginal peoples has been briefly described in an earlier chapter. Not surprisingly, the whalers offered periodic medical assistance to those Aboriginal peoples, primarily Inuit, with whom they had sustained contact.

The journal of whaling captain George Comer provides some insight into medical services made available to the Inuit. Comer was the master of an American whaling schooner operating outside the reach of British and Canadian law in the high Arctic between 1903 and 1905. According to Comer's editor, ships' masters were often called upon to handle a variety of medical problems afflicting crew members, and they were normally equipped with a standard kit of medicines and surgical instruments, even though few had any real medical training (Ross 1984: 100 n8). Doctors were also occasionally assigned to whaling expeditions. Although Comer's journal notes occasional diseases affecting the Inuit they encountered, there is little indication of aid provided to any but the crew, with the exception of Inuit working for the whalers. These, it seems, received a great deal of medical attention, and were treated as if they were ship's crew. For instance, a 1904 entry describes the return of some Inuit families to the temporary ocean-side camp: 'Two families of our natives came back today. One of the women – Shoofly – has a heavy cold on her lungs with quite a fever, had to be helped off the sled and on board the vessel. The doctor from the steamer *Arctic* has been over twice and is now taking care of her' (ibid. 151–2). Over the next two and a half weeks, her progress was periodically charted in Comer's journal. Clearly, she was highly thought of (despite the condescending name ascribed to her by the Americans), since she was visited twice daily by the doctor and was given malted milk and scarce oranges until she was able to return to her family's igloo on shore.

Comer's journal also notes that he provided 'sulphur and molasses' to many of the Inuit suffering from 'the itch' (ibid. 183), and documented the assistance provided to an Inuk named 'Ben,' who was slowly dying despite medical assistance. The latter situation was, apparently, difficult for Comer, as this man had previously saved the captain's life (ibid. 191).

The journal's introduction also notes that the Inuit provided some assistance to the whalers. They hunted, and the fresh meat they supplied was seen by whalers such as Comer as essential to preventing scurvy (ibid. 18). In this sense, the illness of Inuit working for the whalers threatened not only the whalers' economic fortunes, but their physical health as well. Indeed, in his journal Comer makes mention only of medical treatment offered to Inuit in his employ.

THE MISSIONARIES

Like the traders and whalers, missionaries were among the first Europeans to make sustained contact with Aboriginal peoples in Canada. Unlike their commercially oriented European colleagues, however, they hoped to convince the peoples they encountered to undertake radical changes to their cultures and ways of life – or in a word, to become Christian. Inevitably, missionaries found it necessary to provide medical services to Aboriginal inhabitants, from a humanitarian perspective as well as in the hopes of attracting new converts. The historical record suggests that, for a variety of reasons, the missionaries and Indians entered into conflict over the issues of religion, disease, and treatment.

Both Bailey (1969) and Trigger (1985) have documented how Indians in eastern Canada frequently established a connection between the missionaries and their remonstrations on the one hand, and the disease and death of Indians on the other. Baptism, in particular, was seen as both a possible cure for disease, and by some Algonquians and Iroquoians as the cause of disease. Bailey (1969:81) writes: 'Of one thing the Indians were certain: the virulent diseases from which they suffered were the direct result of contact with the Europeans. Moreover, it was useless for the priests to say that baptism was not the cause of the abnormally high death rate. They were baptized and they were dying.'

Among the Hurons, the Jesuits came to be seen not only as the source of disease, but as great and powerful sorcerers. Trigger (1985:246) notes that the various elements of baptism, such as the baptismal water, were seen by the Indians as charms used against their Indian victims. They were seen to have other powers as well, powers that could cause illness among the people. Fear of the Jesuits increased, and some groups resorted to offering gifts to the Black Robes to convince them to stop killing Indians. On the other hand, one Montagnais shaman, noting that the Jesuits did not suffer from the diseases, believed the source of their power to lie in their black socks, and accordingly he recommended the wearing of such to an Indian patient (Bailey 1969:81).

Aboriginal people were quite clearly able to draw the connection between the arrival of missionaries and the development of deadly diseases, although the missionaries were not the sole sources of disease. Nevertheless, they were often viewed as part of the problem, as well as part of the solution through their offering of medical assistance and religious rites. As early as 1637, for instance, the Huron council repeatedly discussed administering the death penalty to the Jesuits (Grant 1984:28). Well known to students of Canadian history are the cases of the Jesuits Brébeuf and Lalemant, who in 1649 were captured by the Iroquois while ministering to the Huron, and who were subsequently killed by Huron who had themselves earlier been captured and adopted by the Iroquois. These Huron, according to Trigger (1985:268), regarded the Jesuits as sorcerers who had caused the destruction of their people. But the execution of missionaries by Indians was not restricted to the east. According to Southesk, writing among the Saulteaux in the Fort Pelly area of Saskatchewan in 1859: 'A few years ago a Roman Catholic priest was killed near this place by the same tribe. Persuaded by his exhortations during a previous visit, the Indians had allowed him to baptize all their children. An epidemic broke out soon afterwards, destroying most of these infants, and the superstitious savages attributed their loss to the mystic rites of the

Church. Ignorant of what happened, the priest after a while returned to his flock in the wilderness, but, instead of welcomes, these lost sheep received their shepherd with blows, and added him to the company of martyrs' (Southesk 1875:342).

Certainly, some Indians were perplexed by the Jesuit's 'zeal for saving souls among the dying' and their apparent apathy towards the living, not an attitude conducive to providing medical services. As Bailey (1969:80) quotes one Jesuit: 'The joy that one feels when he has baptized a Savage who dies soon afterwards, and flies directly to Heaven to become an Angel, certainly is a joy that surpasses anything that can be imagined.'[3] Trigger also notes that, among the Huron, the Jesuits 'were accused of always talking about death rather than hoping for a sick person's recovery, as any decent Huron would do' (1985:246–7). Trigger (ibid. 254) suggests that, after the major smallpox epidemics had waned (around the mid-1600s in Huron country), the Jesuits 'were anxious to avoid a repetition of what they saw as the apostatizing that had occurred during the smallpox epidemic.'

Since the early missionaries were interested in religious conversion, inevitably they encountered some opposition from the Indians' religious practitioners who, frequently, were also healers. Since the traditional healers had no experience with the various epidemic diseases, they were at a distinct disadvantage in a struggle with the missionaries. However, the earliest missionaries found curbing epidemics and restoring the health of sick Indians to be a difficult task. Trigger (ibid. 246) notes that the Jesuits failed conclusively in their attempts to halt the smallpox epidemic of 1636 by conducting rituals in a kind of competition with the Huron shamans. Furthermore, the failure of traditional healing ceremonies had the effect of occasionally spurring the shamans on to more intense efforts to solicit supernatural assistance, thus demonstrating their power; the fact that each round of disease eventually subsided was a positive, supportive sign (ibid. 248–9).

Jesuit efforts to supplant the shamans by undertaking ceremonies to produce rain or cure sickness were also not particularly successful (ibid. 252). Bailey (1969:80) describes an incident in 1633 in which Jesuits remonstrated with a Micmac shaman who had treated in the traditional manner an ill child for whom the Jesuits had recommended rest. The Jesuits were informed by the shaman, 'That is very good for you people; but, for us, it is thus that we cure our sick.'

European medicines, as introduced by the missionaries, seem to have met with mixed responses. French remedies were, in general, opposed by the Montagnais in the early 1600s. On the other hand, a Jesuit hospital in Quebec saw a large patient load in 1640, exhausting its supply of medicines and leading the Mother Superior to note that the Indians had 'no difficulty in taking our medicines, nor in having themselves bled' (cited in Bailey 1969:76). Grant (1984:39), for one, is not surprised that some French medicines, and elements of Catholicism, were accepted by the Indians in eastern Canada, arguing, 'There was nothing in the principles of native religion to limit access to spiritual power to a single cult, and borrowing from the religious repertoire of other tribes was a common practice.' Certainly, the early missionaries' ability to deal with the spirit world was an important part of their acceptance by the Indians, and having medical remedies which appeared to work was important in validating this power. But such powers, those which in the view of the Indians allowed the missionaries to heal, could also be used to cause harm and disease. This explains much of the ambivalence that the historic record suggests existed with respect to Indian acceptance of the medical assistance and proselytizing of the missionaries.

The evidence that the traditional medical systems survived the epidemics is not clear for other groups. For instance, for the Montagnais in the early 1600s, Bailey (1969:81) states, 'As the sorcerers were ridiculed by the priests, and as the imported diseases grew in dimension, they were discredited, having been thought to have lost power over the manitou.'

Missionary success varied from region to region and nation to nation. As European contact increased, and the Europeans' power over the Aboriginal peoples was consolidated, mission success increased. This is particularly true of the Indians of the east coast and along the St Lawrence River. In contrast, Indians farther north and west were less affected, perhaps because 'the system of native medicine was closely woven into the social fabric' (Grant 1984:53). However, certainly a different lifestyle also explains, in part, the reluctance of northern groups such as the Ojibwa and Cree to accept missionaries and their medicines. Involvement in the fur trade reinforced the high degree of mobility of these Indians, and except for the 'Homeguard' who began to settle around the posts, most of the Indians remained mobile and out of effective reach of the missionaries for much of the year. The southern Indians, especially the Huron and Iroquois, lived in villages and followed a horticultural lifestyle; it was comparatively easier for the missionaries to develop a congregation. The Anglicans, in particular, were subsequently accused of creating 'Tobacco Christians,' that is, achieving nominal conversions of northern Indians by means of gifts of tobacco and other provisions, especially in times of need (Grant 1984:113). Ultimately, however, by the mid-1800s even the northern Indians began to accept Christianity, in some instances with a fervour that created a great deal of competition among various Christian denominations; it was believed (with some accuracy) that the first denomination to reach a group would gain a significant foothold (ibid. 114). As we have seen in an earlier chapter, however, while this may have meant some damage to traditional spirituality and medicines, it certainly did not eliminate them completely.

In Labrador, the establishment of missions in the late 1700s and on into the 1800s provided a source of medical care for the Inuit of that region. The Moravians, in particular, found a foothold in Labrador, and although generally lacking in medical training, nevertheless endeavoured to provide what services they could. Nonetheless, from time to time trained medical personnel were available. For instance, in 1897 Rev. Paul Hettasch, trained in medicine, established a temporary hospital in Hopedale (Ben-Dor 1966:185). In 1903 a hospital with a resident physician was built at Okak. When Dr Wilfred Grenfell was appointed to examine conditions along the coast of Labrador, he was ultimately brought to declare, 'There can be no question the Moravians have so far saved the native population for Labrador' (cited in ibid. 185). Grenfell would go on to establish the 'International Grenfell Association,' responsible for medical and educational work in southern Labrador and which, by the 1950s, was officially responsible for services to both Inuit and settlers. By 1959, there was a nurse stationed at Makovik, and the construction of a nursing station followed in 1961 (ibid. 186).

Missionaries continued to be involved in medical care for Indians after Confederation, although, as with the traders, their role in this area declined in the years leading up to the Second World War. One area in which they maintained some control over Indian health was with respect to schooling. Residential schools, in particular, saw Indian children held under the missionaries' charge for up to ten months each year. It is apparent that many of these schools actually lacked proper medical facilities, and that disease, especially tuberculosis, was rampant.

Overall, the conditions in many schools were appalling. Grant (1984:180) describes attempts by Anglicans to explain a high mortality rate at their schools for Blackfoot Indians by referring to high overall Indian mortality rates. But the schools were 'drafty and crowded, food scanty and often unappetizing' (ibid.). Part of the problem was the low government grants provided to the mission societies to operate the schools, and adequate nutritional programs and health services were difficult to attain. Many schools tended to be sealed shut to conserve heat, thus restricting the flow of fresh air (J.R. Miller 1989:212).

Dr Peter Bryce, appointed in 1904 as Canada's first medical officer for the Department of Indian Affairs, issued a report in 1907 exposing the poor sanitary conditions in these boarding schools which led to high mortality rates and indicating that, in the schools' fifteen-year history, 24 per cent of all students who had attended were known to be dead (Bryce 1922:4). Tuberculosis was the main disease which affected students in residential schools. The report resulted in calls to abandon these schools in favour of reserve-based day schools. This course was opposed by many denominations; indeed, in his 1907 report, Bryce commented that 'Everywhere was too apparent the fear that their [tubercular students'] exclusion might lessen the per capita grant' that the schools received (1907:277). So a plan to deal with the poor health conditions was never executed, in part because of the cost, and in part 'because it would have undermined the authority of the churches running the schools' (Grant 1984:193). Although after 1945 the trend towards day schools developed, these changes came too late for many Indian children, as suggested in the words of Duncan Campbell Scott, deputy minister at Indian Affairs in the second decade of the twentieth century: 'It is quite within the mark to say that fifty per cent of the children who passed through these schools did not live to benefit from the education which they had received therein' (cited in J.R. Miller 1989:213).

Under the control of the missionaries, many schools fulfilled multiple purposes, and the children were not the only ones 'educated.' For instance, 'industrial homes' developed in conjunction with many mission hospitals in the Arctic. The first such home was founded at Chesterfield Inlet in 1938 by the Roman Catholics, to be followed within a few years by an Anglican hospital in Pangnirtung and similar establishments elsewhere. These homes provided care for the elderly and infirm, and taught them handicrafts. Medical care was a part of the services offered, and although the number of patients in any given home rarely exceeded twenty at any one time, their role was seen as important (Jenness 1972:69).

The missionaries were also responsible for developing the first hospitals throughout much of Canada. Heagerty (1928:143), in his highly romanticized history of medicine in Canada, identified the logical connection between missionization and medical care: 'The hospital is an expression of Christianity. With the dawning of the era of Christianity there arose the desire for the accomplishment of good works, and this found ready expression in the care of the sick and needy, who abounded in every locality ... Little wonder then that, with such a background, the

French should have been burning with zeal to establish in Canada a hospital for the care of the sick Indians who were reported to be dying by thousands from diseases.' The first such hospital was established in Quebec in 1639, to be followed in 1644 by a hospital in Montreal. Both were operated by the 'Hospital Nuns,' the Ursulines.

It is difficult to document all the hospitals that the various missionary societies and church groups developed. Some were simple tent structures, or were combined with other facilities, and lasted for very short periods. But others were of a more permanent nature, and no doubt made a valuable contribution to the delivery of medical services to Aboriginal peoples. Some of these are discussed in the following chapter.

THE INTRODUCTION OF ALCOHOL

The introduction of alcohol to Aboriginal peoples is often associated with the practices of the fur trade, and our discussion in this chapter would be incomplete if we were not to examine this controversial issue. Aboriginal peoples in Canada at the time of contact lacked a brewing tradition and had no experience with alcohol. With the introduction of the fur trade, alcohol came to be used as a gift item as well as an item of trade. Its use among the Indians created a variety of health and public safety problems, and led to great conflict between the traders and the missionaries, who opposed the use of alcohol.

The French fur trade in eastern Canada introduced alcohol as early as the 1670s, and, as competition between the English, Dutch, and French traders heated up, alcohol became more prominent. The HBC and other fur-trading companies used alcohol in a variety of ways. As Hamer and Steinbring (1980:7) have noted, 'Alcohol was used as an inducement to participate, as a medium of exchange, and as a standard of competitive access.' Presents of alcohol were made to Indians when they arrived at trading posts, and Indians often demanded such, threatening to take their furs to other posts where the alcohol policy was more liberal. According to Ray (1974: 85, 142), lavish gift-giving involving alcohol and tobacco intensified at the height of competition in the mid-eighteenth century; at York Factory, for instance, 864 gallons of rum and brandy were traded in 1753. Traders realized there was a need to stock alcohol to deliver to the Indians, and shortages hampered trading activities. However, it would be erroneous to suggest that ample supply of alcohol alone was required to prosecute a successful trade; indeed, the Indians also demanded a large stock of high-quality trade goods (ibid. 143)

Not surprisingly, traders would use alcohol, especially rum and brandy (invariably cut with water), to entice trappers away from rival company posts. North West Company trader Alexander Henry wrote in 1805 that, 'if they misbehaved at our houses and were checked for it, our neighbours (HBC) were ready to approve their scoundrelly behaviour and encourage them to mischief' (cited in Hamer and Steinbring 1980:9). Alcohol was also used as a trade item itself, along with other items of European manufacture. For instance, in 1744 the HBC had a standard of one gallon of brandy for four beaver pelts. In 1800, Nor'wester Alexander Henry set a standard price on alcohol of two gallons for every ten animals killed by Indian hunters and delivered to the post for food, and refers to one case in which a trapper traded 120 beaver pelts for two blankets, a small mirror, and eight quarts of rum (ibid. 8).

The trade in alcohol had many disruptive effects on the Indians. The Jesuits, who were strongly opposed to the use of alcohol, wrote extensively of the problems it caused among the Indians. They wrote, for instance, that 'Every night is filled with clamours, brawls, and fatal accidents, which the intoxicated cause in their cabins,' and 'It [drunkenness] is so common here, and causes such disorders, that it sometimes seems as if all the people of the village had become insane, so great is the license they allow themselves when they are under the influence of liquor' (cited in Dailey 1968:47). Alexander Mackenzie (Garvin 1927:101) in the late 1700s contrasted the behaviour of Cree Indians under the influence of alcohol with that when sober, noting 'They are also generous and hospitable, and good natured in the extreme, except when their nature is perverted by the inflammatory influence of spirituous liquors.' Similarly, Andrew Graham (G. Williams 1969:152) wrote in the late 1700s that, 'They are much given to fighting and quarrelling when drunk; but at other times are seldom seen passionate or guilty of maiming the person of another.' Daniel Harmon, writing in 1802, lamented his considerable loss of sleep due to constant, all-night drinking parties by the Cree (1911:11). And for a small minority of Indians, the quest for alcohol became serious; George Simpson wrote in 1820 of the Indians 'tormenting us for liquor' (Rich 1938:120).

Assault and murder were just two of a variety of social problems that were caused by alcohol, according to the Jesuits and traders who commented. The variety of social problems also included sexual assault, marriage breakdown, and food deprivation. Indeed, for the periods in which alcohol was consumed, there was a general breakdown in the social norms characteristic of such consumption. Drinking tended to occur over a day or more, until the supply was gone. David Thompson wrote in 1785 of the Cree along Hudson Bay, 'No matter what service the Indian performs, or does he come to trade his furs, strong grog is given to him and sometimes for two or three days, men and women are all drunk and become the most degraded of human beings' (Hopwood 1971:80). Many observers agreed with John Franklin's (1969:56–7) assessment of the Cree, that 'They were formerly a powerful and numerous nation ... but they have long ceased to be held in any fear ... This change is entirely attributed to their intercourse with Europeans; and the vast reduction in their numbers occasioned, I fear, in a considerable degree, by the injudicious introduction amongst them of ardent spirits.'

Alcohol consumption was not a uniquely male activity. Women also engaged in consumption to the point of intoxication. According to Van Kirk (1980:27), many traders noted in their journals that the Homeguard women in particular seemed to become more rapidly addicted to alcohol than the men, and that 'not only did it make them prone to jealous acts of violence and the neglect of their children, but it debauched their morals.' Prostitution of Indian women was one product of this alcohol problem.

It is also important to stress that many Indians abstained from alcohol consumption altogether, and many recognized the social problems it caused. Indeed, some western Indian leaders welcomed the formation of the North-West Mounted Police in 1873 as a means of stemming the American whisky trade. Some trading captains requested that the traders not make alcohol available to band members. Measures were sometimes taken to reduce the carnage wrought by drunkenness, such as restraining individuals by tying them up, or hiding their weapons when they were drinking (Dailey 1968:51). There were also instances where some chose to stay sober, in effect to watch over those that were drinking. And the consumption pattern of most Indians often involved binge drinking at the posts followed by long, even year-long, periods of total abstinence. The consumption of alcohol was primarily a trading post activity; as such, true alcohol addiction was likely rare.

As the competition between the Hudson's Bay Company and the North West Company in western Canada heated up, the availability of liquor increased, and this proved to be a heavy drain on the accounts of both companies. In 1821, when the two amalgamated, the newly reorganized Hudson's Bay Company no longer needed alcohol to propagate the trade. Consequently, in 1825, it passed a new regulation 'that the use of Spiritous Liquor be gradually discontinued' (Fleming 1940:126). The policy, however, did not mean that the trade in alcohol stopped immediately, for the Indians were nevertheless able to keep the liquor flowing to some extent. Indeed, in 1840 the HBC at Cumberland House was warned by one Indian 'that the effects of this new law would be perceivable in the amount of our Return's by next June' (Thistle 1986:91–2). And HBC Governor George Simpson exempted the Plains Indians from the new policy for a time, because these Indians continued to provide important provisions to the company (Rich 1938:303n).

Over the latter part of the nineteenth century, supplies of alcohol to Indians dried up throughout much of the north, aided in part by an *Indian Act* prohibition for registered Indians. Access to alcohol was not completely severed, especially in southern areas, but certainly it became more difficult elsewhere. By the 1960s, some northern Aboriginal communities were resorting to periodic consumption of home brew, referred to cryptically in some areas as 'white lightning' or 'moose milk.' Supplies for making home brew were readily available from local traders, but not all promoted brewing. For instance, a trader at the Cree community of Chemawawin in Manitoba in the 1950s reported that, when he obtained word of brewing activities, he often confiscated the supplies and even called in the police, despite the fact that often he had to pay the fine for the offender (Waldram 1980:56–7). But such cases were an interlude linking the historic introduction of alcohol in the fur trade to the re-introduction of alcohol in the post-1960 years of increasing access to Euro-Canadian society.

CONCLUSIONS

Medical services for Aboriginal peoples in the pre-Confederation era were largely in the hands of the fur traders, whalers, and missionaries. The groups all had some interest in assisting the Aboriginal inhabitants, but despite their efforts, the toll that the epidemic diseases took was significant. Lack of organization and formal medical training and limited access to medical supplies meant that their victories in treating Aboriginal patients were overshadowed by their defeats. When Canada was formed in 1867, the new country demonstrated little concern for the health of Aboriginal peoples, and did not develop strategies for combating disease. As we shall see in the next chapter, the government remained content with the level of service provided by traders, whalers, missionaries, and new government agents in the form of the police and the military.

7

The emergence of government health services

As we noted in the opening chapter of this book, the formation of Canada in 1867 with the *British North America Act* effectively transferred the responsibility for 'Indians and the lands reserved for Indians' to the new federal government. This did not immediately translate into the development of medical services for Indians by the federal government, however; Brett's (1969.521) assertion 'that until the commencement of the twentieth century, the development of medical services in the north was conspicuous by its absence' pertains to most Aboriginal areas of Canada. The Inuit, who were eventually recognized as a federal responsibility, and the Métis, who never were, received organized government medical services even later than the Indians. Missionaries, traders, and government agents continued for many years to provide medical care on an ad-hoc basis throughout most of the new country and territories.

THE 'MEDICINE CHEST' CLAUSE AND TREATY PROVISIONS

One of the most controversial areas of discussion in the field of Aboriginal health care concerns the treaty *right* to free, comprehensive medical services for Indians. Although the issue has been settled in the courts, which have supported the federal government's view that no such right exists, Indian organizations maintain that the treaties, in general, must be interpreted liberally, with an eye towards the 'spirit and the intent' of the agreements. From their view, this means that the right to medical care is a treaty right, notwithstanding any legal decisions.

In order to understand properly the issue of treaty rights to medical care, it is essential first to understand the historic context of the treaties. The first 'numbered' treaty was signed in 1871 in southern Manitoba;

and between 1871 and 1877 a total of seven such treaties were executed. In general, the Indians in the 'northwest angle' in northwestern Ontario, and especially across the southern prairies, were somewhat anxious to sign the treaties. By 1870, eastern settlers had begun to encroach into the west, and the formation of Canada three years earlier foreshadowed a likely westward expansion. Furthermore, many of the Indians in the west were beginning to experience the negative effects of the decline in the bison herds. Starvation and deprivation were becoming more common, and many Indian leaders began to see the treaties, and their provisions for federal agricultural assistance and education, as a means to ensure the future for their people. That these leaders were thinking of the future is clear when one reads Alexander Morris's *The Treaties of Canada with the Indians*, first published in 1880. As Morris was the chief treaty commissioner for many of these first treaties, his observations are pertinent to this discussion.

Unfortunately, when examining the issue of treaty promises, we must appreciate that the Indian side of the story is less precisely documented than the Euro-Canadian side. The best source of information from an Indian perspective comes from the oral tradition, and in rare instances from research undertaken with Indians who were present at the negotiations, or accounts dictated by them. As we shall see, the Indian perspective tends to vary somewhat from the official treaty text and the versions offered by Morris and other Euro-Canadian officials who witnessed the events.

The only treaty which specifically mentions medical care is Treaty Six, which contains two clauses: 'That in the event hereafter of the Indians comprised within this treaty being overtaken by any pestilence, or by a general famine, the Queen, on being satisfied and certified thereof by her Indian Agent or Agents, will grant to the Indians assistance of such character and to such extent as her Chief Superintendent of Indian Affairs shall deem necessary and sufficient to relieve the Indians from the calamity that shall have befallen them.' And, 'That a medicine chest shall be kept at the house of each Indian Agent for the use and benefit of the Indians, at the discretion of such Agent.' It is very apparent from Morris's (1880) description of the Treaty Six negotiations that these two clauses were added into the official text of terms to be offered to the Indians; this represents one of the few instances in which such was the case. These Indians, primarily Plains Cree and Saulteaux, were clearly concerned about the recent turn of events in their region. Morris (ibid. 177) wrote that: 'The Indians were apprehensive of their future. They saw the food supply, the buffalo, passing away, and they were anxious and distressed ... They desired to be fed. Small-pox had destroyed them by hundreds a few years before, and they dreaded pestilence and famine.' In his dispatch of 4 December 1876, Morris recounted the discussions he had had with the Indians which led to the inclusion of these two clauses in the treaty. He wrote at the time: 'At length the Indians informed me that they did not wish to be fed every day, but to be helped when they commenced to settle, because of their ignorance how to commence, and also in case of general famine ... They were anxious to learn to support themselves by agriculture, but felt too ignorant to do so, and they dreaded that during the transition period they would be swept off by disease or famine – already they have suffered terribly from the ravages of measles, scarlet fever and small-pox' (ibid. 185).

The demands of the Indians were clearly articulated to Morris, and these included 'provisions for the poor, unfortunate, blind and lame,' 'the exclusion of fire water in the whole Saskatchewan [district],' and 'a free supply of medicines' (ibid. 185). Morris records his response to these demands as follows: 'I replied ... as to our inability to grant food, and again explaining that only in a national famine did the Crown ever intervene ... We told them that they must help their own poor, and that if they prospered they could do so' (ibid. 186). Morris records no response with respect to the provisioning of medicines.

Less than a week later, Morris met with another group of Indians in the region to sign the treaty. In response to Cree chief Beardy's comments that, 'when I am utterly unable to help myself I want to receive assistance,' Morris once again replied that 'we could not support or feed the Indians ... If a general famine came upon the Indians the charity of the Government would come into exercise' (ibid. 188).

A scribe by the name of A.G. Jackes accompanied Morris and the treaty party and made a record of the events and dialogue leading up to the signing of the treaty with various bands. Here we see some additional insights into the question of medical services. For instance, Jackes quotes Morris as telling one band that 'the fire-water which does so much harm will not be allowed to be sold or used in the reserve' (ibid. 206). Furthermore, Morris stated that 'I cannot promise, however, that the Government will feed and support all the Indians; you are many, and if we were to try to do it, it would take a great deal of money, and some of you would never do anything for yourselves ... [but] that the sympathy of the Queen, and her assistance, would be given you in any unforseen circumstance' (ibid. 210–11). Furthermore, Morris (ibid. 212) suggested that 'some great sickness or famine stands as a special case.' Jackes also records the Indians' request that 'we be supplied with medicines free of cost' (ibid. 215). In response, Morris apparently stated quite clearly that 'A medicine chest will be kept at the house of each Indian agent, in case of sickness amongst you' (ibid. 218).

There is some evidence that health matters may have been discussed at other treaty signings as well, despite the fact that no references to such appear in the treaty documents themselves. For instance, concerns for the health of Indians in northern Saskatchewan and other areas of the north led to requests that treaties be signed with them. Thomas White, super-intendent general of Indian Affairs in 1887, described 'repeated appli-cations ... made by Indians inhabiting the regions north of the boundary of Treaty No. 6,' adding that 'quite recently the Hudson's Bay Company has renewed its solicitations in the same behalf, alleging that serious sickness is now prevalent among the Indians of the Peace River District, and that there is an apprehension of there being an insufficiency of food during the Winter ... The diseases from which they are stated to be suf-fering are stated to be measles and croup.' Indeed, according to White's report, the Hudson's Bay Company took the position that 'the expense of providing and caring for sick and destitute Indians should devolve upon the Government as their natural protectors, and that the Hudson's Bay Company should not charge itself with the same' (cited in Fumoleau 1973:36). Fumoleau (ibid. 37) also described an 1887 *Calgary Tribune* article entitled 'Starving Indians' in which it was suggested that destitute northern Indians needed a treaty in order to alleviate their suffering.

At the negotiations for Treaty Eight, Fumoleau (ibid. 113) argues that the treaty commissioners indeed promised medicines and medical care, citing a 1919 report by D. McLean, assistant deputy and secretary of Indian Affairs, who wrote that the Indians were 'assured ... that the Government would always be ready to avail itself of any opportunity of affording medical service' (cited in ibid. 113). The report of the treaty commissioners apparently suggests that the Indians requested 'assistance in seasons of distress' and that 'the old and indigent who were no longer able to hunt and trap and were consequently often in distress should be cared for by the government' (R. Daniel 1987:98). The treaty commis-sioners 'promised that supplies of medicine would be put in charge of persons selected by the Government at different points, and would be distributed free to those of the Indians who might require them.' Fur-thermore, 'We [the treaty commissioners] explained that it would be practically impossible for the Government to arrange for regular medical attendance upon Indians so widely scattered over such an extensive territory. We assured them, however, that the Government would always be ready to avail itself of any opportunity of affording medical service just as it provided that the physician attached to the Commission should give free attendance to all Indians who he might find in need of treatment as he passed through the country' (cited in ibid. 98).

Fumoleau (1973:114) also notes that medical doctors often accompanied treaty parties after the signings, dispensing medicines and treating Indians. Although inadequate from the perspective of alleviating the widespread ill-health of these peoples, the apparent promises and provision of medical services were, arguably, linked to the treaties themselves.

Fumoleau documents a similar story for the signing of Treaty Eleven. The need for a treaty in the far north was explained in part by the poor health conditions of the Dene Indians who lived in that region. Starvation combined with diseases such as tuberculosis ('consumption'), dysentery, whooping cough, measles, and Spanish influenza were taking a serious toll, and the Indians in many cases appealed to be taken into treaty as a way of ameliorating their suffering.

It is clear, then, that the provision of medical services was either a partial justification for, or entered the discussions of, at least three treaties. Quite likely, similar concerns were expressed at other treaty negotiations as well. The degree to which there is disagreement over the terms of these treaties is profound, and continues to plague government-Indian relations to this day. Indeed, it did not take long for some detractors to begin to argue that, whatever the Treaty Six promise was, it was too much. For instance, in 1880 Manitoba's Dr John Shultz suggested in Parliament that the need to provide food to Indians was 'one of the vicious conditions of Treaty # 6,' and Donald Smith, also of Manitoba, referred to the clause as 'a most unfortunate one and never ought to have been agreed to by the Indian Commissioners' (cited in Ray 1990:41). Prime Minister John A. Macdonald's response to the Treaty Six provisions provides insight into his Indian policy: 'Of course the system is tentative and it is expensive, especially in feeding destitute Indians, *but it is cheaper to feed them than to fight them, and humanity will not allow us to let them starve for the sake of economy*' (cited in ibid. 41; italics ours). Needless to say, the lack of adequate government food supplies was one of the reasons for the Indian 'uprising' during the 1885 'rebellion' in Saskatchewan.

With respect to medical care, the promises can easily be interpreted in many ways. On one hand, the treaty commissioners indicated that medicines would be available, and the provision of free medical services at subsequent annual treaty ceremonies would further cement in the Indians' minds the link between the treaty and medical care. But the treaties also indicate that the provision of such services would be at the discretion of the government, in the person of its agents, and that there were limitations on the extent to which services could or would be delivered. Cost factors clearly limited the government's commitment. W. Morrison (1985:149) describes the anger of Indians at York Factory in 1915 when a physician failed to pay an annual visit, as they believed they were promised by Treaty Five. And there is evidence that the treaty promise as understood today is far from agreed upon even among Indians. So, while authors such as Fumoleau (1973) and R. Daniel (1987) would suggest that the treaty promises regarding medical care have not been fulfilled, at least one Treaty Seven (Peigan) elder interviewed by Daniel (ibid. 142) stated very clearly that 'the only two promises they kept were with regard to medicine and education.'

As the question of treaty rights to medical care attracted attention, especially after 1945, the views of the federal government and Indian political organizations diverged. The federal position was self-serving; for instance, Dr P.E. Moore, superintendent of Indian Health Services, wrote in 1946 that, 'Although neither law nor treaty imposes such a duty, the Federal Government has, for humanitarian reasons, for self-protection, and to prevent spread of disease to the white population, accepted responsibility for health services to the native population ...' (1946:140). The federal government noted in 1957 that medical care was a treaty obligation only under Treaty Six, but that medical services for all Indians were provided on 'humanitarian rather than on legal grounds' (Canada, DNHW 1958:76; cited in Barkwell 1981:9). In 1964, they reiterated that 'the Federal Government has never accepted the position that Indians are entitled to free medical services by Treaty rights' (Canada, DNHW 1965:95; cited in Barkwell 1981:9), and again in 1970 that 'despite popular misconceptions of the situation and vigorous assertions to the contrary, neither the federal nor any other government has any formal obligation to provide Indians, or anyone else, with free medical services' (Canada, DNHW 1971:105; cited in Barkwell 1981:9). In contrast, Indian organizations have taken the view that medical services are, indeed, a treaty right. For instance, the Indian Association of Alberta wrote in 1970 that 'the intent was that Indians should receive from the Federal Government whatever medical care could be made available,' which they interpret to mean the latest technology, medicines, and services (Indian Association of Alberta 1970:33). The Assembly of First Nations has taken a similar position, arguing that 'the Indian treaty negotiators sought, and the Crown negotiators guaranteed, establishment of a free, guaranteed health care package as a perpetual right, to be available to all Indian people, regardless of income or place of residence,' which in effect means *all* registered Indians, whether or not they have treaty status (Assembly of First Nations 1979:3).

The Canadian courts have been asked to rule on the extent of the treaty promise to provide medical care for treaty Indians, and their interpretations have guided recent government policy in this area. The first case occurred in 1935, known legally as *Dreaver v. The King* (unreported case; Barkwell 1981:14). Dreaver was a chief of the Mistawasis Band in Saskatchewan, and under his name the band launched a suit against the federal government to recover monies it had spent on medical supplies between 1919 and 1935. Dreaver had actually been present as a young man at the signing of Treaty Six, and in his testimony argued that all medicines were guaranteed free to Indians under that treaty. Furthermore, evidence indicated that medicines had, in fact, been supplied free from the time of the treaty in 1876 until 1919. The trial judge agreed with Dreaver's interpretation of the treaty.

In 1965, another Treaty Six Indian, Walter Johnston, was charged with failure to pay a 1963 tax under the *Saskatchewan Hospitalization Act*, and he used as his defence the provisions of Treaty Six which gave him tax-exempt status (ibid. 15). Johnston was found not guilty because the act exempted those who were entitled to receive hospital services from the federal government. The judge noted that, 'I can only conclude that the "medicine chest" clause in Treaty No. 6 should be properly interpreted to mean that the Indians are entitled to receive all medical services, including medicines, drugs, medical supplies, and hospital care free of charge' (cited in ibid. 15). However, upon appeal to the Saskatchewan Court of Appeal, the court ruled that a more literal interpretation of the treaty promise was appropriate, and that 'the [medicine chest] clause itself does not give to the Indians an unrestricted right to the use and benefit of the "medicine chest" but such rights as are given are subject to the direction of the Indian agent' (cited in ibid. 16). Hence, according to this appeal judgment, only a 'first-aid' type of kit was required to be provided, and the court agreed with the federal government that it was not the latter's intent to provide comprehensive and free medical services to Indians. Furthermore, even the provision of medicines from the 'medicine chest' was at the discretion of an Indian agent, or other federal representative. The judgment in this case even questioned the validity of the judgment in *Dreaver*.

In 1969 in Manitoba, a member of the Peguis Band claimed the right to free medical care on the grounds that she was a treaty Indian. After an accident, she had obtained monies from the government to cover medical expenses, as she was uninsured and lacked the means to pay. In response, the Manitoba Hospital Commission attempted to recover from her its expenses in treating her. In *Manitoba Hospital Commission v. Klein and Spence* (1969), Judge Wilson noted that there were no provisions for medical care in Treaties One or Two, and that the Treaty Six provision was offered to those Indians by Alexander Morris as lieutenant-governor of the Northwest Territories, and not Manitoba, and therefore the medicine-chest provision could not be extended to Manitoba. Furthermore, Wilson supported the ruling in *Johnston* that a literal reading of the treaties was the most appropriate (Barkwell 1981:17).

The final case to be noted is *R v. Swimmer*, in which in 1969 Andrew Swimmer was charged with not paying a tax under the *Saskatchewan Hospitalization Act* and the *Saskatchewan Medical Care Insurance Act*. The judge accepted that Treaty Six entitled Indians to free medical care, and that Swimmer was therefore exempt from the tax. But on appeal the decision was overturned, in a judgment written by the same judge as in the *Johnston* appeal, and for essentially the same reasons (Barkwell 1981:18).

In essence, the appeal decision in *Johnston* has become the leading case for purposes of interpreting the medicine-chest clause and the question of Indian treaty rights to free medical services. There clearly exist irreconcilable differences between the viewpoints of Indian organizations and the federal government on this issue.

A number of points emerge from this discussion. First, at the time of the signings of at least some of the treaties, the Indians were concerned about their future and expressed a desire for assistance in some form if famine or disease were to afflict them. The fact that by the early 1870s the Indians of western and northern Canada were already suffering extensively from disease and starvation suggests that relief from these conditions was not only on their minds, but that the treaties were seen as a way of improving their lot. Second, the federal government, through its agents, clearly made offers in some instances to provide medical care; the question remains as to the extent of this care. Third, both a literal reading of the treaty and the discussion of the negotiations as described in Morris (1880) suggests that the government intended limits to be placed on medical care, and that it would retain control over such care. Fourth, other evidence suggests that the Indians heard somewhat different promises, perhaps assuming that a 'medicine chest' represented state-of-the-art medical care which would evolve over the years. Fifth, subsequent visits by government officials to pay treaty annuities and other benefits under treaty often included a physician who examined and treated patients at no cost to them, supporting in the Indians' eyes the link between the treaty and medical services.

As a result of these cases, the federal government has been supported in its position to provide medical services to Indians as a matter of *policy*, rather than legal obligation. This effectively allows the government to alter services as it wishes. Indian organizations, in contrast, remain firmly committed to the view that the 'spirit and intent' of the treaties should be honoured, and that the Indian view, as currently evident in the oral tradition, should be accepted as the true version of the promises. Even some scholars accept the premise that Treaty Six 'became the basis for free health care for all Amerindians' (Dickason 1992:282; see also Favel-King 1993), the legal judgments notwithstanding. Yet even if the federal government were to acknowledge that a treaty right exists, such a right would still have to be translated into policy to be implemented (for example, the contents of the 'medicine chest' would have to be defined in a mutually agreeable manner). This would no doubt entail serious negotiations and likely opposition from some sectors of Canadian society, since Canadians in general do not really have a 'right' to specific health care services. At any rate, the whole treaty issue with respect to health care was overtaken by the introduction of universal health insurance in Canada in the 1960s and 1970s.

THE POLICE AND THE MILITARY

The North-West Mounted Police (NWMP), formed in 1873, provided some medical services to Indians, often acting as agents for the Department of Indian Affairs. Established in part as a response to the Indian requests to end the American whisky trade, which was wreaking havoc upon the southern Plains Indians (as well as to demonstrate Canadian sovereignty in the sparsely settled west), their role in controlling the Indians' access to alcohol remained a central activity throughout the force's early history. Even today, in remote areas, the Royal Canadian Mounted Police (RCMP), the successor to the NWMP, continues to deal with alcohol-related problems. But the police provided other services as well. In the Yukon Territory, for instance, Coates (1991:174) suggests that the NWMP surgeons routinely provided services to Indians in the early part of the twentieth century. In 1905, the Department of Indian Affairs had four such doctors on retainer, treating the Indians and charging the federal government two dollars per visit. Medicines and hospitalizations were also made available free of charge to the Indians. However, by 1914 'those [Indians] of means were expected to pay their own bills. When Skookum Jim Mason, co-discoverer of the Klondike strike, fell ill in 1916, the DIA refused to pay the $100 hospital charge' (ibid. 174). The NWMP also played a role in effecting quarantines when diseases struck particular Indian groups.

Fetherstonhaugh (1940), in his tribute to the force, described a number of 'humanitarian' efforts engaged in on behalf of Indians in the prairies. In 1881, in the Fort Qu'Appelle district of Saskatchewan, a constable named Holmes endeavoured to assist Indians affected by smallpox. Having studied medicine and attained some nursing experience, Holmes undertook to vaccinate as many Indians and settlers as possible, and otherwise care for the sick, as there was no doctor available. Fetherstonhaugh (ibid. 123) describes Constable Holmes in rather heroic terms:

This meant travelling many miles on snowshoes, camping in the open with no protection from blizzards and cold other than a hole in some deep drift of snow. It meant days spent in the lodges of the stricken Indians, where sanitation was unknown and the air was foetid with the odour of the disease. It meant all these things and more, but it wrought the district's salvation. Finally, after many deaths, the vaccine took effect. New cases ceased to appear. Immunization triumphed. And Holmes, rewarded only by his pay of seventy-five cents a day, returned to routine duties in the Force as an acting hospital steward.

Fetherstonhaugh (ibid. 123–4) also described the efforts of another constable at Norway House who, when scarlet fever and diphtheria broke out in 1881, 'quietly tackled the grim problem which the epidemics provided,' including caring for the sick and the dying, burying the dead, and disinfecting the tents. When influenza attacked the Inuit and Indians in the Coronation Gulf and Mackenzie River areas between 1926 and 1928, the police offered assistance despite falling ill themselves.

In contrast to Fetherstonhaugh's praise for the force, W. Morrison (1985:143) argues that, at least in the north, the police viewed the Indians 'with a mixture of paternalism and contempt,' perhaps a view conditioned by the 'noble redskin' image many police had of Plains Indians (ibid. 59). References to 'lazy' Indians, for instance, occur repeatedly throughout police reports in the early 1900s, though as Morrison notes, this apparent laziness could have been caused by disease or other factors (if, indeed, the Indians were actually 'lazy'). In Yukon, Morrison notes that 'The attitude of the police towards the Indians they encountered ... was generally that they were a lazy, dirty nuisance, to be given meagre aid if they were actually starving, but to be ignored as much as possible' (ibid. 145). The attitude of the police in the Mackenzie Delta and Hudson Bay 'was much the same.' Some police realized that the Indians were victims of circumstances over which they had no control, however, and the HBC was often criticized by the police for the way it dealt with the Indians (ibid. 146).

For much of the north, both treaty and non-treaty areas, the police acted as agents of the government; this included making treaty payments, undertaking the census, and delivering medical services. Police doctors often provided services to sick Indians but, as Morrison (ibid. 148) explains, the police were sometimes angered over what they perceived to be the Indians' refusal to follow their medical instructions. Morrison (ibid. 148) quotes one police doctor in Churchill in 1915, who stated 'I have repeatedly explained to them the infectious nature of the disease [tuberculosis], how it spreads, and how it could be lessened. My advices seem to have been of very little use, and results have been very discouraging.' The fact that the Indians probably did not comprehend the doctor is suggested by Morrison. The poverty and poor health which characterized many of the Indians living around the fur-trade posts and police stations desensitized the officers, and led them to become callous about the plight of the Indians. In contrast, the force developed more positive views of the Inuit, 'who had all the qualities the Indians lacked,' including thriftiness, cleanliness, and morality (ibid. 152). Nevertheless, by 1910, and especially after 1920, the police found themselves dispensing relief to starving Inuit as well as Indians (ibid. 158). Change, and colonization, had reached into the high Arctic.

The NWMP, then, like the missionaries and traders, provided medical services and relief in varying degrees to Indians and Inuit, in some instances for humanitarian reasons, and in others grudgingly because it was part of their job. Their services to government also included enforcing quarantines, and in this area at least there was some opposition by Indians.

The military also played a role in the delivery of medical services to Aboriginal peoples. In many instances, they simply supported the efforts of others, such as the missionaries in the Arctic; this included providing transportation and delivering medicines. However military doctors were also called upon to provide medical services.

The years following the Second World War saw the military become involved in a variety of medical areas, as a result of military expansion in the north designed to secure Canadian sovereignty during the 'Cold War.' In the high Arctic, radar bases were established as a means of warning against a polar attack by the Soviet Union. These bases collectively were known as the Distant Early Warning Line, or 'DEW Line,' and the military personnel employed Inuit to construct the bases and provide other services. Medical assistance was provided to these Inuit and their families, but the experiences were not always good. Schaefer (1959:81) describes how the construction of the DEW Line base near Davis Inlet on the Labrador coast in the mid-1950s seriously affected the Inuit, many of whom found employment in construction. The resultant noise frightened game away from the area, and Inuit workers became dependent on a carbohydrate-based diet. When the construction ended in 1957 and the Inuit were laid off, the military decided not to further their dependence by administering rations. A series of infections struck their camp, including tuberculosis and measles. By late 1957, almost half of the forty Inuit who had been living in a nearby camp were either dead or had been evacuated south for medical treatment.

Foulkes (1962) has provided a view of military medical services, based largely on his own experiences as a physician with the Royal Canadian Air Force at Fort Nelson, British Columbia, from 1955 to 1957. The first medical services were supplied in this region on an ad-hoc basis, often by U.S. military personnel (attached to the Alaska Highway construction project), or by private physicians under contract to the Department of National Defence. By the mid-1950s, RCAF medical officers had taken the place of these private practitioners. Part of Foulkes's job involved providing medical services to the 'Slave' Indians (a Dene or Athapaskan speaking people also known as Slavey). The living conditions for these people were atrocious, according to Foulkes, particularly for those who lived in the village by the air base. Other Indians lived throughout the region, and Foulkes was required to provide services to these as well. Emergency medical advice was often provided by telegraph. He writes of the Canadian National Telegraph: 'I can recall talking with anxious parents about a sick child, with interpreters who had received a message from an Indian runner about some calamity in the bush, with the consultants in Edmonton and Vancouver regarding an extraordinary case, and with the various individuals within the chain of command for the calling of an aircraft for an urgent air evacuation' (Foulkes 1962a:535). Private citizens were required to pay for medical services, although for Indians the Department of Indian Affairs picked up the costs. The Indian and Northern Health Service of National Health and Welfare also employed a nurse in the region, whose work focused more on preventive medicine.

There were many problems encountered in the treatment of Indian patients. Foulkes (ibid. 548) suggested that 'Treatment, recommended without due consideration of all of the difficulties inherent in the home environment, especially in the Indian settlement, could lead at times either to near-tragedy or to a display of ingenuity.' He describes ways in which Indian patients afflicted with scabies managed to bathe and wash clothes frequently despite a lack of running water, including one who created a bathtub by lining a trench with canvas and heating water on an open fire next to it. Foulkes also notes the continued existence of traditional medicine 'in the hinterland' and mentioned by some of his patients. For instance, he describes seeing patients 'with wounds dressed in obnoxious concoctions of bear grease and assorted unidentifiable ingredients,' which he then treated 'in a more orthodox manner.' He also describes an incident in which parents' fear of hospitals caused one couple to hide their child in the bush for many months; when he was finally found, he was on the verge of dying from what Foulkes describes as 'a once operable tuberculosis in the brain' (ibid. 549).

Indian and other patients were required to share the military hospitals' wards, and Foulkes (ibid. 550) notes that, 'even though the North country is far from free of discrimination and prejudice, there was no loudly expressed objection.' Despite his rather narrow view of Indian traditional medicine, Foulkes presents some enlightened viewpoints on the state of the Indians in the region, including the effects of poverty and other social conditions on their health. For instance, with respect to sexually transmitted diseases, he noted that the major source of the problem lay with the civilian workers and 'their lack of respect for the dignity of Indian girls' (1962b:676).

When the RCAF's Tactical Air Command was dissolved in 1959, the small hospital was transferred to the Fort Nelson community as a civilian hospital. The role of the military in providing medical service in this region was formally relinquished (Foulkes 1962c:750–1).

Grygier (1994) has documented the role that the military played in the detection and treatment of tuberculosis among the Inuit. Their participation included x-raying and transporting patients, and providing other services and facilities. For instance, a Department of National Defence hospital in Edmonton was transferred to the Indian Health Service and opened in 1946 as the Charles Camsell Indian Hospital. The Coastguard ship *C.D. Howe* became the cornerstone of much Arctic screening for Inuit tuberculosis, and some of the medical staff were officers in the RCAF. Given the militarization of the Canadian north after 1945, the role of the military in health as well as other administrative areas is not surprising.

INDIAN AGENTS AND RELIEF MEASURES

The first Department of Indian Affairs was established in 1880, with Prime Minister John A. Macdonald as its superintendent general. This department was not originally concerned with Indian health problems, and initially made no provision for medical services and personnel (Graham-Cumming 1967:123). Some Indian bands voluntarily paid for medical services. Indians were directed to use local physicians and hospitals on a fee-for-service basis.

The Indian-agent system was a quasi-military approach to handling the administration of Indian affairs. Although 'agents' were used by the colonial government prior to Confederation, the era of the 'Indian agent' really commenced after the treaties were signed in western Canada, beginning in 1871. The Indian agents, responsible for virtually all aspects of the administration of Indian affairs and the implementation of elements of the treaties in large 'agencies,' were all-powerful. Often working in conjunction with the police and the missionaries, the Indian agents executed federal policies designed to facilitate the 'protection, civilization and assimilation' of their charges (Tobias 1976). Medical assistance provided to Indians and food rations or 'relief' in times of 'famine or pestilence' were a part of these policies.

Although some Indian agents actually had medical training, for the most part they had little more than lay knowledge of medical matters; indeed, many agency postings were simply political patronage appointments. In the early years, the 'medicine chest' represented the embodiment of medical services available through the agent, but by the early twentieth century government-employed medical officers became more readily available. The government always retained a strong element of control in the hiring of such physicians, and many were placed on salaries rather than being paid on a fee-for-service basis.[1] Private physicians were also utilized, particularly in emergencies or where a government physician was not at hand. A choice of physicians was therefore not readily available to Indians, although Col. E.L. Stone, medical superintendent in the Department of Indian Affairs, was confident that 'The Department does not contemplate that a sick Indian who is genuinely dissatisfied with the regular physician should be denied the services of another' (Stone 1935:84).

One of the problems which faced the new government was the impoverished circumstances of Indians on the western prairies. Disease was rampant on many reserves, and with the collapse of the bison herds many Indians were attempting to make the transition to an agricultural life (the provisions for which were included in the treaties).[2]

The federal government, working through the Indian agents, provided rations to Indian bands, but often under tight restrictions. In some instances, rations were withheld entirely. In 1882, Chief Moosomin of the North Battleford agency in Saskatchewan was brought to write that "There is to-day great distress in my band. The rations are suspended now for 41 days ... It is impossible to work on an empty stomach' (Canada, DIA 1882:195). In other instances, 'able-bodied' Indians were refused rations on the assumption that they could work instead. Indian agents exercised a great deal of autonomy to limit rations and thereby effect savings for the government; conversely, they were often rebuked when their designations of destitute Indians were challenged by superiors. Rations were clearly used as a mechanism of social control: Indians who left their reserves without permission, or who refused to take up agricultural work, could be cut off. Even hungry children, or those suffering from illness, could be refused.

There is also little question that, in general, the rations provided to the Indians were inadequate, and that the Department of Indian Affairs and the Indian agents were aware of this fact. Flour and bacon were the staples of the rations diet, and only occasionally was fresh meat allowed (the government retained tight control over the cattle herds on Indian reserves). Well into the twentieth century, the government went to great lengths to avoid defining any Indian as 'destitute.' Quantities of rations were limited, and the food was of inferior nutritional value. The nutritional health implications of the rations program are clear when one keeps in mind that Aboriginal peoples were undergoing a transition away from a high-protein diet of fresh meat; indeed, some local government administrators often encouraged Indians to keep hunting, despite a formal agricultural policy. By the end of the nineteenth century, some western Indian bands had begun to develop small cattle industries and to grow vegetables, but these endeavours came somewhat late for many Indians who succumbed to diseases while dependent on a rations diet.

FEDERAL INDIAN HEALTH SERVICES

In 1904, Dr Peter H. Bryce was appointed as the first federal official responsible directly for Indian health. As 'General Medical Superintendent,' he proved to be an active and persistent advocate for improving health conditions on Indian reserves.

Bryce had been the secretary of the Ontario Provincial Board of Health prior to his appointment, and had been a leader in the public health movement in Canada (T.K. Young 1984:258). Indian health was clearly a priority for him. In 1903, he had begun to argue that the Indian department required better organized medical services to offset the effects of the many contagious diseases on reserves. But these measures would be costly in the eyes of the Ontario government, an increase in expenditures of between $10,000 and $15,000 each year. His suggestion was turned down (E. Titley 1986:83).

After his appointment to the federal government in 1904, Bryce came into direct conflict with Duncan Campbell Scott of the Department of Indian Affairs, whose own personal mission seemed to focus on reducing government expenditures. For his part, Bryce became particularly concerned with the tuberculosis problem, one which necessitated increasing expenditures. His requests for a special grant of $20,000, to be used for preventive programs among the Indians, was rejected by Parliament in 1907. The seeds for Bryce's downfall were sown, but not before he was able to bring the seriousness of the Indians' health conditions to national attention.

In 1907, Bryce launched an investigation into the conditions at industrial and residential schools on the prairies. The results of his investigations were made available to politicians and the press, and ultimately published in part in 1922 as *The Story of a National Crime: An Appeal for Justice to the Indians of Canada*. He found the schools to be rife with disease and lacking proper medical facilities. According to his data, a survey of fifteen years indicated that from 25 per cent to 35 per cent of all children who had been pupils had died, primarily from tuberculosis but also from other diseases, such as measles (Bryce 1914:137).[3] Bryce even suggested that the Indian schools be transformed into sanatoria, so bad was the health situation! As we saw in the previous chapter, the church officials who operated the schools reacted defensively, but the Indian agents tended to corroborate Bryce's report. Even so, one high-ranking government official accused Bryce of exaggerating the magnitude of the problem (E. Titley 1986:84).

Bryce's plan to improve the health conditions in these schools was reasonable. Each school could employ a health nurse to improve sanitation and environmental conditions, and a program of better exercise and fresh air for the students could be implemented. The churches, Bryce suggested, should not be involved. Realizing that the government was likely to baulk at the increase in expenditures that such a program would entail, Bryce suggested it be tested on an experimental basis in one province. But he failed to get Duncan Campbell Scott's approval for the plan. The churches were very upset with Bryce's report, and would not likely cooperate, according to Scott. Scott's response was to propose improvements in ventilation, exercise, and diet, presumably at a lower cost to the government. Bryce's publication of 1922 contained a critical comment on the way the tuberculosis problem had been handled by Scott and the minister of health, Dr W.A. Roche. With respect to Roche, Bryce scorned his 'transparent hypocrisy' and suggested 'how little the Minister cared for the solution of the tuberculosis problem' (Bryce 1922:8). Invoking the treaties as a last resort, Bryce stated, 'The degree and extent of this criminal disregard for the treaty pledges to guard the welfare of the Indian wards of the nation may be gauged from the facts' of the widespread devastation being caused by tuberculosis.

By 1913, Bryce's railing against the government appeared to render him *persona non grata* among his superiors. His efforts in 1920 to have Indian health removed from the Department of Indian Affairs to a new Department of Health were thwarted. According to Arthur Meighen, then superintendent of Indian Affairs, such a transfer was not possible, in part because it would create a duplication of services, 'and there would be a sort of divided control and authority over the Indians which would produce confusion and insubordination and other ill effects among the Indians themselves' (cited in T.K. Young 1984:259). This meant that Indian health would remain with Indian Affairs for another twenty-five years. However, Bryce was ultimately successful in seeing another of his projects adopted, however: in 1922, a mobile nurse-visitor program was implemented which would see the medical officer's work being complemented by the work of nurses at the community level. The first nursing station was opened in 1930 on the Fisher River reserve in Manitoba. Bryce also introduced some degree of health education for Indians, having circulars on tuberculosis translated into Cree, for instance, as well as issuing a

'Book of Regulations' on medical services to Indian agents. Finally, it was Bryce's idea to fill the obvious vacuum of physician services by contracting local physicians to provide services (Hader 1990:107).

Maundrell (1942; cited in Graham-Cumming 1967:125) suggests that Bryce 'ignored all consideration of money' in his work, a fact which clearly clashed with Scott's acute sense of fiscal responsibility as well as other government priorities. Bryce remained in the position of chief medical officer until he retired in 1921, bitter and disillusioned over the failure of many of his proposals and at being denied the position of deputy minister in the newly formed Department of Health in 1919. His strident, perhaps abrasive, approach left a legacy, however; his position was not refilled until 1927. In the meantime, according to Maundrell (ibid.), 'A study of the reports and correspondence impresses one with the disorganization of the services. The natives received medical treatment but there was little effort to overcome the worst epidemics. The appointment of a Medical Superintendent might have been postponed indefinitely but for the increasing friction between field doctors and the departmental accountant who taxed their fees. Something had to be done to prevent these quarrels ...' Financial concerns, once again, proved to be paramount in these early years of government services to Indians.

In 1927, a medical doctor named Col. E.L. Stone was appointed medical superintendent in the Department of Indian Affairs. Stone had been a physician in the department, travelling throughout Indian agencies undertaking health surveys and treating patients. In 1926 he was a physician at Norway House, Manitoba, and in charge of the hospital there. The hospital served a number of more remote communities, where missionaries acted as dispensers of medicines. But the hospital itself was small, only sixteen beds, and inadequate to meet the needs of long-term patients.

Stone's 1926 report, 'Health and Disease at the Norway House Indian Agency,' provides some indication of his approach to health matters. The Norway House Cree were impoverished, though not necessarily starving, and the rampant tuberculosis they experienced was the result. According to Stone (1926: rpt 1989:246), 'Disease here means one malady, and one only, for all practical purposes. That is tuberculosis. Practically nobody dies of anything else.' But while poverty was a contributing factor to this disease profile, Stone placed greater emphasis on sanitation and personal sanitary habits. He wrote, 'There is no need to go into details about the sanitary habits of these people in their houses. It is enough to say that they are not likely to help limit the spread of infection from the sick to the well.'[4] In an effort to appear as unbiased as possible, he then added,

'And [these sanitary habits] are not much, if any, worse than those of many white people' (ibid. 249). In an oblique reference to the apparent laziness of the Indians, as often reported by the police, traders, and others, Stone wrote insightfully, 'One is often led to wonder what these Indians might be able to accomplish if they were freed, by some miracle, from consumption. There is no doubt that their energy would increase enormously.' But then lapsing into a racial argument common at the time, he adds, 'It must be remembered that they have much white blood, and many of the instincts peculiar to the white race' (ibid. 242). (For a discussion of issues of race and tuberculosis, see also chapter 11.) The ultimate answer to the tuberculosis problem lay with improving the economic fortunes of the people, particularly their ability to earn a living in the trapping industry through better conservation and restrictions on outside trappers. He argued that an increase in rations would not help the population, and that 'the present Medical Services [were] not meeting the needs in that it is dealing with effect rather than cause' (ibid. 256). Nevertheless, Stone had collaborated with Bryce and others in the establishment of a committee in 1924 to investigate the Indian tuberculosis problem, and he ultimately presided over anti-tuberculosis surveys and projects in British Columbia and Saskatchewan (Hader 1990:111,113).

Stone's critical comments pale in comparison to those of Bryce, with whom he had some contact, and Stone was clearly more popular with his superiors. Nevertheless, with his appointment in 1927, Stone was still somewhat of a pioneer. His Norway House reports were taken seriously, and led to the establishment of the Qu'Appelle Medical Health Unit in Saskatchewan to treat tuberculosis patients (Graham-Cumming 1967:125). He also continued Bryce's work in providing circulars on health matters. But, as Bryce had found, the lack of funds provided for Indian health care prevented much progress from being made.

At the time of Stone's appointment, a formal Medical Branch was established within Indian Affairs. Writing in 1935, Stone described the workings of this branch in the *Canadian Medical Association Journal*. The Indian agent retained a great deal of power within the new framework, for as Stone noted, 'The Indian agent ... is responsible for every matter affecting the interests of the Indians under his charge, including ... the administration of the medical and health services' (Stone 1935:82). While some agents were also physicians, most had to rely on branch medical officers to provide services. Nevertheless, the agent's concern was more one of cost, and the medical officers were relatively free to treat patients of their own accord. The Indian agent's permission was required to have a patient hospitalized, and the head office in Ottawa had to consent to a transfer to a sanatorium. The system had holes, but Stone firmly believed 'that no Indian need lack the services of a physician or the advantages of a hospital when he is sick or injured, if by any means of transportation the doctor can be conveyed to him, or he be brought to the doctor or hospital' (ibid. 83).

Stone was not alone in his fight against tuberculosis. In 1928, Dr Robert Ferguson, a pioneer in the treatment of the disease, reported the results of a survey on Indian tuberculosis at an international conference; but despite the alarming incidence of the disease that he identified, federal resources remained relatively slim. Indeed, in its 1933 budget, the medical branch suffered a 20 per cent cutback. As a result, the Department of Indian Affairs was forced to state in 1934 that 'it is impossible to admit to sanatorium more than a very small proportion of Indians who are recommended for such care.' Sanatorium care was to be reserved for the homeless. And in 1935, when a Battleford Agency physician requested a sanatorium admission for a child, he was told that 'The Department is in the unfortunate position of not having sufficient funds to maintain in hospital an increased number of *ordinary* cases of tuberculosis' (cited in Hader 1990:114; italics ours). The government's response in this case was to supply a tent for the child! The problem of shortage of funds was put into perspective in 1937, when a editorial appeared in the *Canadian Tuberculosis Association Bulletin* arguing that 'the facilities for early diagnosis, treatment and prevention that have been used to such good advantage in the White population have never been made available for the attack on the Indian problem' (cited in Hader 1990:117).

In 1935, there were eleven medical officers in the Medical Branch who were employed full time, and eight Indian agents with medical training. Another 250 physicians were employed part time, or as needed, including urban-based specialists; and still others saw Indian patients privately. There was little in the way of dental services, outside of basic services such as extractions. A total of eleven field nurses was employed by the branch, supplemented by others employed by missionary or provincial organizations. The first nursing station had been opened at Fisher River, Manitoba, in 1930, and would be followed by the construction of many more. A network of some 200 hospitals was available, including tuberculosis sanatoria, most of which were quite small and not definable as 'hospitals' *per se*. Stone (1935) states that only seven could be so classed, with the smallest having eight beds and the largest forty. Many of these facilities were operated by provincial governments as public facilities, or by missionary organizations. The revenue accruing to many hospitals as a result of treating Indians was extremely important to their viability.

The costs of medical services to Indians remained an issue throughout Stone's tenure. His efforts to deal with the tuberculosis problem and other communicable diseases and to expand the scope and magnitude of medical services were hampered by a lack of funds. According to Maundrell (1942; cited in Graham-Cumming 1967:126): 'The medical services provided are the more impressive when it is remembered that the Branch has never had at its disposal any more than about one-half the amount per capita expended by the Canadian population at large and that the Indians are relatively a sickly people. In 1934 the per capita cost was $9.60, approximately the same as in 1930, whereas the per capita cost for the white population was $31.00.' It is hard to imagine that medical coverage could have been as good as Stone suggests, given the relatively low expenditures and the fact that the branch was responsible for at least 112,500 people spread over 800 communities.

In 1936, the Department of Indian Affairs was absorbed by the Department of Mines and Natural Resources, including the Medical Division of Indian Affairs and the 'Eskimo' Health Service of the Northwest Territories branch. Stone remained as the medical superintendent, and Dr P.E. Moore became his assistant. When war broke out in 1939, Stone returned to military service and Moore took his place. Moore was ultimately appointed director of the Indian health service in 1945, and when Stone returned after the war the latter concentrated on having a hospital for Indians and Inuit built in Edmonton (Graham-Cumming 1967:126).

Moore, like Stone and Bryce before him, wrote numerous articles on the Indian health service. Writing in 1946, Moore described a health service which had grown somewhat since 1935. Twenty-seven full-time physicians were now employed in the Indian and Northern Health Service, seven of whom were assigned to the Northwest Territories and the eastern Arctic. Some 700 physicians were employed part time, providing services on demand to Indians in their regions. The service was now operating sixteen hospitals in addition to provincial facilities available to Indians across the country, including tuberculosis sanatoria. Twenty-four field nurses were employed, plus many more part-time 'field matrons' and 'field dispensers' who administered medicines, often under the direction of a physician at the other end of a two-way radio. The persistence of traditional Indian medicine, based on 'ignorance and superstition' according to Moore, was still seen as a roadblock in the delivery of medical services, especially in remote areas (P.E. Moore 1946:141).

Physicians were required to travel extensively in this period, and visits to smaller Indian communities were often timed to coordinate with the payment of treaty money. Corrigan (1946), the physician based at Norway House, described accompanying the Indian agent on annual treaty parties, sojourns that took a month. The doctor undertook medical examinations and vaccinations, as well as pulling teeth, while the agent paid out the annual five dollars per capita. In all, some 4,000 Indians were given this whirlwind treatment, and since they were not required to pay for the medical services, it is easy to see how such joint treaty-medical expeditions appeared, to the Indians, to be simply an exercise in fulfilling the treaty right to free medical care.

How did the early physicians view their Indian patients? While most never recorded their thoughts in a manner that would be available to researchers, a significant number could not resist writing of what to them were adventures in the wilds of the country. Their ill-informed (even racist) attitudes, for the most part, can be seen as typical of general Canadian attitudes regarding Indians, as well as formal government policy. William Shaw, a physician among the Kwakiutl of coastal British Columbia, for instance, supported the banishment of the potlatch, arguing 'A new Indian is rising on the ashes of the old, many now have modern houses and motor cars, and are rapidly taking a useful place in the White Man's civilization' (Shaw 1923:659). Wall's report on the Indians along the Quebec-Ontario border noted for one band, 'The Chief here is a careless and indolent man of low mentality, and the mentality of the Band as a whole appears to be lower than the average' (Wall 1926; rpt 1989:269). Cameron Corrigan, the resident physician at Norway House in the mid-1940s, described the Indians there as being 'promiscuous, and amoral,' adding, 'I do not believe an Indian can be treated for any sickness unless he is hospitalized, as he cannot be trusted to take medicine intelligently' (1946:221). The general disdain that most physicians held for traditional medical approaches has been discussed in a previous chapter. In the end, it becomes clear that the physicians believed, as did many in government, that the Indians were clearly threatened with extinction from disease, and that their only hope was assimilation (including intermarriage with non-Aboriginal peoples to strengthen their gene pool).

Racism to some degree was also evident with respect to certain aspects of tuberculosis treatment. Many Indians experienced more or less forced evacuations to northern and southern hospitals for treatment. In Yukon, for instance, tubercular Indians were sent to the general hospital in Whitehorse and, in some instances, down to the Charles Camsell Hospital in

Edmonton in the late 1940s and 1950s (Coates 1991: 105, 215). While efforts to treat and prevent tuberculosis among the Indians were, in part, the result of humanitarian motives, and while quarantining tuberculosis patients was the accepted practice for all, it is also true that 'the regular appearance of disease among the Natives and the perception of non-Natives that such illnesses threatened their communities added support to government and public efforts to segregate the Natives' (ibid. 107). Indeed, as Coates (1991:95) documents for Yukon, racial segregation in the area of medical care was the norm in the 1940s: 'In most centres, the people consistently demanded the segregation of hospitals and refused to share wards with Native patients. The Mayo Hospital, funded by the Treadgold Mining Company, refused to admit Natives to its general wards. Instead, Indians received treatment in a tent to the rear of the main structure ... In Whitehorse, similarly, there was a general hospital and, for a time, a small building "fitted for the infirm and Tubercular Indian patients."'

Some physicians shared the views of the non-Aboriginal public; in 1939 several doctors refused to treat Indians for the same fee rates as for non-Indians, despite the lament of the Department of Indian Affairs that it was 'not prepared to admit that sick Indians are less desirable patients than white people' (Coates 1991:96). Views of Indians as 'dirty' and 'diseased' were widespread, and while the existence of disease among these peoples is not contestable, the underlying attitude at the time that the Indians were inferior certainly is. The link between poverty and disease was clear, and even reports which implied inferiority of moral or physical standards among Indians betrayed the real causes. Coates (ibid. 104) quotes a North-West Mounted Police surgeon, writing in 1903: 'They [Yukon Indians] are a squalid, pitiable looking lot of people. Those who do not exhibit advanced symptoms of disease show signs of the existence of germs. They are particularly unclean in their habits and almost entirely destitute. I declare I have not seen in the different tents I have had occasion to enter, a decent pair of blankets; they have but small flimsy things, and in most cases a mere heap of rags. It is a fact as incontrovertible, as it is deplorable, that disease, actual want and destitution prevail among the majority of them.'

The postwar years saw an increase in the medical services available to Indians. A new federal department, National Health and Welfare, had been formed in 1944, and in 1945 the Indian and Northern Health Service, including services to Inuit, was transferred to it. All other aspects of Indian administration remained with the Indian Affairs Branch, however, and these ultimately were transferred to a new Department of Indian Affairs and Northern Development in 1966, an arrangement that would come to create much frustration among those attempting more holistic health programs. Even at the outset, the Indian agents, renamed 'Superintendents,' retained control over health matters by virtue of their designation as 'Health Officers,' despite the fact that the services themselves were to be delivered by a separate department. As the years passed, however, it became increasingly evident that the poor socio-economic conditions of the Indians, including sanitation and education, were to a large extent responsible for their relatively poor health. Indeed, according to Graham-Cumming (1967:128), officials with the Department of Mines and Natural Resources were upset with the transfer of Indian health matters to the new department, viewing it as a critical comment on their abilities, and hence interdepartmental cooperation was difficult to achieve.

By 1956, National Health and Welfare was operating 18 hospitals (growing to 22 by 1960), 33 nursing stations (37 in 1960), 52 health centres containing dispensaries, and 13 other health centres employing full-time physicians or nurses (83 health centres in 1960) (P.E. Moore 1956:229; T.K. Young 1984:260). Employment had grown considerably, and there were now 39 field medical officers, 43 hospital medical officers, 11 dental surgeons, 106 field nurses, and 232 hospital nurses. Additional services were provided by 63 part-time physicians and more than 1,200 private physicians and 125 dentists. More than $17 million was appropriated for these medical services in 1956.

In 1962, another government reorganization saw the elimination of the Indian Health Service and the creation of a new branch, Medical Services, which amalgamated the services of seven programs: Civil Aviation Medicine, Public Service Health, Indian Health, Northern Health, Quarantine, Immigration, and Sick Mariners' Services. In effect, any Canadian whose medical services fell outside the domain of provincial programs became the responsibility of this new branch. Administration of Indian health services was facilitated by the existence of a region and zone structure across the country (T.K. Young 1984).

The 1960s saw the closure of some Indian hospitals and sanatoria as the need for them decreased; there were only nine hospitals left by the mid-1970s. In contrast, the number of nursing stations and health centres increased to more than 100. Indeed, nursing-station services developed as the backbone of the Medical Services Branch. Overall expenditures on Indian health continued to increase, and by the end of the 1960s the budget was more than $28 million (compared to only $4 million in the

1950s). Hospital insurance was also introduced, and by 1971 all provinces were covered by universal medical care insurance. Questions of medical indigence – or treaty rights to medical care, for that matter – became increasingly irrelevant in a country where everyone had access to medical services. In some provinces, where insurance premiums were implemented, the federal government assisted in their payment by Indian bands. Medical services offered directly to Indians by the federal government were concentrated in the more remote and northern areas; in other instances, Indians sought services from provincial facilities and private physicians, who then billed back to the federal government.

THE DEVELOPMENT OF MEDICAL SERVICES FOR THE INUIT

The Inuit were among the last to be provided with organized medical services by the federal government. The missionaries, traders, military, and police continued to have a prominent role until after the Second World War in some areas.

The first hospitals constructed in the Arctic were operated under the auspices of the churches. For instance, the Anglicans erected a small hospital on Blacklead Island, in Cumberland Sound, in 1902, and another in Pangnirtung in 1929; the Roman Catholics did likewise at Aklavik in 1926 and Chesterfield Inlet in 1929. The Anglicans and Roman Catholics collaborated with the federal government to construct a six-bed facility at Coppermine in 1929 (Jenness 1972:8). These were not always permanent facilities, however, and hospitals often closed only a few years after their construction.

That missionary medical services in these early hospitals were a part of an overall attempt to Christianize the Inuit is clear. One report on the development of the hospitals at Blacklead Island and Pangnirtung reported that the hospitals represented great medical advances, 'since at that time the Eskimo were pagan, and often made it very difficult for the Missionaries to treat the patients properly in their tents and snow huts' (A. Fleming nd:1). This report, issued by the Arctic Mission, concluded by saying: 'The Hospital has been established following the example of the Master Who went about healing the sick and afflicted. Pray that through its means the Saviour may be made known to many – both Eskimo and white' (ibid. 7). As we shall see shortly with respect to tuberculosis treatment, medical care and culture change were often viewed by the Euro-Canadian caregivers to be interrelated.

The medical officers at these church-run hospitals were usually federal employees. The Department of the Interior, followed by Indian Affairs and, after 1935, the Department of Mines and Natural Resources, were responsible for recruiting and employing the medical staff (P.E. Moore 1974:132). Since there were relatively few hospitals in the early years of the twentieth century, however, much medical care still remained in the hands of the missionaries and traders in the more remote areas, and the federal government supplied northern missions with medicines during the early part of the twentieth century (Jenness 1972:44). Between 1918 and 1923, the government spent some $30,800 on relief for the Inuit, most of which was paid to the police and trading companies who provided the aid (ibid. 32). During the years of the Second World War, when relatively few medical personnel were available for Arctic service, the Canada Medical Procurement and Assignment Board posted some medical officers of the Department of National Defence to staff some of the northern hospitals (P.E. Moore 1974:133).

In 1921, the federal government created the Northwest Territories Branch, in the Department of the Interior, to administer the north. It had become apparent that relief measures were required in some Inuit settlements, and that health care required some attention. As Jenness (1972:32) notes, the federal government at that time assumed that it had a legal responsibility to the Inuit, though in 1932 this responsibility was clarified to mean 'they have not the status of Indians, and the provisions of the Indian Act do not apply to them.' Yet, since 1880, in matters of health and education the federal Department of Indian Affairs had made no distinction between the Inuit and Indians in the north. In 1924, Indian Affairs officially took responsibility for the Inuit (through an amendment to the *Indian Act*), extending medical services into the eastern Arctic. In 1928, the Inuit were transferred to the commissioner of the Northwest Territories, and in 1932 the *Indian Act* was amended to delete the Inuit provision (ibid. 33). In 1945, the care of both Indians and Inuit was transferred to the Department of National Health and Welfare, and the Inuit began to receive family allowance benefits for the first time (ibid. 77).

In 1955, the Northern Health Service was established by the federal government, and the responsibility for medical services to the Northwest Territories was placed with the Department of National Health and Welfare. One of the pioneers in the delivery of medical services in the Arctic in this era was Otto Schaefer. The conditions in which he operated were crude, to say the least, and frequently called for innovation and, in the eyes of the doctors themselves, a certain amount of heroism. For instance, here is how Schaefer described one incident that occurred in 1956:

In March 1956, a dog-team came racing into Pangnirtung from a camp 60 miles distant where a woman had suffered a severe haemorrhage associated with an incomplete abortion. The patient had become unconscious and had been regarded as unfit for dog-sled transportation. I rapidly collected blood-grouping sera, transfusion bottles and gynaecological instruments and, with our own dog-team, raced to that camp. There, I grouped and cross-matched a number of Eskimos, transfused 1000 c.c. of blood into the unconscious patient and, after overcoming the shock, proceeded to evacuate the uterus. All these procedures took place in a small, crowded sealskin winter tent, where the low ceiling kept my back bent all the time and the only sources of light were a dim seal-oil lamp and my flashlight. (Schaefer 1959:81)

Schaefer cites other similar incidents, including one in which a missionary, HBC manager, and a 'wise old Eskimo woman' removed the retained placenta from a bleeding woman, under direction of a physician 500 miles away using a two-way radio (ibid. 81).

The consequences of the Inuit's anomalous position *vis-à-vis* Canada are perhaps best demonstrated with respect to the Ungava region of Quebec. As Vanast (1991) has documented, when Quebec gained the northern territory in 1912, it became the only province to contain an Inuit population. Quebec's response was to assume that the Inuit were 'Indians' under the *British North America Act*, and hence a federal responsibility. Canada, on the other hand, believed the Inuit to be Quebec citizens. A battle raged on this issue until 1939, when Quebec achieved a Supreme Court ruling that the Inuit were 'Indians' in law, and hence the responsibility of the federal government. Nevertheless, Canada was slow to act upon its responsibilities until the 1950s, leading Vanast (1991:74) to conclude that while 'There was no conspiracy to keep Ungava's Inuit unfed and unhealthy ... the outcome was not much different than if there had been one.'

One of the easiest ways to reach Inuit settlements throughout the first half of this century was by boat or ship. In some cases, travel facilities were on a modest scale. For instance, in 1930 the physician at Aklavik was provided with a small boat so that he could travel throughout Coronation Gulf. But medical services were also provided by ships which plied the coastal waters. In the 1920s with the advent of the Eastern Arctic Patrol, the vessel *Arctic* travelled the eastern coast with a medical doctor as it replenished supplies at coastal trading posts (later, the *Beothuk* took over this role). When a medical station was established at Pangnirtung in 1924, the patrol doctor managed to examine more than 500 Inuit in the region over two winters (Jenness 1972:44). The Eastern Arctic Patrol ship

CGS *Nascopie*, regularly supplied coastal missions with medicines between 1918 and 1947, and was eventually provided with a medical staff and x-ray equipment as part of the fight against tuberculosis. When it ran aground in 1947, the government was forced to build a new ship, the *C.D. Howe*, which was commissioned in 1950. The *C.D. Howe* was designed with medical work in mind (Graburn 1969:143). However, before the *Nascopie*'s demise, the patrol managed to x-ray more than 1,500 Aboriginal people in 1946 alone. The years from 1947 until the *C.D. Howe* came into use saw the Royal Canadian Air Force and even the U.S. Army Air Force involved in removing tubercular Inuit to Quebec City or the Charles Camsell Hospital in Edmonton for treatment (Jenness 1972:85).

The medical ships in the eastern Arctic had a relatively short season, leaving Montreal at the end of June and returning in late October because of ice threats. For the rest of the year, medical evacuations were undertaken by the RCAF. In some instances where landings were impossible, medical supplies with instructions, and occasionally even physicians, were parachuted into camps (P.E. Moore 1956:232).

The manner in which the federal government attempted to control and eradicate tuberculosis in the north was controversial, and has left a legacy of bitterness among many Inuit to this day. According to Jenness (1972:88):

Very few tubercular Eskimos at that period left their homes willingly; the great majority went in silence, offering no resistance, and their relatives stood silently by and watched them depart without tears. But there were occasions when the Royal Canadian Mounted Police officer had to use his authority, and a number of families deliberately kept away from any settlement when the hospital ship was due to make its annual call. In the south the evacuee, strictly confined to hospital, unable to speak more than a few words of English, could hardly fail to be lonely and depressed, although both the doctors and the nursing staff lavished on him more than usual sympathy and care. His low morale imperilled his recovery and restitution to his home, while his kinsmen in the north, lacking news of him, despaired of ever seeing him again.

The situation as described by Jenness is only partly compatible with that offered by others. For instance, where Jenness describes how government officials provided reading materials in syllabics and facilitated the exchange of letters with relatives back home, it has also been suggested that these officials were so inefficient in their paperwork that sometimes relatives and even spouses were kept in separate wings of the same hospital without anyone's apparent knowledge. There simply was no formal program to keep families together, or keep them informed, until the mid-1950s, ten years after tuberculosis evacuations had begun (La-Pointe 1986:B4). Government attempts to implement a 'disk list' system, a means of keeping track of Inuit whose Inuktitut names were incomprehensible to them, were largely a failure (D.G. Smith 1993). In some cases, families were not informed of the deaths of members until many years later.

The handling of Inuit patients throughout this period was scandalous. It was not uncommon for individuals to board the medical or patrol ships for x-rays, and then be refused permission to return to shore when the results positively indicated tuberculosis. They were simply taken away (Grygier 1994:96). And once in the southern hospitals, according to a federal official whose job it was to reunite families, 'The Inuit people were treated like cattle ... To the bulk of the federal staff in Ottawa, they were just numbers' (LaPointe 1986:B4). But these numbers kept getting mixed up. Another official with the Department of Northern Affairs and National Resources in the 1950s recalled a young boy of perhaps six, speaking only French, who was dropped off by plane in a small northeastern Quebec Inuit village. He was wearing only shorts, sandals, and a shirt, despite the wintry conditions. Having been in the south so long, he was unable to adjust to living in an igloo and eating traditional foods (ibid. B4). Other patients were not even lucky enough to be returned to their families; in some cases they were dropped off at settlements hundreds of kilometres from home, often with little recollection of their families. Some children never returned to the north at all; they were adopted by southern families, or else perished in the hospitals. Not surprisingly, the Inuit came to regard the arrival of the medical ships and their x-ray equipment with apprehension, leading Schaefer (1959:249) to comment in 1959 that, 'many old Indians and Eskimos are still more afraid of evacuation to the white man's land than of death ...'

The potential that hospital treatment had for culture change among the Inuit was clearly recognized at the time; indeed, this was seen as a positive by-product by government. According to Jenness (1972:89), the 'protracted stay in southern Canada has made it more difficult for many Eskimos to return to the primitive conditions of their earlier life.' Some, Jenness argued, were no longer physically capable of enduring the Arctic rigours, as a result of their poor health, while others 'will resent its hardships and privations ... and ... will prefer to remain in the south and enjoy the flesh-pots of our civilization.' Jenness's views are, by today's standards, ruthless. Jenness (ibid. 89) states,

And why, indeed, should they not remain [in the south]? Why should we force them to return, for the rest of their days, to an environment which very few white men are willing to endure for a single winter – an environment in which not many Eskimos can maintain themselves and their families today without continuous help from our government ... Why then should we subsidize our Eskimos to keep them in barren Arctic regions where without our subsidies many of them would die of starvation? Should those to whom we have carried our deadliest diseases, and then brought south to cure them of those diseases – should they not be allowed, even encouraged, to stay among us if they wish, and helped to earn in the south the livelihood that the underdevelopment of the north, and nature herself, deny them today in their homeland?

The Eurocentric biases inherent in Jenness's observations are painful to read today, and they must be seen in the context of his view that all Aboriginal people were destined to be assimilated sooner or later. Nevertheless, it is quite clear that cultural change was an important by-product of tuberculosis treatment which, combined with the separation of families and kin, served to undermine Inuit society to some extent. Medicine and social change do go hand in hand. Indeed, as early as the 1920s, the director of the Northwest Territories Branch, O.S. Finnie, assumed that 'it was the duty of the federal government to civilize the Eskimos and to safeguard their health and welfare' (ibid. 30). Jenness (ibid.) himself argued in his policy paper on 'Eskimo Administration' that 'Integration with other citizens of the Dominion is the only goal possible for Canada's Eskimos.'

A large number of Inuit were taken south for tuberculosis treatment from the 1940s through the 1960s. At the height of treatment, one-sixth of the 9,500 Inuit were being treated for the disease (LaPointe 1986:B4), with an average hospital stay of twenty-eight months (Grygier 1994:83). Although the tuberculosis epidemic which swept the country through these years required serious measures, there can be little question that the Inuit were not treated on a par with the Euro-Canadian victims of the disease.

Many government administrators and doctors were unable to pronounce and spell Inuit names. The Inuit themselves had a low literacy rate, and some had only one name, while others had European surnames, and still others had common or first names which could change over time. In the 1920s, a suggestion was made by one doctor that a universal system of identifying Inuit would greatly facilitate the keeping of medical records and vital statistics. Apparently, other northern government personnel, such as the police, had also thought that a system was needed, and some recommended fingerprinting. As Derek Smith (1993:50) notes, 'A simple and necessary system of medical patient identification had grown into something different and much more comprehensive, if not also much more insidious.' But fingerprinting was quite logically associated by the Inuit with criminal activity, and they were not anxious to participate. It was an unidentified doctor who suggested in 1935 'that at each registration [of vital statistics by the RCMP] the child be given an identity disk on the same lines as the army idenly [sic] disk and the same insistence that it be worne [sic] at all times.' Thus, the 'Eskimo Disk List' system was born.

There was some government opposition to the disk-list system, in which each Inuk would wear a tag around his or her neck or wrist with a unique identification number. In part, this opposition was due to the fact that neither Indians, who had registration numbers, nor any other 'wards' of other dominions wore them. But proponents of the system saw it as an efficient way not only to record vital statistics and medical records, but also to facilitate overall administration of Inuit, including a general hunting and fishing licensing system. But some Inuit refused to wear their disks, some simply threw them away, and even government administrators were sloppy in their use of the numbers. An administrator at Aklavik was brought to lament: 'In trying to sort out hospital accounts and other matters concerning Eskimo [sic – the usual plural at this time] I am encountering more confusion than should be necessary. There seems to be no clear lines exactly as to who is counted as a native Eskimo and thus a charge on the Department and who is of white status and not. I find children of white men with disc numbers and children of Eskimo without. I find at least two cases where Indians also have Eskimo discs' (D.G. Smith 1993:58). Not surprisingly, it was evident by the 1960s that the disk-list system was not working, and it was abandoned officially in the early 1970s with the adoption of 'Project Surname,' an effort to have all Inuit select surnames and standardize the spelling of names.

By 1943, the Northwest Territories had eleven hospitals in operation, nine owned and operated by missionaries and the other two by mining companies; however, the eastern Arctic was considerably less well served, with only 48 hospital beds for 3,762 people, compared to 213 beds for 8,000 people in the west (Duffy 1988:52–3). By 1946, only nine physicians served in the Northwest Territories. The hospitals at Aklavik, Chesterfield Inlet, and Pangnirtung continued to operate throughout the 1940s, although at least one government official referred to the latter as 'disease traps ... unfit for human habitation' (ibid. 57). The federal government began to shift its medical services in a new direction by establishing nursing stations. The first was opened in 1947 at Port Harrison in the eastern Arctic, and the next at Coppermine in the western Arctic. The advent of the DEW Line radar network improved access to medical facilities for some Inuit, particularly employees of the military bases, although the corporation operating the bases was often in conflict with the federal government regarding precisely who was eligible for medical services (ibid. 60–1).

By the early 1960s, twelve major Inuit settlements had nursing stations, the staff of which could service another fourteen smaller outposts, and dependency on the mission hospitals and the ship patrols began to be phased out. The nurses were in contact with physicians via radio (although radio signals were often unclear due to atmospheric conditions). Medical evacuations by plane became more common, with patients often transported to the southern urban hospitals for more comprehensive treatment (Jenness 1972:86–7). The government continued to expand the nursing stations, and by the mid-1960s there were twenty-five in all, supported by federal hospitals in Inuvik and Frobisher Bay (now Iqaluit) and by the Charles Camsell and Moose Factory hospitals, as well as seven smaller mission hospitals (P.E. Moore 1974:134). The nursing-station model was well on its way to being entrenched as the core of the medical services to be delivered to northern Inuit.

There does not appear to have been any great effort to recruit Inuit nurses for these stations at this time; this was a trend that would come later. But one telling incident occurred at Sugluk, where an Inuk nurse was the first hired when the nursing station opened there in 1960. She was not well accepted by the community, who preferred the services of the missionary who had been treating them for more than a decade, and who was 'White'; despite the nurse's training, it was difficult for community members to accept her as being qualified because she obviously did not look 'White' like the other medical practitioners they had experienced (Graburn 1969:149). The change in attitudes required for self-determination was obviously a few years away yet in this community.

THE DEVELOPMENT OF MEDICAL SERVICES FOR MÉTIS

Government services for the Métis in western Canada developed very slowly and in an ad-hoc fashion. This was no doubt due to the anomalous position of the Métis *vis-à-vis* the Indians: the federal government undertook no official responsibility for the Métis, and it was largely left up to the provinces to render medical aid. The provinces, it seems, were reluctant to do so until the Métis population in the west began to experience widespread ill health and were therefore perceived as a threat to the Euro-Canadian population. This seems to have come to a head in the 1930s in Saskatchewan and Alberta. Because of the inadequacy of the data on the Métis, we will examine only some important aspects of the development of medical services for those in Alberta.

By the end of the nineteenth century, many western Métis could be found living on the margins of both Indian and Euro-Canadian societies. Many lived on lands adjacent to Indian reserves; but despite often strong kinship connections to the reserve, they were denied treaty and other benefits and services because of their legal status. Many others lived along road allowances, squatting on provincial lands on the outskirts of Euro-Canadian communities. Even the northern Métis settlements were impoverished, and diseases such as tuberculosis and syphilis quickly became rampant.

In 1932, the Métis Association of Alberta was founded by Malcolm Norris, Jim Brady, and Joseph Dion. Events leading up to its formation included petitions demanding that the Métis obtain rights for, among other things, land, education, and health care. They lobbied for a commission of inquiry into the state of the Métis in Alberta, and were ultimately successful. A royal commission was established in 1934 to examine 'the problems of health, education and general welfare of the half-breed population of the province' (cited in Pocklington 1991:12).

This commission, which became known as the Ewing Commission after its chair, included a medical doctor, Dr E.A. Braithwaite, who had played an important role in organizing public health services in Alberta. Evidence presented by the Métis Association at the commission hearings argued that the Métis were experiencing extremely high rates of infant mortality, tuberculosis and sexually transmitted diseases (ibid. 14). In the process of gathering its data, the Métis Association had obtained testimonials from six doctors and Indian agents in the Grouard area, where many believed the worst health conditions existed. One doctor reported that 50 per cent of the Métis in this area were afflicted with sexually transmitted diseases, but were destitute and therefore unable to pay for treatment (Dobbin 1981:77). According to Jim Brady, in his testimony at the Ewing hearings, 'At a distance of 300 miles from this very spot there are settlements who I don't think ever saw a doctor in their lives' (cited in ibid. 101).

The reliability of the Métis Association's data was challenged by the government in the person of Dr Harold Orr of the Alberta Department of Health. Earlier, Orr had alerted his minister to the political implications of increased health expenditures on the Métis when he advised against sending a doctor to the Grouard area because 'the cost would be prohibitive unless the Venereal Disease Vote was very greatly increased' (cited in ibid. 101). At the hearings, Orr suggested that the prevalence of tuberculosis and sexually transmitted diseases was only slightly higher among the Métis in comparison to the 'Whites.'

When the Ewing Commission report was issued, it ran to only fifteen pages, and it is unclear which way the commission truly leaned on the questions of disease and treatment for the Métis. Nevertheless, the report did agree that the Métis were experiencing serious health problems and identified a number of possible reasons. They noted that many Métis lived far from doctors and nurses and lacked the money both to cover travel costs to consult them and to pay them. Travelling doctors and nurses, who commonly visited Indian reserves, rarely came to these Métis communities. The report also noted the poor sanitary conditions which characterized Métis homes and the lack of proper food (the report implied that some Métis were, in effect, periodically starving). However, in the end the commissioners wrote, 'On the whole, the Commission is of the opinion that while the health situation is serious, it is not, except as to the particular diseases mentioned [presumably tuberculosis and venereal diseases], more serious than among the white settlers' (cited in Pocklington 1991:16).

Clearly, the Alberta Métis were once again victimized by their anomalous legal status. The Ewing Commission made it clear that any assistance provided to them was to be given out of 'considerations of humanity and justice,' but not because the Métis held any special rights as Aboriginal people (cited in ibid. 17). The Ewing Commission did not want the Métis to become wards of the state, like the Indians. However, the commission did recommend that land be set aside for the Métis, parcels which were referred to then as 'colonies' and today as 'settlements,' where small hospitals could be constructed (these colonies were established under the authority of the *Métis Population Betterment Act* of 1938). The Métis living in these colonies would be periodically provided with the services of a travelling physician, with the anticipation that ultimately a resident physician would be hired. It is not clear to what extent the Métis were to be required to pay for these services.

The report of the Ewing Commission was tendered in February of 1936. Subsequently, some efforts were made to deal with the health status of the Métis, especially to provide treatment for tuberculosis. While the systematic treatment of tuberculosis among Indians on reserves had begun in southern Alberta in 1935, the Métis did not receive similar attention until later, primarily in the 1940s, and with the establishment of the 'colonies.' Card and colleagues (1963:25–6) present data that show that, between 1934 and 1939, Métis constituted only 6.9 per cent of the patients discharged from treatment facilities, but this figure began to rise thereafter, until by 1960–1 the Métis constituted 23 per cent of the patients, a disproportionately high number relative to their overall population in the province. Most Métis patients tended to be treated at the Aberhart Memorial Sanatorium, constructed in 1952 to service the northern half of the province. According to Card and colleagues (ibid. 27), the number of 'walk-outs,' or patients leaving hospital prior to the completion of their treatment, began to increase in the 1950s, as Métis patients became more numerous (the implication that these walk-outs were Métis is clear, if not stated directly). This led to a provincial law in 1958 designed to enforce the confinement of 'recalcitrant infectious tuberculosis sufferers.'

The prevalence of disease remained high among the Métis for many years, despite these health programs. Again unlike the Indians, who received regular programs of diagnosis and treatment, the Métis were subjected to only 'irregular' screening. The 1963 report by Card and colleagues, *The Métis in Alberta Society*, provides an interesting snapshot of the perceptions of the Métis at the time. Subtitled 'with special reference to social, economic, and cultural factors associated with persistently high tuberculosis incidence,' the report documented that the Métis tuberculosis rate was, by the early 1960s, about half that of the treaty Indians. These authors appeared to be moving away from simple biological explanations of disease prevalence (that is, that the Métis have high tuberculosis rates because of the ancestral Indian heritage, and therefore a genetic susceptibility). They argued that, 'the major determinants of Métis status, and hence contributing factors to tuberculosis incidence, are economic poverty and what, by all criteria, amounts to a lower-class way of life, not an aboriginal way of life' (ibid. 398). The Métis, they suggested, occupied a class position within the context of the larger Euro-Canadian class structure, and this position was inherently one of poverty. This apparently radical (for the time) observation was tempered, however, by the remnants of attitudes from an earlier era which still influenced the authors, for they suggest that the solution to the disease problem lies in 'extending civilization northward and increasing Métis participation in it,' hence promoting Métis 'individual and group upward mobility' (ibid. 398).

CONCLUSIONS

It is clear from this chapter that there was no grand strategy for the development of government services for Aboriginal peoples. Such development occurred on an ad-hoc basis depending on the region, the legal status of the Aboriginal group in question, and even the personalities of the various caregivers and administrators who, in one way or another, were charged with the responsibility for Aboriginal health. As we shall see in the next chapter, the development of medical services in the contemporary era has not been without its problems either.

8

The organization and utilization of contemporary health services

The previous chapter discussed the constitutional and legislative basis for Aboriginal health services and traced the involvement of the federal government since Confederation. This chapter describes and analyses the way the contemporary health care system 'works' – how services are organized and delivered, how much they cost, and how they are used. Attention is paid to the bureaucratic machinery and health professionals within the system on the one hand, and the users of services – Aboriginal peoples themselves – on the other. The broader political aspects of health care delivery, particularly how health care as an agent of Aboriginal self-determination is regarded and applied, form the subject of chapter 10.

OPERATING THE MEDICAL SERVICES BRANCH

The major government agency in Canada responsible for health services to the majority of registered Indians is the Medical Services Branch (MSB) of the Department of National Health and Welfare. Until the late 1980s, when health services in the Northwest Territories were devolved from the federal to the territorial government, it was also the agency responsible for the Inuit, Dene and other residents in the Northwest Territories. Originally organized in 1962 as a directorate composed of seven independent services which had come into existence with the department in 1944, MSB retains these divisions as identifiable spheres of activity within it. Over the years, new activities have been added, such as Prosthetic Services and Emergency Services, and others, such as Sick Mariners, have been dropped. Like many other federal government agencies, MSB has been afflicted by a penchant for periodic administrative reorganizations – each time associated with an inflation in job classification and titles of the key management staff! This chapter is not intended to be an administrative history of MSB; rather, it describes in some detail the system as it has evolved up to the early 1990s.

It is important to understand the role of the federal health department in Canada, where constitutionally health care is the primary responsibility of the provinces. A federal health department has existed since 1919. In 1928 it became the Department of Pensions and National Health, taking on responsibility for the welfare of First World War veterans. This latter function was given over to the new Department of Veterans Affairs when the present Department of National Health and Welfare (DNHW) came into being in 1944, under the *Department of National Health and Welfare Act*. Health care is no different from many other aspects of Canadian politics, where there have been frequent federal-provincial squabbles about overlapping responsibilities and charges of intrusions into each other's jurisdictions. Some provincial politicians have regarded the existence of a federal health department as unnecessary, by analogy with education, also a provincial responsibility. The federal role in health care has primarily been regulatory, particularly in the areas of safety in foods and drugs, protection from health hazards, and disease control and surveillance. With the introduction of universal hospital, and later medical care insurance, DNHW became responsible for administering transfer payments to the provinces for such programs. The department also sets broad national standards in a variety of public health fields and funds public health research. There remains a mixed group of clients, to whom some direct health services are provided, who are the main responsibility of MSB. Among these special client groups, registered Indians across Canada as well as all residents in the two northern territories (including non-Aboriginal Canadians) receive the complete range of preventive and curative health services. The other groups, such as federal public servants, immigrants, refugees, international travellers, and civil aviation personnel, are provided with only a limited range of services, consisting mostly of health advice, screening examinations, and emergency assistance.

Since its inception, MSB has been administered in a regionalized structure, with regions and zones. Over the years the boundaries have also changed. Initially, the Northwest Territories was divided into zones which were administered along a north-south axis – thus the Keewatin Zone in the central Northwest Territories was part of Central Region, which encompassed also Manitoba and northwestern Ontario. Later, there was one Northern Region, which included both the Northwest Territories and Yukon. The Northern Region eventually split into two regions. By the late 1980s, all MSB regions corresponded to a province or territory, with the exception of the multi-province Atlantic Region. The assistant deputy minister for MSB has overall responsibility for all of the branch's programs. While there are various intervening layers at one time or another, the line authority runs through the regional directors and zone directors. There are also various 'staff' at all levels, primarily health professionals who act in an advisory/consultant capacity to the line managers. While there is a 'director general of Indian and Inuit health services' at MSB headquarters in Ottawa, the incumbent in fact heads only a small professional consultant group. In the branch's financial reporting, expenditures are attributed to various 'activities', one of which is 'Indian and Northern Health Services.' Nevertheless, in operational and organizational terms, there is no such thing as an 'Indian Health Service' in Canada akin to that in the United States.[1]

Until the 1970s, there were usually a base hospital and such peripheral units as health centres, nursing stations, and clinics within each zone. The typical system in more remote zones has been described, for example the Keewatin Zone in the Northwest Territories (L. Black 1969) and the Sioux Lookout Zone in northwestern Ontario (T.K. Young 1981). A 1970 paper in the *Canadian Journal of Public Health* by the then director general of MSB listed a variety of operational problems faced by MSB staff in the north (Wiebe 1970). The sheer geographical expanse of each zone posed immense difficulties with regard to supply and logistics, affecting the cost and timeliness of the construction of facilities, the transportation of patients and staff, and communication with other agencies. On the human scale, there were problems with the insufficient quantity and the poor quality of the staff employed. The conditions of employment, including remuneration, fringe benefits, and general ambience, often made MSB uncompetitive with other health agencies. Furthermore, employees had to recognize and be prepared for the cultural differences and need for mutual understanding between non-Aboriginal staff and Aboriginal clients. Adding to these problems were the legion of 'do-gooders' who volunteered their services to MSB, but often with conditions attached, and assorted short-term researchers and adventurers, whose uncoordinated visits and demands were more trouble than they were worth (ibid.).

Such operational problems still exist today. The decline in the number of MSB hospitals across the country since the 1970s, and the reduced role of those that do remain, has led to the shifting of administrative control from zone headquarters based in such hospitals, usually located on an Indian reserve or close to one, to purely administrative offices located in larger towns. An example is the move of zone headquarters from the Norway House reserve, Manitoba, to the mining town of Thompson in the mid-1970s. By the 1980s, MSB zones with hospitals attached were the exception rather than the rule.

The performance of MSB has been evaluated periodically by the auditor general (AG) of Canada. Some of the auditors' findings relating to specific expenditures are discussed in the next section. In recent years, federal auditing has gone beyond simply checking ledgers and uncovering 'waste' to determining 'value for money' and the internal working of government departments. In 1987, the AG pointed out that 'existing planning, evaluation and management information systems are so deficient that the Department cannot be sure that it is providing an adequate level of health care ... with due regard to economy, efficiency and effectiveness' (Canada, Auditor General 1987: Section 12.43). Where data were collected, they were often not analysed or used. Much of what MSB did was not, or could not be, evaluated. The AG mentioned that an evaluation of the National Native Alcohol and Drug Abuse Program (NNADAP) had gone on for ten years and finally was abandoned due to lack of data. On the positive side, the AG commended the more than 3,000 community health representatives, health liaison workers, and lay dispensers for serving their population well (ibid., Section 12.48–12.50).

In the late 1980s MSB operated some 500 health facilities, including eight hospitals, across the country. The AG reported that four of the hospitals were in an advanced state of deterioration and seven of the eight had such low occupancy rates that they were half empty most of the time (ibid., Section 12.79). While MSB has been keen on 'getting out of the hospital business' since the early 1970s, and has successfully extricated itself in places such as North Battleford, Saskatchewan, many small hospitals are difficult to close due to community pressures, mostly arising from fears that the federal commitment to Aboriginal health care will be eroded and concerns about economic consequences and reduced access to facilities where Aboriginal patients are in the majority. In the case of Sioux Lookout, Ontario, where a small town of 3,000 residents (though serving a catchment population of an additional 15,000) has had two hospitals, one federal and one provincial/municipal, a merger has long been debated. However, little action was taken until the early 1990s, when a quadripartite (Aboriginal, federal, provincial, and municipal) negotiation process was initiated. In the Northwest Territories, MSB contributed substantially to the construction of the new hospital in Yellowknife in the mid-1980s. The successful transfer of the Frobisher Bay (now Iqaluit) hospital to the territorial government heralded the later complete transfer of all MSB activities. This model is to be followed in Yukon, beginning with the transfer of the Whitehorse hospital in the early 1990s.

While the hospital sector shrank, there was a burst of new construction of nursing stations and health centres during the 1980s. The Booz-Allen consultant's report in 1969 recommended a target figure of one nursing station for each community with a population of 400, a target that by the end of the 1980s had more or less been achieved. The auditor general, however, questioned whether this target was still appropriate in view of environmental and technological changes. At any rate, the construction boom revealed some anomalies in the planning process. One station in northwestern Ontario, intended for a population of 390 with fewer than ten patient visits a day, was the exact replica of one built for a community of 950 with three times as many visits, and would be destined to be underused for years to come. Such overcapacity was by no means an isolated incident (Canada, Auditor General 1987: Section 12.85).

FINANCING ABORIGINAL HEALTH SERVICES

It may come as a surprise to many that, to date, no one has determined the actual cost of health services to all the Aboriginal peoples in Canada. Even in the case of registered Indians and Inuit, where the federal government has been the main source of services, accurate attribution of costs has proven difficult. A true, comprehensive picture must also include costs related to services provided by provincial and territorial governments and out-of-pocket costs incurred by patients themselves. The provincial governments, for example, have shared cost arrangements with the federal government for patient care in MSB-operated hospitals in their territory. On the other hand, the federal government also tries to recover from the provincial governments the costs of services provided to non-status Indians and non-Aboriginal residents who live in communities where MSB operates the only health facility, usually a nursing station. Even more elusive are indirect costs and how far one should go in determining what should or should not be defined as health care. Devotees of a broad and all-inclusive definition of health may consider the entire field of human activity to be health-related, up to and including the pursuit of happiness! Furthermore, costing is not simply an accounting procedure, but is influenced by political and social considerations. Critics of a bloated bureaucracy may not consider administrative costs as benefiting the health of those served.

A detailed economic analysis is beyond the scope of this chapter. One can only look at how much MSB spends on Aboriginal health services within the context of overall federal government expenditures. According to the *Public Accounts of Canada* for 1991–2 (which reports on how much was actually spent, rather than what the government intended to spend), the overall DNHW departmental expenditures amounted to some $36 billion. However, more than 95 per cent of these were so-called statutory expenditures (health insurance, family allowance, old age security, pension, and other forms of social assistance and welfare), to which all Canadians are entitled. It is these expenditures that make DNHW a giant among federal departments. MSB's budget of just under $700 million thus represented a minuscule proportion (less than 2 per cent) within the department. (It should be mentioned that, in 1993, the 'Welfare' arm of DNHW was separated from the 'Health' arm. DNHW is now simply 'Health Canada'). Within MSB, activities and programs relating to Indian and Northern Health Services (INHS) accounted for 90 per cent of expenditures. Table 1 shows the rise in expenditures of INHS, within the context of total MSB, total 'Health,' and total DNHW expenditures. Figure 13 shows the trend in the three categories of expenditures attributed to INHS: operating, capital, and transfer payments. It can be seen that capital expenditures (such as construction and renovation of facilities) have declined in the early 1990s from a peak in the mid-1980s, whereas transfer payments and operating expenditures have increased 5 times and 2.5 times respectively. Note that all expenditures are expressed in 'current' rather than 'constant' dollars; in other words, they represent dollars at face value in the year they were spent and are not adjusted for inflation.

The increasing importance of transfer payments in the operation of MSB's programs reflects the shift from direct provision of services to Aboriginal clients to indirect provision, through contributions to the two territorial governments and to Aboriginal governments (such as Band Councils and regional Treaty/Tribal Councils) to provide a variety of health services, which may range from total control of all health services to specific components such as community health representatives, transportation, and support services. Also included under the 'transfer' rubric is the National Native Alcohol and Drug Abuse Program (NNADAP), the Indian and Inuit Health Careers Program (comprising individual bursaries as well as subsidies to universities and colleges), and consultations with Aboriginal associations.

The $654 million spent on Indian and Northern Health Services, instead of being divided into operating, capital, and transfer categories, can al-

TABLE 2
Federal health expenditures, 1984/85–1991/92

	1985/86	1986/87	1987/88	1988/89	1989/90	1900/91	1991/92
Department of National Health and Welfare	25,199	27,612	28,799	30,120	31,640	33,349	35,611
Total 'Health' (excluding 'Welfare')	7,072	7,393	7,324	7,506	7,586	7,139	7,847
Medical Services Branch	398	463	494	495	550	647	697
Indian/Northern Health Services	357	411	449	436	497	601	654

Note: Expenditures in current dollars to nearest million

SOURCE: *Public Accounts of Canada*, relevant years

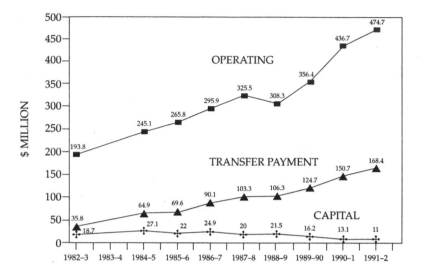

Figure 13
Expenditures on Indian and Northern Health Services, MSB, DNHW, 1982/83–1991/92

Note: Expenditures in current dollars

SOURCE: *Public Accounts of Canada*, relevant years

ternatively be broken down into various subactivities, as shown in Table 3. The lion's share is devoted to expenses under the rubric 'community health.' While the category includes the cost of operation of nursing stations (and thus partly 'illness care') and most public health programs, it also covers many items which are 'community' only in the sense that they are for members of Aboriginal communities. A prime example is so-called non-insured health benefits (NIHBs), which refer to health insurance premiums, patient transportation, prescription drugs, dental care, eyeglasses, and various prosthetic devices and medical appliances.

Of increasing importance in MSB's expenditures, NIHBs generally fall outside coverage by provincial health insurance plans, and for non-Aboriginal Canadians these have to be paid for either out of their own pockets or by third-party insurers. Prior to 1978, MSB provided such benefits to status Indians on reserves and to Inuit on the basis of need. An attempt to tighten fiscal control in 1978, following the release of a *Policy Directive for the Provision of Uninsured Medical and Dental Benefits*, led to widespread protest from Aboriginal groups. The dispute was su-

TABLE 3
Distribution of expenditures on Indian and Northern Health Services, 1991–2 (million $)

Community health	480.7
Management and services	52.7
National Native Alcohol and Drug Abuse Program	52.6
Hospital services	42.5
Services under Indian control	23.5
Environmental health and surveillance	2.5
Total	654.4

SOURCE: Canada, DNHW. *1993–94 Estimates, Part III: Expenditure Plan*

perseded, first by a change in government as a result of the general election, and later by the announcement of the Indian Health Policy in 1979. The policy was widely interpreted in practice to mean the extension of NIHBs to status Indians and Inuit, as an entitlement regardless of ability to pay and often also regardless of place of residence (Canada, Auditor General 1982).

The total cost of NIHBs escalated from $36 million in 1979–80 to $80 million in 1982–3 (ibid. 1982), and $166 million in 1986–7, accounting for 40 per cent of all spending on Indian and Northern Health Services (ibid. 1987). By 1992–3, this sum had grown to $442 million. When adjusted for inflation, and allowing for the growth of eligible population both naturally and as a result of Bill C-31 (which reinstated the status of many Indians, particularly women), the per-capita increase averaged 7 per cent annually in constant dollars (ibid. 1993). The distribution of the 1992–3 NIHB expenditures by benefit type is shown in Figure 14.

When the Indian Health Policy was approved in 1979, the federal cabinet imposed a spending ceiling beyond which MSB had to seek supplemental appropriations. Such annual requests became a regular feature and increased year after year. In fact, non-insured benefits have almost become an open-ended expenditure and a bureaucrat's nightmare – they are deemed uncontrollable because they are authorized by health professionals in the private sector and can be directly accessed by the clients. This fact did not escape the notice of the auditor general. The auditor general's report for 1982 indicated that high staff turnover, the absence of nationally established standards, and the lack of procedural and administrative guidance from branch headquarters to regions and zones

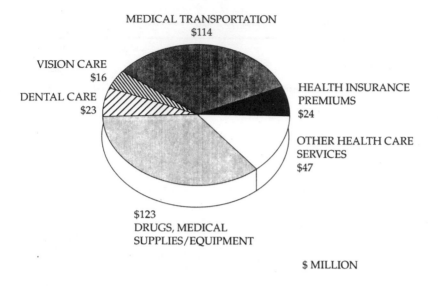

Figure 14
Non-insured health benefits by type, MSB, DNHW, 1992–3

SOURCE: *Report of the Auditor General of Canada*, 1993.

resulted in inconsistent availability of such services across the country. Non-insured benefits also proved a bonanza to health professionals providing services to Aboriginal people. The auditor general's office reported cases of excessive charges which were duly paid by MSB, often without assurance that the services had even been rendered (ibid. 1982:372). Several biennial audits later, in 1993, the report still found MSB 'administering the program without agreement on its exact nature, without complete information on its costs, and without an effective management control framework.' While MSB established national program directives in 1989, the auditors found that had these guidelines been followed, the total 1992–3 NIHB expenditures would have been reduced by 20 per cent. (ibid. 1993:500).

From the Aboriginal perspective, there is solid reason on constitutional and political grounds that NIHBs should be an integral part of the federal government's responsibilities towards Aboriginal peoples. Yet, for NIHBs – which have at best only a marginal impact on the health status of Aboriginal peoples – to constitute such a substantial proportion of total health expenditures on Indian and Northern Health Services, in a climate of fiscal restraint, can only skew and distort overall health priorities. The vast amounts paid to diverse private dentists, optometrists, pharmacists, and taxi companies can surely be better spent on the development of preventive dental programs, vision screening, a formulary of essential and efficacious drugs, and a triage/referral/evacuation policy.

HEALTH PROFESSIONALS IN THE SYSTEM

MSB employs a multidisciplinary corps of health professionals. In the late 1980s, some 2,500 'person-years'[2] can be attributed to Indian and Northern Health Services. The largest of the occupational groups, in terms of both sheer numbers and geographical distribution, is nurses. There are hospital-based and community health nurses – the HOS and the CHNs in the parlance of the public service. Few in and out of MSB would dispute the fact that nurses constitute the backbone of MSB's service-delivery programs. With justification, they are the unsung heroes, often stressed and not very often appreciated. Particularly in the northern zones, the conditions of work are such that in times of high demand Canadian graduates often shun MSB's enticements. Overseas recruitment drives, many of them in Britain, became a regular necessity during the 1980s.

Nurses have been the subject of many inquiries over the years. In the 1970s an Interdepartmental Committee on the Nursing Group (1974), composed of representatives of all federal departments that hired nurses (Veterans Affairs, National Defence, the Penitentiary Service, and National Health and Welfare), perceived a high degree of dissatisfaction over issues of salary, effective utilization, career progression, professional development, management relations, quality of supervision, and the work environment. While none of these are unique to working in Aboriginal communities, the cross-cultural setting and the geographical isolation seem to accentuate these difficulties.

Canitz (1989a, 1989b) examined the factors associated with the high stress and high turnover of MSB nurses, particularly in the isolated North. Life in the nursing-station setting, where the boundary between the personal and the professional is blurred, demands substantial lifestyle adjustments. The expanded occupational responsibilities but decreased professional support, the inadequate preparation and orientation prior to employment, and the lack of direction and support during postings all contribute to dissatisfaction and burnout. A nurse working in Aboriginal communities as an MSB employee is faced with additional challenges. Cultural awareness and tolerance cannot be taught in short order. Gender and age issues are often magnified, when predominantly young, female nurses are perceived to be in positions of authority. Issues of power and control *vis-à-vis* the government bureaucracy, medical dominance, and community pressures all come to the fore in the exercise of the nurses' professional duties. The actual voices of nurses retelling how these issues affect their daily lives are captured in *GOSSIP: A Spoken History of Women in the North* (Canitz 1989b).

Canitz (1989a:178) provides a vivid description of the enormous scope of the northern nurse's daily activities:

Providing medical care, they deal with colds, pregnancy, chest pain, marital problems, depression, employee physicals, and more. They are public health nurses providing pre- and post-natal clinics, immunizations, and home visits to the elderly. They are the resident dentist applying temporary fillings or pulling teeth that can't wait for the next dental visit. At night, they mysteriously turn into an entire emergency room rolled into one person. They are alone to suture, bandage, resuscitate, and console. Northern nurses are x-ray technicians and radiologists through the lens of the primitive x-ray machines they have to use. They are laboratory technicians and pathologists as they draw blood, collect urine, and utilize swabs as a means of pinpointing and identifying the etiology of a disease. They are public health inspectors responsible for the hygiene of all public services.

The idea of nurses working in isolation, diagnosing and treating diseases – activities thought to be the preserve of physicians – often frightened physicians, administrators, and not a few nurses themselves. Yet, a Committee on Clinical Training of Nurses in 1970 suggested that 50 per cent of cases seen in a nursing station were totally manageable by a nurse without additional training, and less than 1 per cent were completely beyond the scope of a nurse even with additional training and available consultation. The rest could be done with training and consultation. While improved skills in physical assessment and case management would better prepare nurses for work in isolated settings, this would be perceived as encroaching upon the realm of practice claimed by physicians. No Canadian medical or nursing licensing bodies have tackled such legal issues head-on. Such grey areas in the remote margins of the country appeared to them to be best left undisturbed. Provincial nursing licensing bodies tend to recognize only what are traditionally considered 'nursing' duties. The issue of liability is further complicated by the transfer of control of some nursing stations to Band and Tribal Councils, which often cannot afford to offer the same amount of insurance coverage formerly provided by MSB. Despite experimental projects in the 1970s, the concept of the nurse-practitioner never did take root in southern Canada. In this respect, MSB can take some credit for having the longest tradition of employing nurses in an expanded role in large swathes of the Canadian hinterland.

In the 1980s, nursing leaders in MSB embraced the rhetoric of health promotion (as did much of the public health profession). Emphasis on clinical training for nurses gave way to talk of the nurses' changing role from one of service provider to 'facilitator, supporter, and resource worker,' and to a shift from treatment to health promotion (Doucette 1989). However, in the communities, nurses continue to be overloaded with acute health problems requiring immediate attention, and the shift from a curative to a preventive orientation remains very much an unrealized goal.

While their number has greatly dwindled, physicians – referred to as medical officers or MOFs – once exercised great authority within MSB. Until the late 1970s, most senior line manager positions, from deputy minister, assistant deputy minister, director general, regional director, down to zone director, were occupied by MOFs. In some zones, the zone director dashed from the operating room to the office, and alternated ward rounds with bursts of bureaucratic chores. As health care became increasingly complex, a managerial revolution swept through all echelons of government. MOFs were considered amateur administrators, and increasingly they were replaced by full-time administrators, many of whom had risen through the clerical ranks. From health practitioners with little or no administrative training, the system was soon taken over by administrators with little or no health background. At senior management meetings, when 'TB' was mentioned, it more likely referred to 'Treasury Board' than 'tuberculosis'!

Physicians who work on salary in the government have traditionally been held in low regard by the rest of the medical profession. The loss of power within the MSB organization would further deter prospective fresh recruits from entering the service. In the early 1980s, the remaining senior MOFs in MSB perceived a crisis with regard to the number, quality, and role of MOFs. A Task Force on Medical Officers was convened in 1983 to make recommendations to reverse the fortunes of the MOFs within MSB. Of great concern to the task force was that its own survey found that at the zone and region level, fewer than 50 per cent of MOFs had postgraduate qualifications in public health. In the early 1960s, MSB MOFs were entitled to one year of postgraduate training for every three years of service, which most took advantage of to obtain clinical upgrading, or spend a year at the University of Toronto's School of Hygiene and acquire the Diploma in Public Health. The trend towards contracting out clinical services to private practitioners and university medical schools meant that the remaining MOFs were expected to function as public health experts, a task many were not able to fulfil. On the management front, the task force recommended the dual track system, whereby key line positions such as regional and zone directors could be staffed by either MOFs or non-MOFs. Little came of the task force. The position of MOFs within MSB continued to be eroded. By the end of the 1980s, few management positions were held by MOFs (with the assistant deputy minister and almost all regional and zone directors being non-MOFs). The 1980s witnessed the burgeoning of the rejuvenated medical specialty of 'Community Medicine.' Compared to provincial and municipal health departments, MSB has not been successful in tapping into this pool of physicians more sympathetic to, and better skilled in, health care management, planning, and evaluation. Within MSB, MOFs constitute a demoralized and disgruntled group, with few real responsibilities, few staff to supervise, and little expertise to offer when consulted.

THE INVOLVEMENT OF ACADEMIC AND PROFESSIONAL ORGANIZATIONS

The crisis in physician recruitment towards the end of the 1960s led to MSB's seeking assistance from medical schools, teaching hospitals, and professional associations. In 1968, the Sioux Lookout Zone had only one surgeon-cum-zone director and a field medical officer serving some twenty-five communities. Similarly the Moose Factory Zone, also in northern Ontario, had one physician serving the James Bay coastal communities. Other zones in the country were not much better off. The poor quality of the clinical staff and their generally short duration of stay throughout most of the 1950s and 1960s was a common complaint of the employer. T.K. Young (1988:104) cited numerous references to the physician problem in the Sioux Lookout Zone from the zone director's annual reports of the period. Such annual reports, often candid to the point of being cruel, were written in the days before their genre became a glossy, public relations affair. One such report from 1962 stated: 'The hospital is anything but satisfactory ... we have not had a single fully competent doctor ... The Civil Service Commission does not seem to check with these doctors' previous places of employment but take all they claim at face value. Medical standards fell ... with the appointment of [Dr X] who had not given satisfactory service at [another Indian Hospital]; and [Dr Y] who had ... been asked to leave from his two previous places of employment. [They] require constant supervision and are indeed not much help in the running of the hospital ...' (cited in ibid. 1988:104).

The medical schools came to the rescue and relieved MSB of the headaches of physician recruitment and retention. This new arrangement is a symbiotic one. The prestige of affiliation with a medical school, generous salaries, benefits, and continuing-education leave, housing subsidies, and the availability of clinical back-up by specialist consultants are seen to be attractions to potential recruits, who generally tend to be young, recent graduates. The universities benefit by gaining access to new community sites where teaching and research can take place in conjunction with the delivery of services. The idea that universities are developing a social conscience and stepping out of the ivory tower to help the impoverished and underserved is also one that universities are keen to foster.

Physician services in various northern zones were contracted out by MSB to the universities: Queen's in Moose Factory Zone, McGill in Baffin Zone, and the University of Toronto in the Sioux Lookout Zone. All these programs are still in existence. The largest of these in terms of staff size, geographical coverage, and budget is the University of Manitoba's Northern Medical Unit, now named the J.A. Hildes Northern Medical Unit in honour of its founder. In 1970 it was requested to assist the hospital in Churchill, and over the years it has expanded into the Keewatin Zone in the Northwest Territories and other northern Manitoba communities. In the 1990s, the relationship is no longer solely with MSB, but also with the provincial and territorial governments, and involves other funding sources.

Most university programs never got beyond the limited role of recruiting general practitioners and rotating medical interns, residents, and consultants. In many ways this is because MSB has insisted that the medical schools remain in a strictly clinical role and has resisted handing over any public health functions. While relationships have mostly been amicable, MSB does perceive some loss of control over a key part of its activities. Reporting relationships between medical staff hired by universities and MSB's own hierarchy are not always clear. Physicians working in the communities also come into conflict with MSB nurses over issues of clinical supervision and decisions about patient care.

A somewhat different type of arrangement for professional support from universities and teaching hospitals is that between the Montreal

General Hospital (MGH) and the Cree Board of Health and Social Services of James Bay (CBHSSJB). Under the regionalized public health system in existence in Quebec until 1994, Départements de Santé Communautaire (DSC), each affiliated with a hospital, were responsible for such functions as disease control and surveillance, and program evaluation. The Cree board was established under the *James Bay and Northern Quebec* Agreement and is responsible for health services to eastern James Bay communities. In 1978 the Cree board requested the Quebec health ministry to designate the Montreal General Hospital, an anglophone institution and McGill teaching hospital, as its DSC. The DSC was also asked to take on responsibilities in recruiting and training staff, arranging specialist visits, and providing patient services (such as transportation, boarding, and interpreters) in Montreal. The MGH-CBHSSJB arrangement thus differs from most other university northern programs in that it has a strong public health orientation and the contractual relationship is with an Aboriginal government directly.

An important consequence of the involvement of universities in service delivery is the establishment of special programs to promote the entry of Aboriginal students into health professional faculties. The University of Manitoba has taken the lead in initiating a Special Premedical Studies Program in 1979 to prepare students for admission into medicine, dentistry, pharmacy, and medical rehabilitation. This program has since been extended to include also a Professional Health Program, as the original students gained entry into, progressed through, and graduated from these faculties (Stephens 1991). While the output is still small – five physicians and two dentists over a ten-year period – a new cadre of Aboriginal role models has been created. Other universities, among them the universities of Toronto and Alberta, have since established similar programs.

In addition to universities, a few professional associations have also taken a keen and sustained interest in the health of Aboriginal peoples, notably the Canadian Pediatric Society (CPS), which in the late 1960s set up an Indian and Eskimo Child Health Committee. In 1970 it produced a discussion paper (labelled 'White Paper') and submitted it to the federal government. It was quite advanced for its day. The recommendations included promoting Aboriginal participation; ensuring a continuing federal responsibility; training nurse-practitioners; involving medical schools in staffing; and specific suggestions regarding family planning, dental caries prevention, injury prevention, tuberculosis control, and nutrition. The last mentioned went beyond dietary education and nutrient supplementation, but included also the protection of hunting rights and the reduction of food costs (Canadian Pediatric Society 1970). The CPS continues to maintain active liaison with MSB and, more recently, has engaged in direct consultations with Aboriginal representatives. The CPS has sponsored conferences on Aboriginal child health, and many of its members have been prominent in university northern programs such as those at Sioux Lookout, Moose Factory, and Keewatin. It functions as an expert advisory group on clinical matters (as well as on health policy issues, although these are less likely to be listened to).

A more short-lived program organized by the Canadian Association of Medical Students and Interns and the Association of Canadian Medical Colleges was the Summer School of Frontier Medicine, usually held in a developing country. In 1967 it was held in Inuvik, where students and faculty spent ten days attending lectures and seminars, seven days doing fieldwork in nursing stations, and finally three days doing summation and evaluation in Edmonton (A. Bryans 1969). Over the years, individual medical schools also offered short elective periods which enabled undergraduate and postgraduate students to work in Aboriginal communities. An early example is Queen's University's program on the Tyendinaga Mohawk reserve (Read and Strick 1969). Many students, thus exposed, later returned for full-time practice as general practitioners, and a few even devoted a considerable portion of their later professional careers to the field of northern and Aboriginal health care.

Canadian faculties of dentistry, notably those at Toronto and Manitoba, also became actively involved in providing services to Aboriginal communities through university MSB contracts. The University of Toronto's dental involvement in the Sioux Lookout Zone dates back to 1970 (K.C. Titley 1973). An evaluation of changes in dental health status after ten years of service in one zone community (as measured by the decayed-missing-filled index) showed little change. While dental manpower woes have largely been overcome, the program's coordinator was honest in admitting that 'until solidly based preventive programs incorporating fluorides, fissure sealants and education become a major component part of the service, the dentist's role in controlling dental disease will be mainly palliative' (K.C. Titley and Bedard 1986).

A unique contribution to dental manpower development – beyond merely supplying southern, non-Aboriginal dentists – is MSB's School of Dental Therapy. The first (and so far only) one of its kind in North America, the school was started in 1972 in Fort Smith, Northwest Territories, but moved to Prince Albert, Saskatchewan, in 1982. Its founding director was seconded from the University of Toronto Faculty of Dentistry to MSB (Davey 1974). Dental therapists can be considered dental auxiliaries with an expanded role in both prevention and treatment. The school's curriculum and training methods have been emulated overseas in such developing countries as Mozambique. Indeed, several African and Caribbean countries began sending students to the school, and these now account for as much as one-third of the student body (Torbert 1990). In Canada, however, attempts to expand into the provinces in the 1980s have been thwarted by provincial dental associations over the issue of licensing and the threat of competition posed by a low-cost, but effective, alternative.

The need for on-site psychiatric consultations to reduce institutionalization at distant mental hospitals has long been recognized. A multi-university team of psychiatrists, for example, assessed mental health needs in the Northwest Territories on behalf of MSB in the late 1960s (Atcheson et al. 1969), and most university northern programs introduced a psychiatry component in the early 1970s: Toronto in Sioux Lookout (Levine et al. 1974), Manitoba in Keewatin, Western Ontario in Moose Factory (Pelz et al. 1981), and the Clarke Institute of Psychiatry, affiliated also with the University of Toronto, in the Baffin Zone (Hood et al. 1993). These programs send psychiatrists and trainees to provide individual therapy to patients referred by local nurses, physicians, and CHRs, conduct interagency conferences and community meetings, and provide continuing education for local staff. The Sioux Lookout program won a merit award in community psychiatry from the American Psychiatric Association in 1978. In the early 1980s, it was one of the first programs to begin the training of Aboriginal counsellors (Timpson 1984). The Canadian Psychiatric Association also established a Native Mental Health section which in 1989 formed its own association, the Native Mental Health Association of Canada.

UTILIZATION OF HEALTH SERVICES BY ABORIGINAL PEOPLES

There is a widespread perception among health professionals and administrators that Aboriginal people use health care services differently from non-Aboriginal people in Canada. Many factors are believed to play a role in accounting for such differences. The health planning literature conceives of *use* as dependent on *supply* (the availability of services), *need* (the burden of ill health), which is expressed as *demand* by those willing to seek or pay for health services to satisfy the need. Thus, the type of services that are made available (or not available) to Aboriginal people, particularly those living in remote areas, would affect utilization. The higher (or lower) prevalence of many health conditions would also affect utilization related to the relief of those conditions. Cultural and socio-economic barriers, even in situations where the need is great, may result in reduced demand and reduced use. On the other hand, the same cultural and socio-economic factors can result in the opposite – apparent over-use.

Many commentators on Aboriginal health have simplistically regarded health service utilization as merely an issue of 'cultural differences' (usually expressed in stereotypes, as in 'Indian time'). Waldram (1990c) referred to a body of 'medical folklore' held by health care practitioners that Aboriginal people underuse or even avoid medical care. On the other hand, there is an equally strongly held belief that Aboriginal people overuse or abuse the health care system – for example, by pestering nurses in off-hours for minor illnesses.

The stereotypes about Aboriginal health care utilization are pervasive. For instance, the 1969 Booz-Allen report, a major review of Indian health services conducted by an international health service consultancy firm for MSB, stated that: 'Many Indians have little understanding of the meaning of good health because of cultural differences and education deficiencies. Indians exhibit little awareness of what is meant by good health and because of this lack of awareness there is a tendency to both over and under-utilize health services ... Indians frequently fail to recognize significant symptoms and delay seeking treatment until they are acutely ill' (Booz-Allen 1969:13). This statement is perhaps typical of the ill-informed, stereotypical, ethnocentric, and simplistic view of Aboriginal health behaviour held by many observers and analysts of Aboriginal health care. There are, of course, few data, either qualitative or quantitative, to support such an assertion; yet such perceptions persist, largely because many researchers have failed to explore the question of Aboriginal perceptions of health, illness, and health care delivery.

Before we discuss what factors are important in determining Aboriginal people's use of health services, we need to establish that differential utilization exists. While there are locally specific case studies, as in Waldram's study of Saskatoon inner-city residents (1990c) – to be discussed in greater detail later – one can look at a variety of data sources at the national and regional level: hospital admissions, visits to ambulatory care offices, and survey-based self-reports of health service use. Another important point which should be recognized is that differential use relative to Canadians in general does not mean that Aboriginal peoples receive 'better' or 'worse' health services, or receive such services more or less efficiently. Using Canadian health services utilization as the yardstick for comparison should not imply that the national level is necessarily the appropriate one.

As all Canadians are covered by universal hospital and medical care insurance, and all hospitals and physicians bill their provincial health insurance agencies for reimbursement, the enormous databases maintained by these agencies can serve as important sources of data on health service utilization. Unfortunately, it is possible to examine utilization by Aboriginal people only in some provinces, namely those in western Canada (British Columbia, Alberta, Saskatchewan, and Manitoba). Furthermore it is only status Indians who are separately identifiable through special coding of their health insurance numbers. In the Northwest Territories, the community of origin may provide some clue as to the likelihood that a particular user is Inuit or Dene.

Data from Saskatchewan in 1985 illustrate that in all age groups, including those over sixty-five, the hospitalization rate of status Indians exceeded that of non-Indians (Figure 15). During infancy, the rates for such conditions as respiratory diseases and infectious diseases were 5 or 6 times higher among status Indians. The higher rate among Indians is not a recent phenomenon, as data from the 1970s show a similar trend (Health Status Research Unit 1989). It is, of course, not possible to tell from these data alone if the high Indian hospitalization rate is due to high frequency of disease. One can argue that, given the level of illness, there should have been an even higher utilization rate, and that Indians underuse hospital services. Alternatively, one can speculate that Indians use hospital services far more frequently than is justified by the level of illness.

Fritz and D'Arcy (1982) examined the use of in-patient and out-patient psychiatric services in Saskatchewan, in both the private fee-for-service sector, and the public sector served by salaried psychiatrists working for the provincial health department's Psychiatric Services Branch and by academic psychiatrists in the medical school. After adjusting for the different age structures of Indians and non-Indians, they found that Indians used more in-patient services than non-Indians, in both the private and public sectors. For out-patient services, the reverse was true: the Indian rate was lower. In general, Saskatchewan residents used the private sector more frequently than the public, and this applied to both Indians and non-Indians. Differences in the prevalence of mental illness cannot account for the divergent trends between hospital and out-patient service

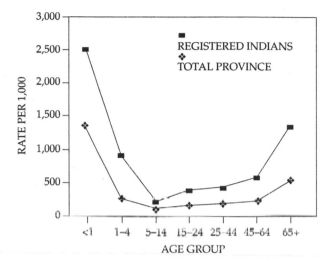

Figure 15

Age-specific hospital separation rate, registered Indians in Saskatchewan compared to total province, 1985–6

SOURCE: Based on data in Saskatchewan Hospital Services Plan, *Annual Report*, cited in Health Status Research Unit (1989)

utilization rates. Organizational and attitudinal factors may be involved – psychiatrists treating Indians may prefer hospital over ambulatory care.

Information on the use of health services can also be obtained in the course of a survey. The 1991 Aboriginal Peoples Survey (APS) included two questions: on consultation with health care providers in the past twelve months, and on the type of personnel consulted. For comparison, one could use the 1978 Canada Health Survey (Statistics Canada and Health and Welfare Canada 1981) and the 1985 General Social Survey (Statistics Canada 1987), both of which covered Canadians in all provinces but excluded Indian reserves and the northern territories.

Table 4 shows that Aboriginal people – particularly the Inuit – consulted physicians less often, and nurses more often, than Canadians in general; this reflects the organization of health services. If we accept that the overall level of illness is higher among Aboriginal people, the higher proportion of Aboriginal people who did not consult any health professional suggests underutilization. This is particularly acute for dental services.

TABLE 4

Percentage of survey respondents who consulted a health worker during the past year
(1978, 1985, 1991)

Type of health worker	Canada		APS (1991)		
	CHS (1978) %	GSS (1985) %	Indians %	Inuit %	Métis %
No one	–	10	27	32	24
Physician	76	81	68	48	72
Nurse	13	10	28	49	28
CHR	–	–	9	4	6
Dental	50	51	36	31	36
Eye	21	–	30	26	28
Pharmacist	5	–	34	13	40
Counsellor	3	–	3	2	2
Traditional healer	–	–	5	1	2

Notes: CHR – community health representative
         Dental – dentist, dental therapist, dental hygienist
         Eye – optometrist, ophthalmologist
         'Counsellor' includes social worker and psychologist in the CHS; and alcohol
         worker in the APS.

         Categories are not mutually exclusive and do not add up to 100 per cent.

SOURCES: CHS – Canada Health Survey
         GSS – General Social Survey
         APS – Aboriginal People's Survey

Table 5 shows that within the Aboriginal population, health care utilization varies according to such demographic and socio-economic factors
as age, sex, income, and education. The pattern is similar to those observed in other populations. Thus, women tend to use health services
more frequently than men, and the elderly more than the young. Those
with postsecondary education use health services more than those with
a lower level of education, while those with an annual income of less than
$10,000 use health services the least compared to the other income
groups. Table 5 also compares Aboriginal people living in urban areas
with Indians living on-reserve. Overall, urban Aboriginal residents are
more likely to have used health services in the previous year than on-
reserve Indians. This differential exists in all age, sex, education, and
income subcategories as well.

It is important to balance such national/provincial perspectives on the
use of health services with more in-depth inquiries at the local/regional

TABLE 5

Percentage of Aboriginal people who used health services during the past year (1991) by categories of age, sex, income, education, and residence

	All Aboriginal people %	Urban residents %	Indians on-reserve %
Total sample	73.5	77.5	68.0
Sex			
Male	65.2	69.5	60.7
Female	80.7	83.6	75.9
Age			
15–24	69.2	74.7	60.6
25–54	73.7	77.5	68.3
55+	84.4	87.8	83.1
Income			
< $10,000/yr	72.2	77.0	66.7
$10,000–19,999/yr	75.2	78.6	70.7
≥ $20,000/yr	75.0	77.6	69.8
Education			
≤ Grade 8	71.2	77.5	68.1
Grade 9–13	71.9	75.5	64.7
Some postsecondary	77.8	80.2	74.0

Notes: 'All Aboriginal people' and 'Urban residents' refer to Indians, Métis, and Inuit.

SOURCE: Special tabulation from the *Aboriginal Peoples Survey* of 1991 by Statistics Canada

level. Thouez, Foggin, and Rannou (1990) surveyed the Cree and Inuit in northern Quebec and found that, as expected, functional incapacity and perceived morbidity variables were linked to the degree that primary health care and hospital services were used. However, they also found that negative perceptions about the services provided and doubts about the physician were also significant determinants of health service use.

Waldram (1990c) surveyed inner-city residents in Saskatoon and compared the pattern and determinants of visits to physicians by Aboriginal and non-Aboriginal patients. To his surprise, he found little difference between the two groups. Just under 80 per cent of Aboriginal people indicated that they had a regular physician, and were able to provide that person's name. A similar proportion reported having consulted their regular physician at least once in the previous three months, while 57 per cent had undergone a physical examination within the last year. These differences were not statistically significant compared to the proportions reported by non-Aboriginal patients, and thus contradict the conventional wisdom that Aboriginal people in the city had a tendency to avoid physicians.

The study further demonstrated that long-term urban residents, people with children, women, and married people were the most likely to have a regular physician and to have had a recent contact with that practitioner. While Waldram did show that only 33 per cent of the Aboriginal patients had arrived with an appointment on the day of their interview, compared to 59 per cent of the non-Aboriginal patients, he also found that only 29 per cent of the Aboriginal patients had telephones, compared to 82 per cent of non-Aboriginal patients, and that most patients with telephones had made appointments.

The use of health care services should also be viewed in the political context, particularly that of the power relationship between Aboriginal 'clients' and predominantly non-Aboriginal 'providers.' (The conventional use of such terms is in itself problematic). The pattern of health service use can be profoundly altered in those communities which have assumed control of their health care delivery. The William Charles Band, located at Montreal Lake in Saskatchewan, was the first band in Canada to obtain control over health care delivery under the Health Transfer Agreement of MSB (see chapter 10). Before the transfer of control, amid a high level of physical and social health problems, the community practised little self-care and home management of minor childhood illnesses. Immunization rates were low. Some residents, particularly seniors, avoided contact with the nursing station, while others made constant demands on the nurses after hours. After the transfer of control in 1988, this pattern of behaviour changed dramatically (M. Moore et al. 1990).

O'Neil (1986, 1990) studied the provider-client relationship in the Arctic and how it could be affected by personalities. Nurses and physicians who are sensitive to cross-cultural differences, and who have a high degree of commitment to community issues, generally find it easier to develop satisfactory relationships than those with rigid ideas about their professional role and little interest in community life. O'Neil believed that the existing structure of federal health care tended to frustrate the efforts of sensitive and committed practitioners and reward practitioners with an aloof, detached, and 'colonial' approach.

Health care encounters involving non-Aboriginal medical practitioners and Aboriginal people are often affected by ingrained racial stereotyping. Sherley-Spiers (1989) documented the perceptions of Dakota patients in southwestern Manitoba. In their view, seriously ill patients were often assumed to be intoxicated by the attending physicians. Physicians often scolded mothers for not taking proper care of their children and for bringing them to the clinic either too early when they were not sick enough, or too late when the illness was too far advanced.

While many Aboriginal people will express their views of the health care system only in the course of private conversations, or in response to health care researchers, there have also been numerous community meetings across the country where dissatisfaction with the health care system is aired, sometimes in anger, sometimes in sorrow. Common concerns range from systemic ones such as the infrequency of doctors' visits, the inaccessibility of nursing stations after hours, the lack of Aboriginal health personnel, inflexible referral and evacuation policies, and inadequate boarding arrangements, to highly personal accounts of insensitive treatment, misdiagnosis, and delayed evacuation. Similar issues are sometimes brought up in highly publicized official or semi-official inquiries, such as in the Keewatin region in 1980 (Ruderman and Weller 1981), or during the New Democratic Party's Task Force on Northern Health Issues whirlwind fact-finding tour (1989). The so-called Scott-McKay-Bain Health Panel was convened by MSB and the Nishnawbe-Aski Nation of northern Ontario in response to a hunger strike by Aboriginal leaders in the Sioux Lookout Zone Hospital in 1988. It was the most extensive inquiry with an exclusive (though broadly defined) health focus ever, and involved hearings in many communities. On the national scene, the Royal Commission on Aboriginal Peoples during 1991–4 also invited Aboriginal communities to voice their concerns about health care, among other issues.

In summarizing the personal accounts of the health care system by 'clients' who made presentations in community hearings to the Scott-McKay-Bain Health Panel, Madeline Beardy wrote: 'The Native women of the Sioux Lookout Zone had a lot to say about the present health care system. They expressed views about the nursing stations, hospital experiences, nurses, doctors, transportation and communications. Often when people are asked what their views are on medical matters they associate the question with pain, discomfort, frustration and some anger. Also the family and friends of people involved in health problems face fear, anxiety, confusion and shock' (Scott-McKay-Bain Health Panel 1989a:4–5). For example, some women reported:

Why people have to be practically in their 'death-bed' before they are referred for proper treatment. (ibid. 9)

We try to convince the doctors and nurses who come to the community that the people who come to the nursing station are actually in need of medical attention. We have elders in the community who know when a person is really sick. (ibid. 9)

It is my hope that there would be a doctor here who would be very experienced. Who would examine patients and know where to refer them ... (ibid. 10)

People are often sent out to the hospital and sent back without the doctors really knowing what is wrong with them. Sometimes the doctor himself is still in training. (ibid. 11)

The nurse is in at 1:00 and leaves at 3:00 p.m. She doesn't get to see all the patients. She just rewrites prescriptions. (ibid. 13)

THE FUTURE ROLE OF GOVERNMENTS

What role will the federal government play under the coming era of 'new relationships' with Aboriginal peoples? Early in 1994, the minister of Indian Affairs announced in the House of Commons the government's intention to dismantle the Department of Indian Affairs and Northern Development, beginning with Manitoba as a pilot project. The federal role in providing services to Aboriginal peoples is increasingly viewed as one of 'funder' rather than 'provider.' Similar thinking can also be found within MSB. In 1993, MSB conducted a 'business line review'[3] which reviewed all direct health services provided by the department to determine if it should be in the business of doing so at all. It came to the conclusion that, within five years, all MSB program- and service-delivery responsibilities should be transferred to Aboriginal groups, other federal departments, and the provinces. As is already evident from Figure 13, the role of transfer payments will become predominant. Only a residual role is envisaged for MSB in strategic policy development, information management, and financial accountability. All current zone and regional structures will be taken over by the Aboriginal peoples. While it remains to be seen if such a scenario will materialize, there is a strong likelihood that the MSB as we have known it will no longer exist.

A new relationship is emerging, one in which the provincial/territorial governments are increasingly interposed between the 'special relationship' that has governed the federal government and Aboriginal peoples. Provincial governments have traditionally shied away from involvement in the direct provision of health services to Aboriginal people on reserves, preferring to let the federal government worry about them (and pay the lion's share). Aboriginal organizations have also insisted on dealing only with the federal government, in accordance with a 'nation-to-nation' mode of discourse, except when it comes to eligibility for provincial services. The truth of the matter is, however, that provincial governments have become a significant player in Aboriginal affairs. In health care, provincially administered universal health insurance plans cover Aboriginal people within their respective jurisdictions, including registered Indians. In recognition of the multijurisdictional nature of Aboriginal health care, a Tripartite Working Group on Aboriginal Health was struck in 1991 as a result of a meeting between the federal, provincial, and territorial health ministers and the leaders of the four national political Indian, Inuit, and Métis organizations. This working group reported to the Conference of Health Ministers in 1993, bringing to the national level the recognition, if not the solution, of structural barriers to the delivery of Aboriginal health services.

Within several provincial health ministries, small tentative steps have been taken to include Aboriginal health in the organizational structure. Ontario has proceeded the farthest, a consequence of the government's Statement of Political Relationship of 1991, which recognized the inherent right of self-government for Aboriginal peoples and committed the province to further negotiations to articulate that right. An Aboriginal Health Office was established within the Ministry of Health. After extensive consultations with Aboriginal organizations, which undertook their own community-level consultations, a draft Aboriginal Health Policy was prepared in 1993, the first of its kind in the country.

CONCLUSIONS

This chapter began with a description of the Aboriginal health care system, primarily from a technocratic viewpoint. It ends with a prediction about the changing role of the various levels of government. A health care system has many components, but the most important of these are the 'providers' and the 'clients.' Yet 'clients' as a term is inadequate to depict the central role played by Aboriginal peoples in such a system. No longer satisfied to be passive consumers of services, albeit services generally competently delivered and at great expense, Aboriginal peoples in the 1980s and 1990s have entered a new era of self-determination. This will be the subject of chapter 10. An Aboriginal health care system not only has Aboriginal people as 'clients,' but Aboriginal people as 'providers,' and everything in between as well.

9

Aboriginal medicine in the contemporary context

As we suggested in chapter 5, Aboriginal medicine and healing approaches began to re-emerge (from the perspective of non-Aboriginal observers) in the 1980s. By this time, many Aboriginal communities had experienced significant losses of traditional healing knowledge, and there were relatively fewer healers than in the past. These are but part of the legacy of colonialism, epidemic diseases, missionization, residential schools, and government policies of assimilation (including the outlawing of some healing-related ceremonies, as we saw in chapter 5). But not all was lost. It might be just as accurate to say that most aspects of Aboriginal healing and spirituality were shielded from the scrutiny of non-Aboriginal people, including law-enforcement officials. For instance, predictions of the demise of the Midewiwin and shaking tent were simply wrong, and these activities have continued to this day. The sweat lodge is currently experiencing a resurgence, and is being introduced back into communities where it has been absent for generations. The Sun Dance and the potlatch are very much a part of Aboriginal traditions on the Plains and Northwest Coast, respectively. In recent years, these and other healing and spiritual ceremonies have been opened up more to non-Aboriginal people, to the extent where we are now hearing calls to incorporate elements of Aboriginal medicine into biomedicine, even to the point of formal collaboration between the practitioners in the two systems. The issues surrounding these movements are complex and are linked to a reversal of the processes of deculturation and despiritualization, and the current shift towards self-determination in health. In this chapter, we will examine elements of the Aboriginal healing traditions as they exist today, and critically examine these new initiatives.

TRADITIONAL HEALING IN A CONTEMPORARY CONTEXT

There are many examples of the re-emergence of traditional Aboriginal medicine. We will concentrate here on 'public' efforts, that is, those that are documented in the literature and the media, or are otherwise made known to non-Aboriginal people.

It has become fairly common in hospitals in certain parts of Canada (particularly the west) to see an Aboriginal healer undertaking a ceremony for a patient. This development really accelerated in the early 1980s, as hospital administrators grappled with the complexities of having so many culturally different patients who were going to consult healers with or without hospital involvement. Accommodating healers required flexibility. For instance, the simple act of holding a sweetgrass ceremony violated hospital regulations against 'smoking' in the wards, and the proposed solution of disconnecting smoke detectors was not always well received, for obvious reasons. Tension often occurred around the issue of drugs and medical devices, such as intravenous tubes; many healers demanded that patients be free of all biomedical accoutrements. Nevertheless, through compromise and dialogue, accommodations have been made.

One of the best examples of the complexities of having an Aboriginal healer working within a hospital may be found at the Lake of the Woods Hospital in Kenora, Ontario. A plaque in the lobby of the hospital states, 'We believe traditional Native healing and culture have a place in our provision of health care services to the Native people' (cited in Gagnon 1989:176). Beginning in 1980, the Ontario Ministry of Health provided funding to hire a healer to work within the hospital. The move was a controversial one, with some Aboriginal people arguing against it. According to a report on this program (Seaby 1983:2), the following complaints were made:

the hiring of a single healer did not recognize that healers, like physicians have areas of specialization;

it was breaking traditional practice for the government to pay for the services of the healer as it is the responsibility of the person who is consulting the healer to provide payment;

the flurry of media attention at the outset of the program has detracted from the healer's credibility within the native community;

the location of the healer in the hospital did not meet the approval of the Elders.

When the healer died suddenly, within a year of his appointment, some observers were led to believe that this was a sign that the experiment was inappropriate. Nevertheless, soon after, a program coordinator was hired to arrange healer services for patients according to family preferences and the specialization of the healer. Efforts were made to have more Aboriginal input into the program as well, to prevent the type of conflict that arose under the first program. By the mid-1980s, more than half of the hospital physicians were referring patients to healers for a variety of treatments (D.E. Young and Smith 1991:45). Subsequently, a healer was hired within the hospital's Department of Psychiatry.

In Winnipeg, an initiative to develop a medical interpreters' program at two hospitals led to the introduction of Aboriginal healing into the hospitals themselves (Kaufert and Koolage 1985; O'Neil 1988). These Aboriginal interpreters found that, among their many duties as they developed with the program, there was a need to facilitate traditional healing for some patients. Since many of these patients were hospitalized far from their communities, they lacked connections with the urban Aboriginal network. The interpreters helped to identify healers and worked with the hospital physicians and administrators to make the necessary arrangements so that healing could occur in as culturally appropriate a manner as possible.

In a more recent development, the Battlefords Union Hospital in Saskatchewan announced plans to construct a traditional healing room as part of the hospital's renovation plans. Initial plans called for the room to be used for prayers and traditional smudging ceremonies, but the prospects for actual healing activities in the future are good (Saskatoon Star-Phoenix, 11 August 1993, A8).

Insofar as the biomedical system has accepted Aboriginal healing, there has been a tendency to marginalize it somewhat within the realm of 'mental health' programs. One of the pioneers in this area is British Columbia psychiatrist Wolfgang Jilek, who has worked successfully since the 1970s with Aboriginal healers in the treatment of patients with alcohol problems and other psychiatric disorders that are perceived to have a cultural component (Jilek 1982b; see also Jilek 1978, 1982a, and Jilek and Jilek-Aall 1982, 1991). In particular, Jilek has documented the therapeutic effectiveness of Coast Salish 'Spirit Dancing' as a treatment strategy, especially for alcoholism. However, in general the psychiatric profession in Canada has not been particularly open to Aboriginal healing approaches.

Aboriginal communities themselves have taken the lead in promoting traditional healing approaches for their people. Perhaps the best known case is that of Alkali Lake, British Columbia, a community which was rife with alcoholism and its attendant problems (violence, sexual abuse, suicide, etc.) that turned itself around to become almost totally alcohol free (York 1990; Johnson and Johnson 1993; see also the band-produced video *The Honour of All*). This transformation was accomplished with the assistance of a non-local traditional healer, who was asked to help the community rediscover the sweat lodge and other traditional healing approaches.

Throughout Canada, and especially in the west, 'healing circles' are becoming common. These are therapeutic sessions organized by Aboriginal people to deal with such problems as the effects of residential schools, sexual abuse, and alcoholism. In general, there has been an extensive revitalization of the sweat lodge as a general treatment approach for a wide variety of physical and mental health problems (as well as for social and spiritual purposes), an approach which also has the effect of reintegrating individuals into their cultures. In many cases, the sweat lodges are being reintroduced with the assistance of elders and healers from other communities, and often other cultural traditions.

There have been some official non-Aboriginal pronouncements recognizing Aboriginal medicine in recent years which pay at least lip-service to its continued existence. A 1980 report issued by the Medical Services Branch (MSB) advocated 'a closer working relationship between traditional healers and physicians' (cited in Gagnon 1989:176), and in 1983 the then minister of Indian Affairs, John Munro, told a 'National Indian and Inuit Health Conference' that 'Health and Welfare Canada fully recognizes the value of traditional Native medicine' (Munro 1983:7). In a submission to the Special Committee on Indian Self-Government (the Penner Committee), National Health and Welfare's position was clearly articulated: 'We have come to appreciate very much the relevance and the utility of traditional approaches, particularly to mental health problems – approaches which address the suicide rate, approaches which address addiction problems. We believe that in areas such as those the application of traditional medicine and native culture perhaps can be more successful than anything we could offer in terms of contemporary psychiatric approaches to those kinds of problems' (cited in Penner 1983:35).

Throughout the 1980s the MSB funded the provision of traditional medical services for Aboriginal peoples throughout western Canada (Gregory 1989). This often took the form of paying the costs of having healers travel to communities to treat patients, as well as sending patients to healers. Conferences between Aboriginal healers and biomedical practitioners are becoming more common, as the two groups seek to understand each other better and to facilitate collaborative relationships. One such conference was held in The Pas in 1986 (ibid. 1989). The purpose of this conference was to seek the advice and assistance of healers in the development of curricula for a new northern nursing program. In 1993, a conference of healers was held at the Regional Psychiatric Centre (Prairies) in Saskatoon, a federal correctional facility which offers a variety of psychological treatment programs. Healers from across western Canada attended with correctional psychologists and psychiatrists in an effort to facilitate a more traditional approach to the healing of Aboriginal offenders. One positive outcome of this conference has been the holding of two healing sessions for Aboriginal inmates/patients. Lasting about eight days each, the sessions were undertaken by a Cree healer from northern Alberta. The area of corrections in general has shown slow but steady progress in recent years, and the soon-to-be-opened Aboriginal 'healing lodges' in Maple Creek, Saskatchewan (for female offenders), and Hobbema, Alberta (for male offenders), will include traditional approaches.

More recently, the Ontario government released a policy paper on Aboriginal health which included as a fundamental principle that 'Traditional Aboriginal approaches to wellness, including the use of traditional resources, traditional healers, medicine people, midwives and elders, are recognized, respected and protected from government regulation. They enhance and complement healing, as well as programs and services throughout the health system' (Ontario 1994:15). The implications of this sweeping policy principle will be briefly addressed later in this chapter.

There has also been some significant new research into various aspects of Aboriginal medicine. Much of this research has focused on the persistence of cultural beliefs about health held by contemporary Aboriginal people, and how this affects their strategies for seeking health care from both the traditional and the biomedical systems. Garro (1987; 1988a; 1988b; 1990), for instance, has documented the knowledge and attitudes about diabetes, high blood pressure, and other illnesses among *Anishinaabe* (Ojibwa) communities in Manitoba. She has also described the manner in which traditional medicine is utilized by these people.

In another study, Garro (1991) documented 468 illness case histories, of which 4 per cent involved requesting an *Anishinaabe* healer for a remedy, and 17 per cent involved requests for a diagnosis. The total of 21 per cent of the illnesses which resulted in a consultation with a healer was in contrast to 48 per cent where physicians were seen. In 7 per cent of the cases, a healer was consulted without also consulting a physician. Overall, of the sixty-one households studied by Garro, some 62 per cent reported having visited a healer over the six to eight months of her research. She also documented the extensive use of herbal medicines by these people.

In a different vein, David Young and his colleagues have attempted to determine the efficacy of a traditional treatment for psoriasis by employing the testing and validation measures of biomedicine (D.E. Young, Swartz, Ingram, and Morse 1988). This is a difficult and politically dangerous type of experiment, since it requires the removal of the treatment from its proper cultural context and evaluation using standards other than those for which the treatment was devised.[1] Working with northern Cree healer Russell Willier, Young and his associates documented his treatment of non-Aboriginal patients; they utilized both videotape and still cameras, and employed biomedical practices in judging the outcome (for example, measuring the size of the psoriasis scabs). Some of the herbal medicines used by Willier were even analysed in the laboratory.

From yet another perspective, Waldram (1993) has described how Aboriginal spirituality programs in prisons should be viewed as a form of symbolic healing: that is, a process of healing involving the identification and manipulation of culturally specific symbols (such as the sweat lodge, the sacred pipe, tobacco, and sweetgrass) by elders in a manner that promotes healing among offenders. Many Aboriginal offenders are suffering from a process of despiritualization and cultural identity problems. Involvement with elders and healers re-establishes their spiritual and cultural identities as Aboriginal people, which in turn not only contributes to their own healing (for instance, in resolving alcohol and drug problems), but also makes them more amenable to the messages of the biomedical/psychosocial treatment programs.

The scientific study of Aboriginal healing is contentious. There are some Aboriginal people who feel that their medicine is a gift from the Creator, and that as a result there is no need to 'prove' its efficacy according to scientific principles. But there are others who believe that limited scientific study is essential to having Aboriginal medicine accepted by Aboriginal and non-Aboriginal patients and by health care administrators and funding agencies.

THE IMPLICATIONS OF MEDICAL PLURALISM

'Medical pluralism' refers to the practice of utilizing the medical services of more than one medical system. A recent study in the United States discovered that more than one-third of respondents had utilized at least one form of therapy that was not scientifically based (defined in the study as those therapies not taught widely at American medical schools) (Eisenberg et al. 1993). In the case of Aboriginal peoples in Canada, they have access not only to biomedical services and various other alternative, non-Aboriginal treatment modalities (such as chiropractic, acupuncture, homeopathy), but also to their own medical systems. The continued use of traditional medical services after the introduction of biomedical services is a global phenomenon (see Press 1969; Schwartz 1969; Garrison 1977; Woods 1977; Asuni 1979; Waldram 1990b). The literature suggests that patients move fairly easily from one system to another, for as Welsch (1983:34) accurately notes, people move between alternative *treatments*, and not alternative systems, and according to Asuni (1979:37), 'He [the patient] will use both ... with or without the knowledge or approval of either.'

It is widely known that some Aboriginal patients will seek treatment simultaneously from a physician and a traditional healer. In such instances, two cognitive processes may be at work. First, the patients' 'explanatory model,' or their subjective conceptualization of their symptoms, etiology, and need for treatment (see Kleinman 1980) may include a bifurcated notion of etiology and symptomatology. In other words, they may seek out physician treatment to alleviate the symptoms, and the traditional healer to eliminate the cause. Second, they may be simply employing a shotgun approach to treatment, seeking the assistance of practitioners from both medical systems to ensure that all possible causes and symptoms are addressed. It is also known that some Aboriginal people will utilize the two medical systems in a serial fashion, seeking treatment solely from one until a certain subjective point of dissatisfaction is reached, whereupon the services of the other are obtained. In the case of long or problematic illnesses, this pattern can repeat itself many times over.

Kennedy (1984) has written about the extended medical history of one Okanagan (Interior Salish) man as he sought treatment for leg ulcers over a sixty-seven-year period. His case is no doubt extraordinary, for during this period he utilized the services of traditional Aboriginal healers, physicians, Chinese traditional doctors, a variety of self-treatments, and even the Shaker church. As he moved from treatment to treatment, his views of the illness (his 'explanatory model') changed. At times he thought the problem was due to poisonous plants, at other times to sorcery or 'bad medicine,' and at still other times to a combination of etiologies. Kennedy notes that the severity of the particular episode of illness conditioned his response; he often went to physicians and hospitals when the symptoms were most severe. She also notes that the patient's adherence to the prescribed treatment of any practitioner was greatest when the explanatory model of the patient and healer were most similar.

Garro (1990;1991) has also provided a good description of *Anishinaabe* views of treatment and illness. She notes that there are two broad categories of illness, 'White Man's Sickness,' for which a physician's treatment is sought, and '*Anishinaabe* sickness' for which a healer's treatment is sought. Most patients will seek out the services of a physician first when they fall ill, for according to Garro (1991:215), 'unless there are indications to the contrary, it is generally assumed that an illness is not an *Anishinaabe* sickness.' She continues: 'People go to see physicians both because there are no costs associated with their use and because the physician's treatment is judged efficacious. Indeed, treatment by physicians is often seen as offering a higher likelihood of cure in cases that are not due to "*Anishinaabe* sicknesses." This is reinforced by the medicine man referring patients to physicians in many cases of illness which are not seen as being "*Anishinaabe* sicknesses." ' But Garro emphasizes that the healers do not constitute a treatment of last resort, when the physician's treatment has failed. Rather, those individuals whom she documents as being treated by healers tended to point to features of the illness which implied '*Anishinaabe* sicknesses.'

The significance of medical pluralism as a treatment strategy needs to be drawn out. From the patient's perspective, it actually empowers the patient, who, through the choice of medical system and practitioner, has a measure of control over his or her own health. Likewise, the availability of significantly different alternatives further provides for choice should the encounter with one system prove unsatisfactory. Cultural understandings of illness and treatment are validated, since Aboriginal medicine can be sought, yet the patient can also use biomedical services to treat the same problem, or a component of that problem. In effect, medical pluralism allows the patient to retain both control and the cultural context of healing.

From the perspective of the practitioners, some problems are evident. It would be safe to conclude that most physicians do not question their patients with regard to the use of alternative treatments; many do not even enquire if home management has been attempted. For many physicians, Aboriginal medicine lacks credibility to such an extent that they regard even questions about it as ludicrous. However, if the patient is seeing or plans to see a traditional healer, then some conflict can occur. For instance, the healer may require the patient to discontinue medication in order to undergo a healing ceremony. There are anecdotal stories of diabetic patients suffering as a result of directions to discontinue insulin. The fact that a patient may be consulting with two different medical systems, without the knowledge of either, may empower the patient, but may also lead to contradictions in treatment and possible medical complications (an issue of relevance in all cases of medical pluralism).

It should be made clear at this point, however, that most Aboriginal healers have a very well-defined understanding of their abilities, knowledge, and limitations. Like physicians, when confronted with a problem for which they are not 'qualified' they will make a referral, either to another healer or to a physician. Some physicians have also been known to make referrals to Aboriginal healers. Usually, this takes the form of general referrals, that a patient should consult with a physician or Aboriginal healer in general, without specifically naming an individual. Indeed, this system of informal referral is the most common model of 'collaboration' between the two medical systems.

ABORIGINAL MEDICINE AND URBANIZATION

When people think of Aboriginal medicine, they often visualize the context of a reserve or remote community, where the healing traditions are integral parts of, and supported by, the culture. However, since more than one-third of Canada's Aboriginal people now live in urban areas (and the urban population is growing quickly), a new context needs to be addressed. Characteristically, in cities Aboriginal people from different cultural traditions live side by side with Euro-Canadians and residents from other parts of the world. Is Aboriginal medicine left behind when migration takes place, or are the cultural beliefs about this form of healing transplanted to the urban context? This question is particularly pertinent since, in the city, Aboriginal people are surrounded by biomedical services and facilities.

There have been relatively few studies of traditional Aboriginal medicine in the city in North America. An early 1970s study in San Francisco determined that urban 'Native Americans' who had difficulties using biomedical services were more likely to use traditional medicine, but that much of the latter was done on the home reservations and not in the city itself (Fuchs and Bashshur 1975). The study also demonstrated that traditional medicine persisted in the city, and that variables such as economic status and level of education did not seem relevant in predicting the use of traditional services.

A project undertaken by Waldram (1990a, 1990b) examined the issue of traditional medicine in the urban context in greater detail, in a study of health care utilization in Saskatoon. Overall, he found that traditional Aboriginal medicine was maintained by urban dwellers, that socio-economic variables explained little, and that the utilization of Aboriginal medicine did not detract from the use of biomedical services. However, in contrast with the findings of the San Francisco study, utilization of Aboriginal medicine was not related to problems in gaining access to biomedical services. The most important explanatory variables were those pertaining to language. For instance, individuals who spoke an Aboriginal language were more likely to seek out traditional healers and to believe in the superiority of Aboriginal medicine over biomedicine for certain health problems. Hence, it was determined that urban Aboriginal people in this study continued to believe in and utilize traditional medical services for reasons largely unrelated to the existence of biomedical services or problems in utilizing those services. Aboriginal medicine remains important for cultural reasons, including beliefs in efficacy.

Waldram's (1990a, 1990b) study also examined issues relating to access to Aboriginal medicine in Saskatoon. Given the persistence of beliefs in this medicine, is it accessible in the city? The study found that only a small fraction of the Aboriginal respondents knew a healer in the city, and slightly less than half believed they would not be able to find one if they tried. Not surprisingly, therefore, some 60 per cent responded affirmatively to the question, 'Would you like to see an Indian healer available in a clinic?' Even those most firmly anchored in their Aboriginal culture (as indicated by language variables) were supportive of this kind of formal access to Aboriginal medicine. A clear need for better access was established in this study. As health care consumers, Saskatoon's Aboriginal urban residents wanted access to a full range of health services in the city, not just biomedical services, and they were unconcerned with the many implications that such formalization would entail (see the next section for a discussion of these issues). By comparison, it has also been noted that the demand for access to services provided by Aboriginal healers and elders at the Anishnawbe Health Centre in Toronto has been overwhelming (George and Nahwegahbow 1993:242). As we saw in the previous section, Aboriginal people, like all people, want such a full range of services, and see no incompatibility in using them, regardless of what the various medical practitioners think. As Kleinman (1980) notes, the patient's explanatory model or understanding of his or her illness is often different from that of the practitioner; significantly, the extent to which the explanatory models of both are compatible explains to a great extent the patient's assessment of the therapeutic encounter, compliance with a particular treatment, and likelihood of seeking treatment from elsewhere.

THE FORMALIZATION-COLLABORATION DEBATE

Recently, there has been a great deal of discussion regarding the formalization of Aboriginal medicine to make it more readily available, and about the need for collaboration between Aboriginal medicine and biomedicine. We will briefly detail some of the issues that any increased formalization of Aboriginal medicine, including collaboration with biomedicine, would entail.

1 Epistemological and philosophical issues

Although both traditional Aboriginal medicine and biomedicine seek to heal patients, there are some fundamental differences in epistemology and philosophy which inhibit formal collaboration. Aboriginal medicine is based on *tradition*, which is to say that, as a medical system, it accepts that the medicines, techniques, and knowledge of the past were effective because they have been time-tested and, in many instances, shared with humans by the Creator. In a sense, while new approaches to treatment are incorporated, this medicine is primarily informed and guided by the traditions of the past. Practitioners gain their knowledge to heal very slowly, so that most are relatively old and the oldest (elders) are the most revered. Medical knowledge exists only within the oral tradition. There is also a great degree of individualism and idiosyncrasy in the practice of traditional medicine. Current users are less concerned with questions of efficacy, because of their faith or belief that traditional medicine works. In contrast, biomedicine is empirical and positivist, based on a philosophy of scepticism. Something must be proven to work before it is accepted, and the method by which such proof is attained is scrutinized carefully. While biomedicine is also informed by tradition, it tends to be constantly seeking new medical knowledge, which in turn is scrutinized and verified. This means that medical knowledge changes rapidly. Relatively young practitioners experience a brief but intense period of training to become competent, and it is often difficult for older physicians to remain in touch with the latest medical developments. Nevertheless, a physician's knowledge is fairly standard no matter where the person was trained, and is derived from both oral instruction and written texts.

In a sense, then, the issue is one of science versus faith. This is particularly problematic because science, in effect, developed in response to faith as a means of independently verifying knowledge in an objective manner. Science and faith have been at odds for centuries, and the most central debate, that of creationism versus evolution, remains topical today. The philosophical underpinnings of science render it unlikely to accept traditional medical traditions which are not verifiable through the scientific method. Science is rigid, and hence it will either demand that Aboriginal medicine be examined scientifically or else will reject it as faith – that is, as inherently unscientific.

Of course, it is not appropriate to paint all biomedical practitioners with one brush when it comes to Aboriginal medicine. It is apparent that numerous examples exist of physicians and nurses working in conjunction with Aboriginal healers in one form or another. Two studies emanating out of Manitoba are particularly insightful. Gregory (1989) has documented the existence of cross referrals between Aboriginal healers and MSB nurses in northern Manitoba. Indeed, 52 per cent of the nurses he interviewed responded that they had made referrals to elders and healers, and that the MSB had even provided some funding to bring healers into communities from elsewhere. Such a collaborative relationship requires an understanding on the parts of both traditional and biomedical practitioners, but the situation is particularly enlightening because nurses are involved. The authors are also aware of many other anecdotal cases of local nurses working with local healers, sometimes publicly but often very quietly.

In contrast to Gregory's (1989) study, Gagnon (1989) found quite contradictory views among physicians and medical students working at the Lake of the Woods Hospital in Kenora, Ontario, as well as at the Northern Medical Unit at the University of Manitoba. Given the nature of these two groups and the extensive exposure to Aboriginal patients and issues which is, in part, their *raison d'être*, one would expect them to be among the most open-minded of the biomedical practitioners. Gagnon found that 'most respondents are in favour of some form of collaboration *but indicated a reluctance to relinquish control'* (ibid. 181; emphasis added). Some 90 per cent believed that traditional healers played an important 'psycho-social' role (but not necessarily a *medical* role), and only 55 per cent stated that they would actually allow a healing ceremony to be held in their hospital. Furthermore, 73 per cent stated that traditional medical practices should not 'interfere' with biomedicine. Traditional healing, it seems, was something to be done in the community, but not within bio-medical institutions. The isolation of the physicians from the community level was apparent from the fact that only 15 per cent of them had ever referred a patient to a healer.

We might speculate that the responses of these physicians and medical students were conditioned as much by concerns of political correctness (not to offend Aboriginal cultures) as by their knowledge and tolerance of Aboriginal medicine. Certainly the nurses, whose practices are more grounded at the community level where most traditional healing takes place, proved to be much more receptive to issues of collaboration. But clearly, in the end, biomedical practitioners demonstrate a reluctance to accept traditional medicine as a viable alternative, primarily for episte-mological and philosophical reasons. Where traditional medicine might be included, it would clearly be subservient to biomedicine. Because of the uniqueness of their samples, the studies by Gregory and Gagnon likely *overestimate* the knowledge of and support for Aboriginal medicine that exists within the biomedical system in Canada.

A central issue to be considered here is one of efficacy. Does Aboriginal medicine 'work'? We believe that this question is central to any discussion of barriers to collaboration, for, as we have seen in previous chapters, there is a long-standing tradition among biomedical practitioners in par-ticular, and non-Aboriginal people in general, of viewing Aboriginal medicine as quackery. Not surprisingly, this is one question that few seem to want to address directly; non-Aboriginal people in particular fear being accused of racism if they bring up such an issue. We will not skirt our responsibilities here.

The efficacy of traditional medicine must be seen within its proper social and cultural context. What constitutes an illness differs from society to society (with intrasocietal variation as well), and it is best to think of 'illness' as socially and culturally defined. Therefore, what constitutes an effective treatment for an 'illness' will also be socially and culturally defined. To use an Aboriginal example, victims of 'bad medicine' are 'ill' as defined by their Aboriginal cultures; whether biomedical science can discern any disease is not relevant. The culturally appropriate means of dealing with 'bad medicine' is to seek out a traditional healer, who will perform the necessary healing ceremonies. The patient is healed insofar as the patient, and his or her significant others, subjectively believe that the 'bad medicine' has been removed. But the issue is not as simple as this sounds, since it has been suggested that within Aboriginal healing traditions 'illness is not necessarily a bad thing,' and that 'It is often sent to help people re-evaluate their lives' (Aboriginal Nurses Association of Canada 1993:14). Hence, illness might be viewed as a significant indication of personal breaches of the moral order of the society, simultaneously calling for proper rehabilitation of that breach and for reinforcing the norms and values of the society.

Questions of efficacy are most commonly raised with respect to the use of herbal medicines, possibly because this is one area that biomedicine can objectively (that is, scientifically) examine. But it is necessary to keep in mind that even the preparation and administration of herbal medicines is often steeped in spirituality, and the removal of the spiritual component in a scientific search to see if a herbal preparation 'works' may violate the proper cultural context. David Young and colleagues (D.E. Young, Swartz, Ingram, and Morse 1988) report on an experiment with northern Alberta Cree healer Russell Willier, whose treatment for psoriasis was scientifically examined, at his request. Willier allowed one of his herbal medicines to be analysed in the laboratory (using a pseudonym to protect its identity from the chemists), and some antibacterial agents were found. The overall treatment experiment was successful to some degree, especially given that Willier's patients had essentially given up on biomedical treatments of their problem. But the success rate as defined by Willier was not as good as he had anticipated, which was explained in part by Willier as the result of the unusual circumstances in which he was required to function (that is, in an Edmonton clinic with non-Aboriginal patients who were required to administer herbal remedies in their own homes). Our point here is that biomedical scientists often fail to comprehend the cultural context of such healing, and look instead for purely clinical evidence.

The question 'Does it work?' is an important one. There is all kinds of evidence within the oral tradition and histories of Aboriginal people of the healing of terminal diseases, especially cancer, through traditional medicine. Aboriginal healing traditions purport to have cures for all kinds of disorders, but it is rare indeed when these are shared with non-Aboriginal people. There is a genuine fear that non-Aboriginal people will steal the recipes for herbal medicines, for instance, and sell them for money; this is not an unreasonable fear, given that the pharmaceutical industry has a history of looking to traditional peoples' medicines for new drugs. As it stands now, Russell Willier remains one of a very few Aboriginal healers who have allowed scientific evaluation of their treatments, and scientific practitioners will not likely endorse any Aboriginal healing approach that it cannot verify with its own methods. We believe that there are many benefits to traditional medicine, when viewed both biomedically and within the proper cultural context. As non-Aboriginal researchers, we are limited by the degree to which we can observe these healing traditions in order to learn more about them. But the simple fact that so many Aboriginal people believe in their medicine makes the question of efficacy an important one.

2 Validating Aboriginal healers

The biomedical and traditional Aboriginal systems are in conflict with respect to methods of validating healing knowledge and practitioners. With biomedicine, practitioners receive formal education, must pass rigorous exams, and must continue to practise efficiently while under the scrutiny of licensing and professional associations. Canadian law protects the patient from exposure to unqualified medical practitioners, and will assist patients who are harmed as a result of medical incompetence. In contrast, Aboriginal medical knowledge is often handed down from generation to generation to individuals selected by existing healers. Ultimately, as Alberta Cree healer Russell Willier has said, the power to heal comes from the Creator (D.E. Young et al. 1989). Healers in the Aboriginal tradition are culturally validated; they are accepted by community members as healers, and those who wish to avail themselves of a healer's services follow the culturally prescribed method of requesting assistance. There are no licences, and no regulating bodies. In general, people know who the good healers are, and will attempt to avoid those who are considered to be incompetent or are known to deal in 'bad medicine.' Furthermore, it has been suggested that an underlying assumption exists that 'fraudulent healers will be taken care of by a natural or metaphysical process' (Aboriginal Nurses Association of Canada 1993:15). Uncertainty pervades this issue, even at the community level. For instance, Garro (1990:428) has documented a lack of consensus among Anishinaabe in Manitoba about who is a legitimate healer and who deals in 'bad medicine,' and about the degree of competency of practitioners in the various traditional healing specialities.

From a purely cultural perspective, the validation of Aboriginal healers is generally effective, though not unproblematic. Once we begin to talk about making Aboriginal medicine more formal and, more readily available, and about developing collaborative programs, then the question of validation becomes more difficult. It is not easy for most non-Aboriginal people, and even many Aboriginal people who have little traditional cultural knowledge, to distinguish true traditional healers from others whose knowledge lacks cultural or community validation. Indeed, there is a whole growth industry, related to current 'New Age' trends, in promoting and selling Aboriginal medicine and philosophies. Charlatanism is a serious issue. It is so serious, in fact, that the Traditional Elders Circle of the Indigenous Nations of North America passed a resolution in 1980 warning that many so-called 'medicine people' lack the proper knowledge and authority to heal and to carry sacred objects, such as the pipe (Alberta elder Peter O'Chiese was a signatory to this resolution). A key issue was the use of traditional medicine for profit, often involving non-Aboriginal clients. Subsequently, the American Indian Movement, a U.S.-based activist organization, passed a resolution condemning charlatans, and went so far as to name specific individuals. Prominent on the list was Sun Bear, a 'plastic medicine man' who has developed his own series of books and workshops, and even his own 'tribe' of followers (Churchill 1990).

In Canada, we have recently seen a variety of travelling Aboriginal healers who move from community to community in a manner reminiscent of the medicine shows of the last century. Two characteristics above all typify these individuals: they are fluent in English and they know the ways of bureaucracy. Many could well be graduates of Dale Carnegie or Toastmaster's courses, so compelling are they as speakers. In effect, they are successful because they can, and will, deal with bureaucracies, sign contracts to deliver their services, keep records of expenses, and, above all, tell people (invariably non-Aboriginals) what they want to hear. Some of these are appropriately validated healers, others are not.

True Aboriginal healers, those with cultural validation, are most likely to speak their Aboriginal language and be, at the most, bilingual. They are also humble about their abilities. One would not normally hear a healer pronounce that he or she is in fact a healer; this is a status that is ascribed to them by others. Some are also still afraid of legal prosecution, a legacy of the past. Furthermore, many operate under constraints preventing them from disclosing fully their medical traditions, for fear of losing their powers (Aboriginal Nurses Association of Canada 1993:15). It is not surprising, therefore, that the biomedical system and the Aboriginal healing systems find it difficult to work together. Indeed, if many traditional healers will not even admit that they are healers (as is the cultural protocol), then some serious cross-cultural communication problems are evident.

The authors know of many Aboriginal people who are considered to be charlatan healers by other Aboriginal people. But the issue is more complex than this, because even well-respected healers may have their detractors. Furthermore, even charlatans have the potential to heal *if* the patient has faith in the healer's powers. In the absence of clear avenues of certification, it is hard to imagine that biomedical practitioners will be able to decipher this complex, cultural issue. Many have responded by simply ignoring the issue altogether when working with a healer (no doubt hoping that there won't be an incident), while a common strategy employed by those who wish to have some formal collaboration is to hire an Aboriginal person and let him or her manage any crisis that may erupt. Perhaps the Navajo model makes the greatest sense, since the family of the ill person, and not an institution or biomedical practitioner, has the responsibility to select the healer. The Indian Health Service hospital at Chinle, Arizona, provides a traditional healing hogan within the hospital itself, but beyond that the family is responsible for arranging traditional healing ceremonies. A 1990 report on health care in Saskatchewan would agree, stating that, 'Because of the very personal nature of the medicine man's services, it would be inappropriate to suggest he become part of a highly regulated and organized health care system' (Murray 1990:210). A round table on the issue of collaboration, organized by the Aboriginal Nurses Association of Canada on behalf of the Royal Commission on Aboriginal Peoples, was unable to develop a consensus on the types of collaborative models that should be invoked, and even whether collaboration should be sought. According to their report, 'It was the belief of many traditional practitioners that the best that could be attained was respect for and acceptance of the differences' (Aboriginal Nurses Association of Canada 1993:16).

3 Legal issues

It seems as though very few observers wish to tackle openly the legal aspects of formalizing Aboriginal medicine, perhaps because they are complex and pose a direct threat to the integrity of the Aboriginal cultures themselves. Certainly a central question in any discussion of legal aspects is, 'Does Aboriginal medicine work?,' a question whose corollary, 'Can Aboriginal medicine do harm?,' no one seems to want to discuss. Related to these questions is another one which is linked more directly to the legal framework of the country: 'Do Aboriginal healers practise medicine without a licence?' In terms of the Constitution, we could ask, 'Is Aboriginal medicine an Aboriginal right under Section 35?' The answers to these questions will not come easily, but we believe they must be addressed before any significant change to the status quo can occur.

Robb (1988) has provided an interesting legal viewpoint on Aboriginal medicine. In general, Robb sees the problem as one of a lack of Aboriginal sovereignty, since, under the current system, even on-reserve Aboriginal people are subjected to provincial laws of general applicability, in addition to being under federal jurisdiction by virtue of Section 91 (24) of the *Constitution Act*. The federal *Food and Drug Act* 'makes it an offense to advertise any food, drug, cosmetic, or device to the general public as a treatment, preventative or cure for any diseases, disorders, or abnormal physical states' as defined in the act, including alcoholism, gout, depression, diabetes, gangrene, influenza, and obesity (Robb 1988:135). Provincially, Robb identifies Alberta's *Medical Profession Act* as a problem, for it makes it an offence for anyone except a registered (licensed) physician to practise medicine. According to Robb, the definition of 'practise medicine' is 'breathtaking in its scope,' and includes prescribing or administering any treatment, performing any operation or manipulation, applying any apparatus or appliance, or advertising (including uttering statements) with respect to 'the prevention, alleviation or cure of any human disease, ailment, deformity, defect or injury' (cited in Robb 1988:136). So broad is this definition that even a parent administering to a child is in violation, but Robb notes that the act tends to be enforced when the professional monopoly of the biomedical practitioners is challenged. It is Robb's legal opinion that this act does not apply to reserves, but does for any off-reserve practitioners.

Robb also identifies issues of criminal and civil liability. Criminally, the law states that parents, guardians, or spouses must provide the necessities of life, including medical treatment; the courts have established that medical services in accord with a person's faith, religion, or belief are not reasonable in this sense. The Criminal Code also states that anyone who provides medical services must have reasonable knowledge and skill. Clearly, these criminal provisions threaten Aboriginal healers as they currently practise. In terms of civil liability, the law states that medical practitioners are not expected to guarantee successful treatment, but that they must possess the necessary skill and knowledge to practise according to accepted standards (such as those that would be expected given the locale of the practice). According to Robb (1988:137), these legal issues raise some fundamental questions, such as: Can an Aboriginal healer obtain liability insurance? and Can one be employed by a physician and covered by the latter's insurance? Perhaps the most significant question, however, is: 'Will the medical profession permit doctors to employ traditional Aboriginal medical practitioners' as assistants or, indeed, in any other capacity? Clearly there are implications for both the Aboriginal healer and the physician in any formal collaborative relationship. In effect, if Aboriginal healers are practising medicine as defined in Canadian law, then they are doing so without a licence. If it is something else that they are doing, if it can be said they are involved in a *cultural* practice, then it seems that some legal protection, or at least a constitutional clarification, is still required. Culture is an amorphic entity and, as we saw in the introductory chapter of this book, Aboriginal cultures are extremely diverse; intracultural variability is extensive, and there are those who simply do not follow Aboriginal cultural customs. To rely on culture to validate healing will inevitably lead to legal problems. The following example highlights this.

In 1992, the British Columbia Supreme Court issued its judgment in the case of *Thomas v. Norris* ([1992] 2 C.N.L.R.]). Mr Thomas was initiated against his will into the Coast Salish Big House Tradition called the Spirit Dance. Thomas was a member of the band, but had lived off-reserve for many years and did not identify with the Coast Salish culture. His wife at the time, believing that initiation into the Spirit Dance would heal him of his alcohol problem and repair their marriage, requested that he be initiated. According to Coast Salish custom, the collective right of the people to force an individual such as Mr Thomas to undergo Spirit Dancing in the interests of the community at large was paramount over Mr Thomas's individual rights. Justice Hood disagreed, stating that Mr Thomas's individual rights, in this case guarantees against 'assault, battery and false imprisonment,' prevailed within Canadian law. Furthermore, the judge ruled that Spirit Dancing was not an 'aboriginal right' under Section 35 of the Constitution. The judge also stated of the plaintiff that, 'He lives in a free society and his rights are inviolable. He is free to believe in, and to practice, any religion or tradition, if he chooses to do so. He cannot be coerced or forced to participate in one by any group purporting to exercise their collective rights in doing so' (162).

According to the judgment, Mr Thomas was 'forcibly seized' in 1988, and taken to the Semenos Long House of the Cowichan Indian Band. Over a four-day period, Mr Thomas was periodically 'lifted up horizontally by eight men, who then took turns digging their fingers into his stomach area and biting him on his sides' (142). He was given only a cup of water each day, but no food. Stated the judgment: 'At one point he was taken to a creek, stripped naked and forced to walk backwards into the water and to "go under three times." He was then whipped or beaten with cedar branches, hard enough to raise welts on his skin' (142). Finally, Mr Thomas began to suffer from a pre-existing ulcer, and was taken to hospital for treatment. The attending physician testified that he was suffering from 'dehydration and multiple contusions' in addition to the peptic ulcer (144).

Two of the defendants in the case were elders, whose responsibility was to ensure that the initiation was properly carried out according to custom. One elder testified that it was culturally appropriate to 'grab' an intransigent potential initiate at the request of another band member, and he stated that they decided to make the initiation easier for Mr Thomas in comparison to what they themselves had experienced in the past. He personally observed the ceremony to ensure that no harm would be done. He also acknowledged that, earlier in 1988, an initiate had actually died during the ceremony. By the judgment, the plaintiff, Mr Thomas, was awarded $12,000 in damages for 'assault, battery and false imprisonment.' Clearly, what we have here is a clash of cultures and legal traditions.

Spirit Dancing is easily misunderstood when stripped of the proper cultural context as described in the judgment (as any biomedical practice or European religious service would be). A proper understanding of this cultural context (see Jilek 1982b), as expressed by the elders, provides a very different view of the process of initiation into the dance which Mr Thomas underwent. But, as was pointed out, Mr Thomas did not believe in this aspect of Coast Salish culture, and the courts supported his assertion that the initiation was nothing more than a kind of torture. The lessons in this case for Aboriginal medicine are clear: there are inherent legal dangers, since not all Aboriginal people are equally supportive of their heritages. While we are unaware of any legal cases involving an Aboriginal healer charged with practising medicine without a licence, or with endangering a life, it would seem inevitable that some will occur. Indeed, the most common of healing ceremonies, the sweat lodge, entails intense physical stress, and sooner or later someone may die while participating in one. Biomedical practitioners are legally protected in the event that a patient dies while under their care, as long as they have followed accepted medical procedure in a competent fashion. Aboriginal healers do not appear to have that protection.[3]

One hospital, St Mary's in Tucson, Arizona, has apparently attempted to deal directly with the problem of malpractice. In an 1989 interview with one of the authors (Waldram), an Aboriginal healer who is on staff at the hospital stated that the administration had taken out malpractice insurance on his behalf, but not at his request. We are unaware of any other such cases in Canada or the United States, though they may exist.

Within this context, the position adopted by the Government of Ontario in its new Aboriginal health policy is perplexing (Ontario 1994). The policy statement, while indicating that traditional Aboriginal healing will be 'protected from government regulation,' is remarkably vague. It is not clear if separate legislation to protect Aboriginal healers will be passed, or if changes will be made to the Criminal Code (a federal statute). It is also not clear if Ontario is guaranteeing both Aboriginal healers and patients protection from civil lawsuits, and if in so doing it is denying individuals the rights of protection and redress under the law, both civilly and criminally. Ontario's policy opens up a complex issue with little evidence that these complexities have been thoroughly understood and addressed.

THE THREAT TO ABORIGINAL HEALING TRADITIONS POSED BY FORMALIZATION AND COLLABORATION

Chapter 5 described the manner in which Aboriginal healing traditions were embedded within their host cultures. Indeed, one must view this form of healing as inherently cultural, where definitions of illness and modes of treatment, issues of efficacy, and the transmission of medical knowledge are all culturally determined. Chapter 5 also concluded by examining the historic threats to Aboriginal medicine and culture posed by government policy and church actions. Few would consider that the recent trend towards a spiritual revival among Aboriginal peoples, including the movement to accept traditional medicine often to the point of making it more formally available and even collaborating with bio-medicine, is actually a threat to Aboriginal cultures.

That current trends pose such a threat is evident from a critical examination of the issues. The study by D.E. Young and colleagues (1989) is particularly useful in this regard, as it is an excellent documentation of the activities of one healer (Russell Willier) who, at the time of their study, was openly contemplating establishing a clinic to make Aboriginal medicine more readily available to both Aboriginal and non-Aboriginal people. Part of his concern was that Aboriginal healing traditions were disappearing, there were few healers left, and most young people were not interested in learning these healing arts. Willier's healing methods were clearly traditional: they involved prolonged, intensive treatments using both spiritual and herbal means. In some cases, patients essentially moved in with Willier and his family, and treatments took many days. Custom dictated that Willier could not charge for his treatment, but that patients would offer a gift of some sort according to their own conscience. Let us speculate what would happen if a healer was able to formalize his or her medical services through the development of a clinic.

Formalization would bring with it an increase in demand for the healer's services. Both Aboriginal and non-Aboriginal people would be made aware of the healer's abilities and willingness to treat patients. There is a significant non-Aboriginal population which generally uses a variety of alternative medical systems (Eisenberg et al. 1993), and they would likely place a strong demand on the healer. Given this increase in demand, a number of questions become pertinent. Would the healer have enough time to treat each patient in the culturally appropriate, time-consuming manner? In Willier's efforts to treat non-Aboriginal psoriasis patients, he was frustrated by his lack of control over the patients, and subsequently indicated that the treatments would have been more successful had he been able to treat them on his reserve, rather than in an Edmonton clinic. But even here, he was treating a *group* of patients, not a usual traditional approach. Would the increase in demand require that healers use more group approaches? Would they have to take short cuts? Would they have enough time to prepare the herbal medicines? Indeed, would there be an overwhelming demand placed on the plants such that they would be overharvested? Would the healer be required to turn people away who requested help, something that traditionally was not appropriate for a healer to do except for good reason (such as an inability to help with a particular problem). And finally, with an increase in demand, would the healer be able to rely on the traditional form of payment to support self and family? These are not merely academic questions. In fact, in Willier's case, he set up a non-profit organization to raise funds to establish a traditional healing clinic on his reserve (D.E. Young, Ingram, and Swartz 1988). In a more recent development, Willier has installed a telephone answering machine (and fax) in Edmonton to record calls from potential patients; he visits the city for a few days each week, checks his calls, and then follows up on the cases with home visits (D.E. Young personal communication with Waldram, 1993). These are new initiatives which are most certainly a departure from traditional healing practices.

Given that there is a relative shortage of Aboriginal healers practising in Canada and that an increase in demand would invariably follow any formalization of traditional medicine, the cultural underpinnings of the healing traditions would be threatened. Healers and other spiritual people already working with large Aboriginal populations are under a great deal of stress because of overwork. For instance, elders who work in federal prisons generally find that the individual needs of inmates far exceed the time and resources available; as more Aboriginal inmates continue to rediscover their spiritual roots, the workload increases. Traditional Aboriginal medicine works according to its own time framework, and the assembly-line medical treatment characteristic of biomedicine is foreign to it. But any increase in demand for traditional Aboriginal services would lead to intense pressures to alter the mode of delivery and would, in effect, result in a change in the nature of those healing traditions. The cultural implications are clear.

CONCLUSIONS

Aboriginal medical traditions are alive and well in Canada today, and they appear to be undergoing a revitalization as their forms of treatment are recognized as those most appropriate for many of the health and behavioural problems experienced by Aboriginal people. Traditional approaches to healing may prove to be the most effective in the areas of alcohol and drug abuse, forensic treatment, and psychosocial distress, the areas in which they are now employed. The linkage of healing and spirituality with cultural identity is evident in these various healing initiatives developed by Aboriginal people, as the historic processes of deculturation and despiritualization are reversed as part of a broad movement towards the 'healing' of the Aboriginal population. Medical pluralism provides both empowerment and culturally appropriate treatment for patients, and it too is likely to continue into the future. There is still some concern regarding the relative lack of healers, and the lack of interest of younger people in learning about traditional medicine. Various initiatives to make Aboriginal medicine more formally available, including the development of models of collaboration, will likely continue. These issues are best left with the Aboriginal community to determine, since any change in the current situation of traditional Aboriginal medicine will result in other, broader cultural changes. However, it is incumbent upon biomedical practitioners and researchers to learn more about traditional medicine, and for Aboriginal healers to overcome their reluctance to discuss their medical approaches, so that the best interests of those who are ill can be served. The current movement towards self-determination in health provides perhaps the greatest opportunity to resolve some of these complex issues.

10

Self-determination and health care

The 1990s will no doubt go down in Canadian history as the decade in which Aboriginal peoples made significant strides towards becoming self-determining peoples. The road to self-determination has been long, and fraught with difficulties. One of the stumbling blocks in recent years has been the problem of defining self-determination in a manner acceptable to all the Aboriginal groups, all provincial governments, the federal government, and Canadians in general. This problem has also pervaded the self-determination movement in the area of health care. Our intent in this chapter is to examine this movement critically. There is much in the area of self-determination of health that warrants praise and holds promise, but the road is hardly clear.

Health, in general, has never received the kind of attention that other aspects of self-determination have garnered. For the most part, lip-service has been paid to matters of health care, with the demands for 'Indian control of Indian health' competing with other demands, such as those for control over education and social services, especially child welfare. Because the urgent need to improve the economic situation of Aboriginal peoples logically underlies all other questions, it has attracted the greatest attention, and one can argue that improvements in health, through changes to the health care system, are not likely to be dramatic in the absence of more basic changes in the socio-economic position of Aboriginal peoples. But, while economic and constitutional matters have made the headlines and occupied the Aboriginal organizations to a great extent, there have also been some interesting and significant changes with respect to health care.

THE SIX NATIONS IROQUOIS: AN EARLY EXAMPLE OF SELF-
DETERMINATION IN HEALTH CARE

The issue of self-determination in health care is not exclusively a recent development. Historically, Aboriginal peoples were not simply passive recipients of European and Euro-Canadian medical care and the culture change that often accompanied it. Such care was actively sought out when deemed necessary, but Aboriginal peoples retained a strong measure of control over their health care by retaining important elements of their traditional medical systems. The case of the Six Nations (or Grand River) Iroquois, as documented by Weaver (1972), demonstrates the extent to which one Aboriginal group was willing to go to ensure local control of developing medical services.[1]

In 1784 and 1785, some 1,600 Iroquois (mostly Mohawks, but also including the Oneida, Onondaga, Seneca, Cayuga, and Tuscarora) came to the area along the Grand River in southwestern Ontario where they were to settle following the American Revolution, in which they had supported the British. Government assistance was provided to the Iroquois from the outset as payment for their role in the war, and under Joseph Brant they began a new life in what would become Canada. Brant believed strongly in the sovereignty of the Iroquois, and this was a view also held by many of his followers. Sovereignty was an issue that pervaded Iroquois relations with the British and, subsequently, Canadian governments, relations that included arrangements for the provision of medical services.

In the period 1784 to 1850, medical assistance was offered by itinerant physicians, including physicians in the employ of the New England Company and local physicians from neighbouring towns such as Brantford. When smallpox threatened the community in 1842, the Iroquois made arrangements to be vaccinated, contracting with a local doctor and agreeing to pay him one dollar per head for vaccination. As Weaver explains, this was a period in which physicians were largely the last resort during episodes of illness, and the traditional medical system of the Iroquois was still dominant.

By the mid-nineteenth century, the Six Nations people began to have medical care provided by resident physicians, who were paid monthly salaries out of the Indians' band funds (plus a sum for the purchase of medicines). Although these physicians were appointed through the Indian Department of the colonial government, the Six Nations were held to be responsible for actual costs. Along with this responsibility for costs came the right of the Six Nations to control physician services. Such control was one element of the expression of their autonomy.

The first resident physician, Dr R.H. Dee, was appointed medical officer of health for the reserve in 1853, and enjoyed the support of the people until his retirement in 1889. Most of the medical services were delivered at the physician's office, although 'house calls' were also made, which afforded the opportunity for the physician to demonstrate various medical practices. Nevertheless, traditional medicine remained influential, especially among the Longhouse people, the traditionalists who eschewed the Christianity of some other Iroquois. One physician, writing in 1898, stated the following about Longhouse supporters, whom he referred to as 'pagans':

Among the Pagans it is quite common to find a patient's bed surrounded by curtains to keep him or her from being defiled by contact with the outer world. The sick person may be kept for days in this seclusion and fed on *white* chickens and *white* beans, this diet being symbolical of purity. The Indian medicine women ... administer some medicine, usually herbs or roots, in the efficacy of which they themselves have no faith, but put all their trust in superstitious ceremonies, and invocations to the Great Spirit. A physician is only called after this method of treatment has proved to be of no avail, or after some intelligent advisor has succeeded in getting the patient's consent to have the doctor. (cited in Weaver 1972:43; italics in original)

By the 1890s, considerable pressure was being placed upon the Department of Indian Affairs and the Six Nations Band Council to improve medical services. A hospital had been opened in Brantford in 1885, and it immediately began receiving Iroquois patients, but a medical officer for the band, Dr L. Secord, argued that more biomedical services were required to stem the tide of tuberculosis and other problems. He lobbied for the construction of a hospital on the reserve, and the establishment of a local Board of Health, both of which were ultimately approved despite the reluctance of both the band and Indian Affairs. Dr Secord himself was under suspicion by the Iroquois for 'improper practice' at the time, and hence his influence with the band was waning. Part of the problem stemmed from Secord's refusal to accept the power of the band, which felt it had the right to hire and dismiss physicians by virtue of the fact that it paid for these services out of band funds. Indeed, it is apparent that a struggle between the doctor and the Band Council developed when

Secord, acting alone, dismissed an assistant physician. The band's response was to demand that Indian Affairs reinstate the individual. The band was also angry that Secord refused to live permanently on the reserve, and that he pushed change on the people too quickly.

Although the Band Council paid for the medical services out of band funds, it is apparent that the notion of self-determination also operated at the family level. It was the family's responsibility to pay for the costs of some medical treatments, such as hospitalization or specialists' services, that were obtained off-reserve, and the band occasionally withheld a family's annuity if medical accounts remained outstanding. However, if a family was unable to pay, particularly where illness prevented the breadwinner from working, then the accounts would be paid out of band funds. Nevertheless, general physician services were the responsibility of the band in general.

In 1900, the band passed the *Six Nations Public Health Act*, further expanding its control over the delivery of medical services on the reserve. Concomitant with the new act was the development of the Board of Health, which functioned from 1901 until 1924 (when it was replaced by another body). The board was given a broad mandate, and many of its activities were in the domain of public health. For instance, the inspection of food, dwellings, and water systems and the handling of other health hazard complaints were assigned to the board. The board was also given the power to declare quarantines in cases of infectious disease. The ultimate effectiveness of the board, however, is debatable; for instance, there is evidence that only once during its existence did it attempt to inspect ice and food sold on the reserve, and it handled only a few complaints about health hazards. It was considerably more active in assisting in the control of infectious diseases; for example, it assisted in the fumigating of houses in which diseases had been found.

In 1908, the Band Council approved the construction of a tent hospital on the reserve and formed a Hospital Board to manage the facility and to deal with Indian Affairs on hospital matters. The original intent was to treat tubercular patients, although many other problems were also attended to. A permanent facility, the Lady Willingdon Hospital, was built in 1927, partly with Six Nations money. Not surprisingly, the community therefore felt it had some degree of control over the facility, and one chief even attempted to restrict the hospital to Six Nations patients only (excluding other Indian patients); he was unsuccessful.

The medical affairs of the community and the people's relationship with the federal government in the early twentieth century were conditioned by the increasing interference of the government in Six Nations

internal matters. Most significant of these was the government's determination to destroy the hereditary system of government and replace it
with an elected Band Council. The elected system was established in 1924,
but the tensions between the hereditary council and its supporters and
adherents of the elected system continued throughout the twentieth century and still affect the Iroquois communities today. In the medical sphere,
the deteriorating relations between the federal Indian department and
the Band Council continued; between 1900 and 1927, five doctors in
succession were hired as medical superintendent for the community, four
of whom were ultimately dismissed by the council after being called upon
to respond to various charges. Secord, for instance, was dismissed for
refusing to reside on the reserve. The political struggle between the council and the federal government is clearly evident in a 1910 resolution
dismissing another physician:

The Council after hearing the Petition and charges against the Medical Supt.
Doctor Holmes read decided that he be dismissed from the position of Medical
Supt. of the Six Nations upon the grounds as set forth in the petition fyled [sic] by
the warriors charging him with negligence of his duties and a lack of regard and
attention in cases where he is summoned to visit patients, also upon the grounds
that he refused to come before the Council when officially summoned by it to face
his accusers, and answer their charges. There are also other charges which were
read to the Council and have not been refuted.

The Council is of the opinion that, as Doctor Holmes is paid out of the funds of
the Six Nations, he should at least have been courteous enough to the Six Nations
Council to have attended the meeting when summoned instead of writing an
insulting letter to it in which he refused to come.

The Council is alive to the fact that there must be sympathy between patient
and the Doctor and as there can be none exist between the petitioners and him
his efficiency and usefulness will be utterly gone in so far as they are concerned.
(cited in Weaver 1972:50)

In each of the five cases, a question arose regarding the authority of the
council in this matter, and the dismissals did not receive immediate sanction by Indian Affairs. However, the physicians eventually resigned anyway.

The Band Council also argued with Indian Affairs regarding the appointment of new physicians, stating in 1911 that 'The Council claim that
the appointment of Medical Supt. of this Reserve belongs to this Council
and will therefore insist that they must have something to say in the new

appointment that is going to be made now' (cited in ibid. 52). When a short list of physicians to be considered was not provided to the council, a delegation went to Ottawa to argue the band's viewpoint, whereupon the council was given the authority to write the contract for the position. Nevertheless, the government's continued refusal to allow the council to select its own physicians remained a source of tension for many years.

Politics on the Six Nations reserve remained volatile into the 1950s and 1960s, characterized by unsuccessful attempts in 1959 by some Mohawk Warriors and Longhouse supporters to depose the elected Band Council and replace it with the traditional hereditary system. The Mohawks in particular seemed aggressive in their assertions of sovereignty, and many refused to register for mother's allowance and other social welfare benefits that developed in this period.

With the expansion of hospital services in the 1950s, many Six Nations residents began to find employment in the medical sector. The Six Nations and some of the other Iroquoian communities are renowned today for the number and variety of professional people who have their roots there. At Six Nations, since 1950, most of the hospital nursing staff have been local people, as were most of the laboratory technicians and effectively all of the support staff. Some reduction in hospital staffing and services occurred after 1961, when the federal government began to redirect resources to facilities in surrounding towns. There were also changes in the administration of medical services. When in 1956 hospital accounts were directed to individual patients, many residents saw an emerging threat to the essentially free health care they had been receiving. The idea of hospitalization insurance was also not well received. When the Indian Health Service attempted to undertake a survey of residents in anticipation of extending health insurance, the council refused to appoint the surveyors; it took the position that the Six Nations are not financially responsible for their medical care. In particular, it argued that the Six Nations previous financial investment in the Lady Willingdon Hospital rendered them exempt from hospitalization costs of any kind, and further that many residents could not afford to pay for medical care. It also noted that the *Indian Act* contained no provision requiring them to pay for such services. An attempt by the government to carry out the survey anyway was unsuccessful. As Weaver (1972:87) indicates, at the time of her study in 1963 and 1964 it was widely believed on the Six Nations reserve that medical bills could not be legally collected, and individuals were left to their own consciences to decide whether they were liable or whether the government was responsible for settling accounts. Nevertheless, little by little, compulsory hospital insurance was extended throughout the community.

The Six Nations Iroquois, and indeed other Iroquoian communities, have continued to assert their sovereignty in many areas for more than two centuries. In the medical sphere, their efforts to retain control have been to a great extent successful, though not without much conflict both internally and with the federal government. They provide an excellent case study of local control of medical care, demonstrating continuity of approach over a long period. For them, local control is not only an Aboriginal right, but a right which they have historically exercised, with some success.

THE ROAD TO SELF-DETERMINATION

As we have seen in previous chapters, Aboriginal peoples have retained many elements of their traditional medical systems, and this fact alone suggests that they have also retained some measure of self-determination. As long as some options were available, Aboriginal people dissatisfied with the services rendered by a physician could seek out a traditional healer (or vice versa). Aboriginal people as *consumers* of health care have constructed a coherent, complex system out of disparate biomedical and traditional services, and therefore practise self-determination (or empowerment) on the individual level. The main focus in the movement towards self-determination in health care has been on a different level, however – that of the delivery of biomedical services and the role of traditional healing within the context of those services.

In 1979, the federal government unveiled its new Indian Health Policy. Central to this new policy was the belief that a simple increase in health programs and services would not result in a substantial improvement in health status. What was required was increased input by Aboriginal peoples themselves. Furthermore, the policy emphasized that spiritual health was as important as physical health, thus setting the stage for the re-emergence of traditional healing services. In that same year, the federal government also endorsed the Alma-Ata Declaration of 1978. This declaration was signed by 134 countries, under the auspices of the World Health Organization, and reiterated the definition of health first published in the preamble to its 1948 constitution. This definition states that 'health is ... a state of complete physical, mental and social wellbeing, and not merely the absence of disease,' a definition which, while broad, is still considered paramount today (World Health Organization 1978:2). In anticipating 'Health for All by the Year 2000,' the declaration endorsed the 'Primary Health Care' (PHC) movement, with a focus on the meeting of basic human health needs, such as the need for safe water, nutritious food, maternal and child care, immunization, local disease control and medical services, and health education. In proposing that health be considered a fundamental human right, Alma-Ata presented a blueprint for the development of local, community-level services with, implicitly, some measure of local control. Canada, by virtue of signing the declaration, explicitly agreed.

In 1980, Thomas Berger[2] submitted the report of the Advisory Commission on Indian and Inuit Health Consultation (Berger 1980). This may seem somewhat unusual in that the consultation began *after* the announcement of the new Indian Health Policy in 1979, and hence was unable to inform the development of that policy, but in the history of government-Indian relations, this is not so surprising. The intent of the commission seems to have been to develop a method for enacting a community consultation process as a step towards identifying the shape of the new institutions that would be required to implement the health policy. The report recommended that funds be allocated to various Aboriginal organizations 'to develop the consultative process,' and that the commission in effect be made into a permanent, Indian-controlled, national health organization. The latter recommendation was not implemented, but the subsequent health transfer process appears to have benefited to some extent from Berger's detailing of community participation. Overall, the report seems to have had little impact, no doubt the result of its timing, which meant that some of its recommended initiatives were already being considered by the federal government.

The 1983 report of the Special Committee on Indian Self-Government (also known as the Penner Committee after its chair, Keith Penner), added its voice to increasing demands for changes in Aboriginal health care. Although only a small portion of the report dealt with health matters, it emphasized the need for a more holistic approach to health care, incorporating traditional approaches as well as biomedical ones and emphasizing preventive health programs. Interestingly, the report stated that 'witnesses did not specify how health care services should be provided. The emphasis was on control of the system rather than designing new systems' (Penner 1983:35). Aboriginal control, the witnesses argued, should be flexible when implemented, allowing for negotiations with federal and provincial governments and agencies, as well as private enterprises, to develop an integrated model of health care services.

For registered Indians, health transfer began in 1982 with the Community Health Demonstration Program, a plan to allow bands to experiment with different models of delivery and different degrees of control. Thirty-one such projects ultimately received funding. However, it became apparent that other transfer initiatives were slowed or stalled while these 'experiments' were undertaken (D.E. Young and Smith 1991:19). A critique of the program by Garro and colleagues (1986:281), focusing on the experiences of Sandy Bay, Manitoba, suggests that many Aboriginal organizations asked a fundamental – and quite reasonable – question: why was a 'demonstration' of Aboriginal control necessary? Furthermore, they wondered what would become of the projects when the two-year funding was terminated? Apparently, the project's objectives were not well thought out, and its principles not uniformly applied. Hence, projects were funded that did not even propose the transfer of health services; in fact, only seven actually dealt with the transfer issue (ibid. 282).

The Sandy Bay proposal represented a continuation of past efforts to improve nursing and other services by hiring a health coordinator on the reserve, an initiative that was stymied by a lack of federal funding until the Demonstration Program was announced. The proposal also dealt with the transfer of health services to the band. According to Garro and colleagues, the project allowed the band to undertake a health-needs survey and develop a local Health Committee, and to refine administrative policies. The band was also able to initiate more prevention programs. However, there were some problems. Apparently, the community members were not easily involved in health matters, and they tended to retain a view of the nursing station as primarily a place for treatment. Furthermore, there were some problems in developing the Health Committee to a point where it could offer guidance to the health centre. Some progress was made in these areas towards the end of the two-year project, but obviously the short time span was insufficient to mobilize and empower the community fully in the complex area of health matters. As Garro and colleagues (ibid. 283) note, it was the fact that the band had some previous experience of working in health areas that allowed it to accomplish what it did. In general, the Demonstration Program did not allow sufficient time for communities to hire, train, and mobilize.

In their paper, Garro and colleagues were quite critical of the approach to health transfer taken by the government in the Demonstration Program. Indian organizations, while consulted, were not made aware that only communities funded under the Demonstration Program would be allowed to transfer health services to local control. This was, in these author's views, 'a breach of the consultation process proclaimed in the

1979 Health Policy,' and represented 'a unilateral decision [which] does little to engender trust and cooperation between government and Indian groups.' Furthermore, the Demonstration Program focused on the band level, prohibiting a 'unified expression of Indian interests in the field of health care.' Indeed, this approach to self-determination, stressing band-level initiatives and the transfer of some federal powers, was part of the broader federal approach, one that continues to be much criticized by some Aboriginal groups.

THE INDIAN HEALTH TRANSFER POLICY

The Community Health Demonstration Program was effectively terminated in 1985. In 1986, Indian bands in Canada were told of the formation of the Program Transfer and Development Directorate to direct the new Indian Health Transfer Policy. The basic premise of the policy is that Indian bands can move slowly, by stages, to the point where they ultimately obtain control over the delivery of health services. According to the federal government, the policy was developed 'after much discussion and consultation within and outside' the Medical Services Branch (MSB) (Lynch 1991:174). The approach emphasized a federal perspective on self-determination, to be implemented on a community-by-community basis. A 1987 booklet published by the Department of National Health and Welfare outlined the steps that bands were required to take in the process of gaining control. These steps would prove to be complicated and frustrating.

Three main steps were identified in the transfer process. The first is 'Pre-Transfer Planning.' This planning process involves assessing the current state of health care delivery, identifying the most important needs, and examining how the health care budget should be organized to meet these needs. This stage requires the development of a 'Community Health Plan,' a document designed to explain how the community would manage health resources. Funding to develop a plan is available after a funding proposal has been prepared and accepted by the MSB (Canada, DNHW, *Health Transfer Newsletter*, Spring 1989:2), but there is a two-year limit on the duration of funding. The Community Health Plan is then submitted to a review committee, a group with substantial government representation. Included in this committee are the assistant deputy minister of the MSB, plus the directors general of Program Transfer, Policy and Planning, and the Indian and Northern Health Service. If successful, the community is allowed to move to the next stage, that of 'Negotiation.'

The process of negotiation begins with acceptance of the plan by the

MSB, which retains the power to return plans approved by the review committee to the community, for instance where MSB determines that more information on some aspect of the plan is required. Once the plan is accepted by MSB, then a 'Memorandum of Understanding' is drawn up, outlining the negotiation process leading up to a Transfer Agreement. The Transfer Agreement, once approved, has a duration of three to five years, after which a review of the implementation of the Community Health Plan is undertaken in preparation for a renewal of funding (ibid.).

With the effecting of health transfer, the chief and council of the band become responsible for the plan and all health matters. They are required to keep their band members informed of the progress of the health plan, but are accountable to the minister of national health and welfare for executing the terms of the transfer agreement.

Some Indian leaders expressed reservations about the health transfer program. At a national conference in 1989, Georges Erasmus, then National Chief of the Assembly of First Nations, argued that 'it is not possible to consider health transfer in isolation from all other developments taking place in Indian communities' (Canada, DNHW, *Health Transfer Newsletter*, Special Issue 1990:2). In fact, the whole idea of the 'transfer' or devolution of any services to Indian bands did not fit with Erasmus's view of self-determination, focused as it was on having the 'inherent' right to self-government accepted in the Canadian Constitution. Nevertheless, he was forced to accept that those bands who saw health transfer as a way to meet their own needs and goals had a right to participate in the plan. Indeed, it quickly became apparent that many bands were willing to run the gauntlet of the health transfer process; by the fall of 1989, fifty-eight pre-transfer projects were under way, involving 212 Indian communities across the country (Canada, DNHW, *Health Transfer Newsletter*, Fall 1989:1). Most were at the earliest stages, but their numbers clearly indicated that this was one initiative that many bands were willing to take seriously. Some opposition still remained, however, including that offered by the Union of Ontario Indians and the Assembly of First Nations, who argued that the health transfer process was an abrogation of the federal government's responsibilities for Indian health.

The 1989 health transfer conference also brought calls from Indian delegates to remove some of the constraints built into the process. The two-year limit on funding for the development of Community Health Plans and the limited funding for health-needs assessments were two areas that generated much discussion. Staff training also required greater funding. There were also calls for giving Indians the opportunity to take control of existing MSB facilities, such as the Sioux Lookout Zone Hospital, as part of the transfer process (although these hospitals would ultimately be phased out).

By the fall of 1990, eight transfer agreements had been signed, and some sixty-seven bands were involved in pre-transfer planning. These agreements were signed both with single bands and with larger tribal councils representing multiple bands (D.E. Young and Smith 1991:20). The first agreement was signed with the William Charles Band at Montreal Lake, Saskatchewan, followed by the Sandy Lake and Matthias Colomb Bands in Manitoba, the Nuu-Chah-Nulth Tribal Council in British Columbia, and the River Desert First Nation in Quebec. Two years later, at the end of 1992, there had been twenty-three transfer agreements signed, representing seventy-one different bands in British Columbia, Saskatchewan, Manitoba, Quebec, Newfoundland, and New Brunswick (Canada, DNHW, *Health Transfer Newsletter*, Winter 1992:5).

The Matthias Colomb Band was the first to create a Health Authority Board, under the *Indian Act*, responsible for the delivery of community health services, personnel and financial administration, policy development and implementation, operation of the nursing station, and contract negotiations with health care providers. The health board concept was developed in conjunction with the initiatives of the Swampy Cree Tribal Council, which, through the formation of the Cree Nation Tribal Health Centre, was able to coordinate the development of proposals and plans for implementing transfers for six bands (Connell et al. 1991:44). The philosophy of the tribal council with regard to health transfer is guarded, and perhaps characteristic of that of many groups involved in the process: 'Overall, this policy direction had been criticized as an attempt to abrogate treaty rights and have Indian people administer their own misery. Nevertheless, we entered the transfer process – but with our eyes wide open. We saw transfer as a way to achieve some of our objectives and we felt we could look after ourselves in dealing with the government' (ibid. 44).

THE MONTREAL LAKE CASE

The William Charles Band, located at Montreal Lake in Saskatchewan, is not only the first band to have obtained control of health care under the transfer policy; it is also the best-documented case. Although an overall evaluation of the transfer policy across the country has yet to be undertaken, the Montreal Lake case gives an idea of the kinds of changes that local control has engendered.

The William Charles Band consisted of a total membership of 1,800, with close to 800 living on the reserve, located 100 kilometres north of Prince Albert. In 1984, the band commenced a feasibility study for a new health facility on the reserve, in conjunction with the MSB. The study indicated that the living conditions on the reserve were poor: only five houses had running water and proper sewage disposal, and most were overcrowded. Economic conditions were also poor, with most families reliant on welfare for at least part of the year. There was a serious alcohol- and drug-abuse problem, and the rate of family violence and sexual abuse was high. The people suffered from high rates of respiratory diseases, gastro-intestinal diseases, and skin infections. The study also documented a lack of health care knowledge, poor self-care, and a lack of reliable medical service. The community was serviced by a half-time nurse and two community health representatives. Three individuals worked in ad- dictions. Most medical treatment was obtained in Prince Albert (M. Moore et al. 1990:153–4; Bird and Moore 1991:47).

The study determined that there was a need for a new facility for primary health care under band control with better access to physicians and nurses, so that health care could be delivered to the people, rather than people being moved to health care facilities in Prince Albert (in 1984, travel costs for medical reasons were $236,000). The band's actions on this front actually predated the Health Transfer Program, and therefore there was some foot-dragging by the federal government. But in 1987 the MSB accepted the band's proposal, and they entered into the negotiating phase.[3]

According to the band representatives involved, 'the negotiation pro- cess was very stressful, partly because such detailed agreements had never been drafted before in Canada and all parties were learning as we went along' (Bird and Moore 1991:47). The transfer agreement which emerged from these negotiations was comprehensive and demanding. For instance, it committed both the federal government and the band to ensuring that the quality of health services would not diminish under band control, and allowed the federal government to 'intervene to stabi- lize the health service in times of emergency or institutional difficulty' (ibid. 48). Nevertheless, both parties were committed to work together to achieve the aims of the health plan. Not surprisingly, the agreement also noted that it did not prejudice treaty rights and future claims (the band taking the position that health care is a treaty right).

After three years of planning, the new William Charles Health Centre was opened on the Montreal Lake reserve. The health centre was designed to provide a wide array of services. Many of these services were educational and preventive in orientation. Among them were school-based health education; immunization programs; alcohol education, referral, and follow-up; prenatal health education; and health promotion and education for chronic disease patients. The new centre also provided more consistent medical treatment, calling for a physician to visit the community one day each week, a dentist once a month, and full-time community nursing services (M. Moore et al. 1990:154). The original hope to formally include traditional medical services was put on hold while the health centre personnel investigated the legal implications of such action.

To date, an epidemiological investigation of the outcome of the process of local control for Montreal Lake has not been undertaken, but anecdotal information and the observations of health centre staff indicate that there have been some important changes. In general, the band members have come to feel more secure about their health, as a result of having better qualified personnel available on a more regular basis. Emergencies that would have required evacuation to the city are now more likely to be handled at the community level. In some cases – with childbirth and coronary attacks, for example – the availability of immediate medical service has been rewarded. The educational component of the centre has encouraged more people to attempt home management of minor illnesses (especially management of children's illnesses by parents), and has led to a reduction in after-hours calls at the nursing station. Some elders, who previously tended to avoid the nursing station and city medical facilities, have become more comfortable with the services provided at the centre, perhaps partly because it allows them to use their Cree language; as a result, more elders have become amenable to periodic medical examinations. Indeed, according to Moore, Forbes, and Henderson (1990:157), cultural and linguistic compatibility has been an essential ingredient in the health centre's success. 'The feeling of just being a number in a "White" medical clinic where English is the only language has been replaced by being served by people who know the name, family members, customs and language of the Elders. People living on a trapline with no washing facilities can come directly to the health centre knowing they are welcome and that staff are accustomed to seeing people in such circumstances. Instead of feeling a sense of shame and uncomfortable visibility, people feel at home. Translation is never a problem as all but three staff speak Cree, and many translators are available.'

The preliminary reports also indicate that the number of immunizations of children increased substantially after the centre was opened. An examination of patient charts for the first quarters of 1989 and 1990 indicated that some changes have ensued in health status. For instance, whereas there were fifteen hospital admissions for ear infections during the year prior to the opening of the centre, in this period in 1989–90, there were none. There is some suggestion that hospitalizations for upper-respiratory infections have declined. However, these data are incomplete and in no way represent a legitimate epidemiological inquiry. The perceptions of the nurses nevertheless suggest that, while the centre received a 'backlog' of patients when it first opened (individuals reluctant to seek care under the former system), after a year there was a noticeable decline, and a corresponding increase in the numbers of those seeking treatment at earlier stages of illness. Health centre physicians have also noted a decline in emergency out-patient visits (ibid. 161).

There is no question that the creation of the William Charles Health Centre and the transfer of control over health care to the band have resulted in an important shift in attitudes and practices. According to Moore, Forbes, and Henderson (ibid. 163), this represents one of the more intangible benefits of the transfer process:

Before the health centre, the community fabric was disintegrating. Residents lived in considerable fear, isolation and despair. The relations among health service providers and other community services reflected this isolation as well as contributed to it. The staff and to a lesser extent the health committee have begun to recreate the sense of community. They have discovered ways to support each other and work together, yet maintain separate identities. They provide a role model for the concept of community for the people whom they serve ... It is perhaps this element of the spirit that causes the health centre to be seen as a 'community centre' ... People have a greater sense of 'belonging' – an element that has been missing.

Conclusive epidemiological data supporting these observations may yet emerge; as health researchers we would encourage such inquiry. Whether health transfer in and of itself will actually result in improved health and health care is still very much an open question, based as it is on faith in the idea that local control inevitably leads to better health practices. And the health transfer concept still has many critics.

A CRITIQUE OF THE HEALTH TRANSFER PROCESS

As we have already suggested, some Aboriginal groups were sceptical of the health transfer process. The Assembly of First Nations (1988) suggested that transfer was ultimately designed to assist the government in reducing its spending on Indian health, and therefore abrogated treaty rights and the federal government's fiduciary responsibility to Indians. In the light of the government's own exercise in determining where budget allocations could be cut across all federal programs (as evidenced in the so-called Nielsen Report, see Weaver 1986), it appears that the fears that there was, indeed, a 'hidden agenda' behind the health transfer program may have been well-founded.

Dara Culhane Speck (1989:207), in her critical analysis of the transfer policy, argues in favour of the hidden-agenda hypothesis, stating that the policy 'does not represent a positive departure from the past or a funda-mental change in position by the federal government' with respect to Indian health care. Particularly problematic for her is the government's continued refusal to accept a legal responsibility for Indian health, and what she sees as the attempt ultimately to transfer the responsibility for Indian health to the provincial governments (a step also recommended in the 1969 White Paper's proposals to terminate Indian status and turn over program administration to the provinces, a change the Indians have generally resisted). Culhane Speck even argues that the transfer policy is inherently assimilationist and that government simply parrots the rhetoric of self-determination while unilaterally diverging from the Indian meaning of the concept (a critique advanced by Georges Erasmus, among others).

Culhane Speck identifies a number of flaws in the transfer process. The transfer agreements do not include non-insured benefits, such as prescription eyeglasses, dental work, and transportation costs for medical services. Also excluded from transfer is funding for up-grading and clinical training for outpost nurses, and such federal programs as the National Native Alcohol and Drug Abuse Program. Indeed, according to Culhane Speck, the exclusion of training funds is particularly problematic, since training under band control 'is fundamental to designing culturally and locally appropriate services' (ibid. 200).

Another problem with the policy is that there exists a 'no enrichment' clause, which Culhane Speck argues means there will be no additional funding for communities taking control: their budgets will effectively be frozen as of the date of the transfer. In effect, this would mean that bands would be attempting to introduce new programs to combat the health problems on reserves, but would have to do so by reallocating from existing sources while maintaining the level of health services. In other words, they would have to do more with less. This problem is further compounded by the fact that non-reserve members are not accounted for in the budgeting, and neither are newly reinstated Indians under Bill C-31. Since many of these people will still spend varying amounts of time living on the reserve, and some may move there on a permanent basis (especially if conditions were to improve, which of course is a goal of the transfer process), they will put a strain on the existing services.

Finally, we should note Culhane Speck's view that there are no guarantees that the federal government will continue funding at the band level after the three- to five-year period in which a plan is approved; and, given that the government does not accept a legal or fiduciary responsibility to provide health care, it leaves future funding vulnerable to fiscal restraint programs or shifts in policy. She also questions the fate of those bands who decide not to accept transfer. This is particularly problematic for the future, if the majority of the bands take control and the MSB chooses to vacate the treatment services role.

Despite the problems with the transfer process identified by Culhane Speck, the fact remains that many bands and tribal councils across the country have entered into the process. Before a final judgment can be offered, we need more time to gauge the government's response to the expiration of the first agreements and the need to renegotiate. Will more funding be made available, or will more restrictions be placed on these bands? Furthermore, from a purely health perspective, has transfer truly affected the health status of band members? Health, like other matters, is a component in the political game being played by Aboriginal groups and governments in Canada. 'Control' is the catchword of the current era, built on the faith that positive change will result. In the area of health, the jury is still out on this one, but the signs look positive.

THE NORTHWEST TERRITORIES EXPERIENCE

In preparation for health transfer, in 1982 the federal government transferred the MSB hospital at Iqaluit to the Government of the Northwest Territories (GNWT) (referred to as 'Baffin Phase I'), and in 1985 the GNWT Devolution Office was opened. In 1986, the 'Baffin Phase II' plan was initiated, involving the transfer of the Baffin Zone of Medical Services to the GNWT, followed in 1988 with the transfer of health care throughout the entire Northwest Territories to the GNWT (D.E. Young and Smith 1991:17).

There was, then, some degree of devolution of health services in the Northwest Territories before the implementation of the health transfer program. Emerging from its frustration with the administration of health services by the federal government, the Inuit Tapirisat of Canada supported the transfer of these services to the GNWT. Subsequently, in 1981 the Baffin Regional Hospital Board was created, responsible for administration and patient accommodation in Iqaluit (the location of the Baffin Hospital). MSB retained responsibility for the nursing stations and staff in each community, and for other aspects of medical care. There was broad-based Inuit input into the new board, with Inuit holding seven of eleven positions. When the board was expanded to fifteen members in 1986, the Inuit captured thirteen positions. At that time, the board was renamed the Baffin Regional Health Board (O'Neil 1991). The mandate of the board includes setting broad policies regarding the delivery of health services in relation to community needs, the hiring of staff, the provision of safe patient accommodation, and the administration of the health services budget.

Political issues have intruded into the operation of the board, a common occurrence in the other case studies we have so far discussed. When it became known that some individuals within the region had tested HIV positive, the board debated disclosing the names and communities of these individuals as a means of protecting others. O'Neil (ibid. 52) suggests that this was a cultural response, based upon Inuit concerns to protect the group as a whole, though not without consideration of the rights of the individual. Non-Aboriginal administrative staff held the biomedical view that the confidentiality of patient information should be protected. As a result of further discussions, the board decided to publicize the names of the communities, but not the individuals involved. The Department of Health in Yellowknife requested that it wait until the minister had considered the issue, but were surprised when, a few days later, the existence of the HIV-positive cases in the Northwest Territories was announced on the radio. Subsequently, the board announced that there were precisely three cases in the region, but did not mention actual communities. The GNWT's minister of health responded by stating that the Baffin Regional Health Board would be disciplined for breaking confidentiality. O'Neil (1991:53) concludes that, 'If a primary goal of devolution and the transfer of health services to local control is to facilitate the development of a health care system sensitive to local cultural expression and needs, planners must be willing to consider some cultural principles with which they disagree.' The conflict between 'cultural expression and needs' and emerging public health concerns and knowledge is significant; insofar as traditional cultural views will remain opposed to recent public health initiatives, conflict will continue.[4] This example also suggests that, even with this form of control, some ambiguity still exists with respect to who ultimately controls health policy.

Again, in this case as in the others, it is difficult to examine outcomes critically. O'Neil (1990:190) has suggested that 'devolution of health services has had only minimal impact at the community level in the Baffin region.' But the problem seems to lie not with the services themselves, but with the fact that the extensive bureaucracy that has been established is not working coherently; particularly problematic is the conflict between the region and the territorial levels regarding their approaches to the devolution issue. Politics, again, appears to be interfering with the establishment of true local control.

OTHER EXAMPLES OF SELF-DETERMINATION

Some Aboriginal groups have developed a degree of self-determination in health care through means other than the health transfer process. It would be useful to examine a few such cases.

The first group to sign a comprehensive land claim agreement in Canada in the contemporary era were the Cree and Inuit of James Bay. Under the terms of the *James Bay and Northern Quebec Agreement*, signed in 1975, a Cree Board of Health and Social Services was established in 1978. The overall agreement has apparently led to the development of a Cree regional society in northern Quebec (Salisbury 1986), and the development of a health and social services board can be viewed as fitting within this framework. The mandate of the board is expansive, encompassing all the responsibilities of any health board in Quebec as well as the responsibility to deal directly with health and social services for the Cree. But, despite the agreement, the Cree received considerable opposition to their formation of the board, being forced to undertake legal proceedings and other political action to obtain control, and even then there was an attempt to place the Cree Board of Health under trusteeship in 1980 (Bearskin and Dumont 1991:123).

What makes the Cree situation different from that of many Indian groups in the country is that the *James Bay and Northern Quebec Agreement* removed the federal government's responsibility for much of Cree life, and transferred it to Quebec and the Cree. Hence, the Cree Board of Health is one of many such boards under the auspices of the Quebec government. The Cree have retained all their benefits as Indians, but these are now administered through Quebec. The board itself contains three representatives from each of the nine Cree villages, representatives of the clinical and non-clinical staff, a representative from the parent governmental organization (the Cree Regional Authority), and a representative from the Department of Community Health at Montreal General Hospital. The board oversees the operation of a regional hospital at Chisasibi, and through it the Cree have control over the hiring of health care staff through the village and regional levels. This means that some strides have been made towards developing more culturally appropriate health care, including the establishment of a new nursing program. But, as Bearskin and Dumont (1991:125) note, the Cree Board of Health has been challenged by newly developing health problems, such as heart disease, diabetes, and substance abuse. The lack of availability of Cree professional staff is still an issue as well (Moffatt 1987). Somewhat surprisingly, some Cree view the board as a non-Cree organization, and Bearskin and Dumont (1991:125) candidly point out that such a board is a new entity for the Cree, and that 'It is distant from the traditional organizations that the Cree are used to. So enough time must be given for the Cree to get to know how such an organization functions and to integrate it smoothly into their society.' Obviously, there is more to the issue of local control of health care than simply gaining political control.

For the Cree, the battle to gain control has been a difficult one, fraught with tense negotiations with the Quebec government in particular, and accusations that sufficient funding as called for under the agreement has not been made available. As with other examples, there are as yet no concrete data on the outcome of the Cree experience with the control of health. For instance, Thouez and colleagues (1990:32) have suggested that the Cree harbour a dissatisfaction with the delivery of health care services in their region, primarily because of negative perceptions of the health care personnel. But these authors make no effort to address the question of whether health status has improved since the 1975 agreement. Robinson's (1988) data are not much better; she documents a decline in infant mortality for the Cree, from 49.7 per 1,000 in the 1975–7 period to 22.2 in the 1981–3 period. Post-neonatal mortality and neonatal mortality have also declined appreciably. But there is no evidence to suggest that these changes have occurred as a result of Cree control over health. Furthermore, while anecdotal information suggests that infectious diseases are declining among the Cree, they are being replaced by chronic diseases such as diabetes and alcoholism. Despite this general lack of data, Robinson (ibid. 1611) supports the idea that control of health is important, though adding that 'this control needs to be extended by the training of board members and of Native health professionals and administrators at all levels.' The Cree situation is complicated, however, by all the other social and economic changes which have accompanied the James Bay hydro project.

There have been other initiatives with respect to the process of gaining control over health care. The Alberta Indian Health Care Commission (AIHCC) was established in 1980 to act as a provincial health board for all Alberta Indians, and a local board of health was established on the Blood reserve, the largest in Canada (Nuttall 1982). The objectives of the AIHCC included promoting of local or regional health boards, and planning and developing health care programs and services for reserves. The Blood board essentially has the same objectives, but for the community level. Among other things, the AIHCC has created an urban Community Health Representative (CHR) program in Edmonton and Calgary. Such urban initiatives, though still quite rare, are obviously needed, given increasing rates of urban migration. The Alberta program involves the CHRs in assisting and advocating for urban patients.

In Saskatchewan, the Battlefords Indian Health Centre (BIHC) was opened in 1979. Its mandate is to facilitate the delivery of health care services to a number of reserves in the rural region surrounding the town of North Battleford, and its focus has been primarily preventive. Only a handful of the member reserves had Community Health Representatives, and most people obtained physician services in North Battleford. The centre does not offer clinical physician services, and indeed there was some controversy when the centre attempted to recruit a physician. While two physicians were interviewed for the position, they received a hostile reaction from local doctors, who feared that the health centre would cut into their patient loads. The Saskatchewan Medical Association even ran an ad in a British medical journal discouraging physicians from applying, and one potential physician was told he would not obtain admitting privileges at the local hospital. Eventually, the health centre was forced to reorganize and to drop the idea of providing physician services.

The shift towards more preventive and educational services resulted in the development of a variety of new programs at the BIHC. School-based health programs, public health, dentistry, and nutrition programs have been implemented. A CHR program provides various preventive and education programs on the member reserves. The health centre operates an alcohol and drug abuse program, under the National Native Alcohol and Drug Abuse Program (NNADAP), and a hospital liaison program, wherein a health centre employee works at the local hospital as a patient advocate and interpreter. This role apparently engenders some conflict, since the hospital tends to think of her as a hospital employee, and tends to refer to her almost everything that pertains to Indians. For instance, she has been called upon to assist hospital staff with intoxicated patients who present themselves at the emergency department.

The BIHC has been faced with a number of challenges in delivering its programs. In order to facilitate hospitalization for maternity patients, health centre staff will work over a number of months to complete the required forms and orient the patient to the hospital experience. Physical examinations of children are sometimes done over a number of physician visits, since some parents do not like comprehensive exams where the physician appears to be looking for something wrong. Community-based nurses are encouraged to visit patients first, before attempting home-care programs. And the hospital liaison employee has managed to arrange for the sprinkler system in her office to be disconnected, so that traditional sweetgrass ceremonies can be performed for patients. At the band level, the community nurses work with local elders to facilitate the holistic healing of patients; but the centre lacks the funds to direct such a program, and leaves it up to the nurses to make ad-hoc arrangements with the elders.

The MSB contracts with the member bands to maintain the health centre. NNADAP and Canada Employment also provide some funding for programs. The centre is governed by a board consisting of the chiefs of the eight reserves, and represents another example of a degree of Indian control over health programs. Most of the member bands also have councillors with health portfolios. Efforts have been made to include local people – through health committees, for instance – to make the health centre's programs more responsive to the band members overall (Cardenas and Lucarz 1985).

The final example we wish to examine is that of the Anishnawbe Health Centre in Toronto. Urban institutions designed exclusively for Aboriginal people and under some Aboriginal control are relatively rare. This centre was established in 1988. It had its roots in late-1970s initiatives to develop a program to deliver health services to Toronto's increasing Aboriginal population and in a Native Diabetes Education Program begun in 1981. The centre offers culturally appropriate clinical and educational programs and employs mostly Aboriginal people, overseen by a mostly Aboriginal board. A holistic approach, encompassing cultural education and the teachings of the Medicine Wheel, informs all aspects of the programs offered. Indeed, according to centre personnel, 'Many of the problems faced by Natives these days are related to the loss of self-esteem and pride in their Indian heritage, loss of dignity as a result of racism and prejudice, and loss of their identity as a Native person due to the historic erosion of traditional cultural and religious ceremonies' (Anishnawbe Health Toronto 1990). Hence, cultural and historical education plays an important role in the centre's programs (George and Nahwegahbow 1993). Funding is provided primarily by the Government of Ontario, perhaps reflecting the fact that the centre assists clients of all Aboriginal cultural and legal backgrounds. A small budget for the traditional healing program is made available by the federal MSB.

The Anishnawbe Health Centre also offers a street-patrol program similar to those in other centres such as Kenora and Winnipeg. Staffers and volunteers patrol areas of the city where there is a concentration of Aboriginal people, offering assistance to those who may be homeless or intoxicated (McClure et al. 1992:16).

EDUCATION AND TRAINING: THE KEY TO SELF-DETERMINATION

Not surprisingly, there are relatively few Aboriginal health professionals in Canada. One source places the number of practising Aboriginal physicians at between eighteen and twenty-five in Canada (Stephens 1991:136). The numbers are increasing, especially those of community health representatives and nurses, and more slowly at the level of physician, dentist, lab technician, and so on. Despite improvements, however, much of the actual health care delivered under Aboriginal control still involves non-Aboriginal staff. In the next section, we will look at this issue more closely, simply noting here that the training of Aboriginal health professionals is considered a priority by Aboriginal organizations and that, with assistance from a number of government and educational institutions, some progress is being made.

Major impetus for the development of health careers programs came with the formation of the Indian and Inuit Nurses of Canada (IINC) association in 1975. A core group of forty individuals met to form the association, working from a list of eighty such individuals that was developed only with a great deal of work. The road to achieving acceptability was difficult, as it seems all cases of self-determination have been. The association was discouraged by the federal government, and 'a national Indian political group' blocked one early federal funding initiative (Cuthand Goodwill 1989:119). When funding was obtained from the Native Women's Program of the secretary of state, one program officer objected to the fact that the first chair of the association was male. Later, in the early 1980s, MSB began to fund the association, putting it on a more secure footing.

The association, now the Aboriginal Nurses Association of Canada, has many broad objectives, including promoting and lobbying for better health and health care for Indian and Inuit people, encouraging and facilitating 'culturally appropriate' health care, and assisting in the process of self-determination in the area of health care.[5] Central to its mandate are its efforts to promote educational opportunities for Aboriginal people in the health professions. Its lobbying efforts have contributed to the development of a number of health career programs for Aboriginal students.

The federal government sponsors a broad program known as the Indian and Inuit Health Careers Program (IIHCP). This program was begun in 1984, with the assistance of the IINC, and is an MSB program designed 'to encourage and support Indian participation in educational opportunities and provide a learning environment designed to overcome many of the social and cultural barriers that culturally inhibit the Native students' educational achievement' (cited in D.E. Young and Smith 1991:35). It provides bursaries and scholarships, as well as funding for professional development (such as conferences), job training, and community educational initiatives. Funding has also been made available for day care and for cultural activities – including elders' services – associated with health care institutions. This program is viewed as a support for the Health Transfer Program.

The National Native Access Program to Nursing (NNAPN) began in 1985 at the University of Saskatchewan. Funded by the MSB, this is a pre-nursing program designed to help Aboriginal students gain admission to university (degree-granting) nursing schools. Students normally obtain a conditional acceptance to a nursing school, and then attend a nine-week spring course at the University of Saskatchewan campus. Individual students, often supported financially by their bands or communities through other federal or provincial programs, are given the opportunity to experience the university environment, upgrade skills and knowledge, and learn about study skills, exam writing, and library research. Clinical observations and fieldwork also provide the student with some idea of what it means to be a nurse. Upon successful completion of the course, the students move on to their individual nursing schools to enter the nursing program. The program has achieved an excellent success rate to date. Beginning with just eleven students in 1986, enrolment in the last few years has varied from between sixteen and twenty-five, and a total of ninety students have taken the program. Some do decide that nursing is not what they want and, of course, some simply fail to achieve the necessary grades to continue. Overall, 73 per cent of those enrolling have been subsequently recommended to continue in nursing. By the fall of 1992, of those who had completed the program, four students had completed their Bachelor of Science in Nursing degrees, two had completed Registered Nursing degrees, and four had completed degrees in other areas. Overall, forty-six students who had completed the program were still attending college or university, including nineteen in a BSN program (McNab 1993).

Other nursing programs include Memorial University's Outpost Nursing and Nurse-Midwifery Program, Dalhousie University's Northern Nursing Program, the University of Manitoba's Northern Baccalaureate Nursing Program, operated in conjunction with the Swampy Cree Tribal Council (Thomlinson et al. 1991), and the Native Nurses Entry Program at Lakehead University (Roberts 1991). Some of these are exclusively for Aboriginal students, while others have a focus on Aboriginal health care issues and are open to students of all backgrounds.

There have been other university-based initiatives as well. The University of Manitoba established its Special Premedical Studies Program for Manitoba Aboriginal students in 1979. This program combines elements of affirmative action with academic support services and financial assistance. A paper by the first graduates of the program suggested that, in general, Aboriginal students of medicine experienced a variety of problems, including relatively poor preparation in maths and sciences, and cultural differences (such as a lack of assertiveness), as well as a general lack of confidence (Bartlett et al. 1988). Students are linked up with the university's Northern Medical Unit to gain practical experience in delivery services to Aboriginal communities. The success rate of the program has been estimated at 40 per cent, having produced five physicians, two dentists, and other health professionals by 1990. Curiously, despite the fact that this was the first and most successful of the university-based Aboriginal physician training programs (there are others at the universities of Toronto and Alberta), the federal government withdrew its funding in 1989, arguing that the program was too expensive; the Manitoba government stepped in to cover the additional costs (Stephens 1991).

Finally, we should note that there are now a variety of Community

Health Representative (CHR) training programs in Canada. For instance, there is the Labrador Inuit Health Commission CHR Program (Allen 1991), the Northern Community Health Representative Program at Confederation College in Thunder Bay (Roberts 1991), and the Community Health Representative Program at the Yellowknife campus of Arctic College. These programs demonstrate varying degrees of Aboriginal input and control.

The CHR program dates back to the early 1960s, and has undergone significant changes since then. It was originally intended as a means of giving support to the non-Aboriginal nurses who dominated the delivery of MSB health services, and of providing a mechanism for liaison between the nurses and the community. In the early years, however, CHRs received relatively little training, and tended to be marginalized within the context of nursing services – for instance, by being restricted to such activities as clerical work and community sanitation initiatives. The program clearly smacked of tokenism, since at the time there were no efforts to train Aboriginal people for the more advanced medical positions. More recently, however, the training has improved, to the point where CHRs provide clinical services in smaller communities without the services of resident nurses. As part of the health transfer initiative, the role of CHRs has been redefined to some extent to encompass more community health and education activities.

The Nechi Institute in Alberta is a unique facility for training individuals (primarily Aboriginal) in addiction counselling. It is the training wing of Poundmaker's Lodge, and represents an attempt to combine both traditional Aboriginal and biomedical/psychotherapeutic techniques in a holistic, and intense, program of instruction. It has achieved the paramount role in Canada for such training, and is considered essential by both Aboriginal and other governments.

There are other programs as well, too many to discuss in the space available. It should be clear at this point, however, that there are many special, Aboriginal-oriented health career programs in Canada. Most are relatively recent, and we are only now beginning to see the effects as Aboriginal professionals graduate and enter the workforce. Of course, Aboriginal people are not required to enter these special programs, and some do choose to enter the regular medical programs. Unfortunately, concrete assessments of various initiatives are rare, but clearly they are viewed as essential to the process of health transfer and the development of self-determination in health care.

DOES ABORIGINAL CONTROL LEAD TO A DIFFERENT STYLE OF HEALTH
CARE?

The movement towards self-determination in health care has been influenced by two factors: the general move towards self-determination, in
which all aspects of Aboriginal life are being defined and rights to 'control'
asserted; and the observation that the health of Aboriginal peoples is far
worse than that of other Canadians, and that changes in the health care
delivery system are required. As we will assert here, the two factors are
intertwined. There can be no significant improvement in health unless
the broader socio-economic and political issues are addressed. In the first
chapter of this book, we outlined the contemporary socio-economic conditions experienced by Aboriginal peoples as a group; improving health
care, by no matter what method, can lead to only marginal changes in the
health status of these peoples. This is a lesson which, nationally and
internationally, we have already learned. So, when Aboriginal peoples
gain control of the health care system, do their efforts produce a noticeable
improvement in health status, or are their efforts frustrated by problems
within the larger socio-economic world within which they live?

So far in this chapter we have presented some hints as to how things
are different under Aboriginal control. Perhaps the most common theme
of Aboriginal control is the desire to make treatment more community-
oriented and 'holistic,' with a focus on both treatment and prevention.
Currently, there are many models of Aboriginal control that we can examine to address this issue, but perhaps the most interesting are the
facilities for alcohol- and drug-abuse treatment.

There are a great many programs for alcohol- and drug-abuse treatment
being operated by Aboriginal groups, on reserves, in rural areas, and in
cities. The flagship program, without question, is Poundmaker's Lodge,
just outside Edmonton. The fundamental principle underlying treatment
at Poundmaker's, and the other facilities, is that a culturally sensitive
environment must be created in order for the whole person – mind, body,
and spirit – to be healed. Heavy emphasis is placed on Aboriginal cultural
education, including seminars in cultural traditions and Aboriginal history. The loss of a cultural identity is considered to be a root cause of an
individual's substance-abuse problems.

At Poundmaker's, all patients are required to attend sweetgrass ceremonies morning and evening; at many other programs, only one such
session is held. Sitting in a circle, individuals are allowed time to pray in

their own way and their own language, and time is made available for them to talk, in turn, about what may be on their mind. Unlike some non-Aboriginal programs, this one applies no overt pressure to talk, although the group dynamic tends to bring most individuals into the fold. Sweat lodge ceremonies are also made available at these programs, although rarely are these mandatory.

Elders, who may or may not be healers, are invariably involved in the programming. Some programs employ elders on a contract basis, others access local elders through a more traditional approach, and a few have elders on staff. Poundmaker's Lodge is one example where staff elders work with the patients. One of us (Waldram) interviewed one elder in 1989, and his perspective was quite clear: he sought to help patients reconnect with whatever Aboriginal culture they were from. Although Cree himself, he did not force the Cree way on any residents, but tried to have them accept the underlying principles and values which he, like many elders, believes are common to the various Aboriginal cultures. Emphasis is invariably placed on the need to respect both oneself and others, and to demonstrate humility and altruism while acknowledging the central role of the Creator in life. It is the cultural programming that sets these Aboriginal programs apart from those offered for non-Aboriginal people. However, while this part of the programming is seen as the core of treatment, and while most staff are Aboriginal and the centres themselves have an architectural component that is 'Aboriginal' (such as the central, teepee-style inner room at Poundmaker's where the sweet-grass ceremonies are held), much of the treatment is derived from similar, non-Aboriginal programs. Alcoholics Anonymous (AA), Narcotics Anonymous, Al-Anon, and so on, have been accepted with only minor modifications. At Poundmaker's, for instance, the twelve-step AA program has been translated into Aboriginal languages, and made more culturally acceptable (for example, by referring to the Creator instead of God), but the basic model remains intact. Patients undergo intensive, classroom-style instruction and participate in various group-therapy exercises. These are residential programs which, in effect, capture the patients for periods of up to ninety days in some instances; while patients are free to leave, if they do so on their own they are not welcomed back. Emphasis is placed on the individual to take responsibility for his or her problem.

A key issue for the staff of these treatment programs is the lack of support services in the communities. No matter how effective the treatment has been, when individuals return to their communities they are faced with the same problems as before: unemployment, peer pressure to drink or sniff, and the general sense of hopelessness that pervades some Aboriginal communities. In many communities, support groups have developed which help recovering abusers, but the resources for these are limited. None of the treatment programs visited by one author (Waldram) were able to offer any statistics on the 'success' rate, however defined, and it was apparent that, while these programs are absolutely essential, recovering abusers still face many obstacles on the road to maintaining their sobriety.[6]

It is clear, then, that Aboriginal control over health care does not mean a complete rejection of biomedical and psychosocial treatment programs and methods. Rather, where possible, these are made culturally more appropriate, and traditional approaches to healing are brought in to augment, but not necessarily replace, biomedical approaches.

CONCLUSIONS

The process of self-determination in health care is irreversible, linked as it is to the broader struggle for self-determination of Aboriginal peoples in general. While this is a new process, the evidence to date suggests that some significant changes are occurring. Nevertheless, control over something as potentially serious and costly as health is not without its problems. The relative lack of Aboriginal professionals has led to a continuing reliance on non-Aboriginal people who, although under the employ of the Aboriginal groups, are still seen as temporary. Funding remains a perennial problem; all programs have experienced shortages, and funding seems to be becoming more difficult just as progress is being made. Current government thinking seems to be pointing in the direction of reducing the role of the Medical Services Branch and transferring resources to Aboriginal communities and organizations. Indeed, in October of 1994, the federal government announced a $243-million, five-year funding program for Aboriginal health, of which $87 million would go towards Aboriginal-controlled community-based health programs.

With local control, Aboriginal groups seem to be willing to keep the best of biomedicine and complement it with more traditional programs. Whether there is any significant change in health status is another question, one which the lack of data prevents us from addressing. While the issues of *control* over health care and *improved health status* are intertwined in the discourse, they are somewhat separate in practice. The issue of control is within the realm of the political, and represents the legitimate aspirations of Aboriginal peoples to have control over the delivery of health services within their communities. We do not argue with this process. But it is often assumed that improved health status will follow logically from such control. We believe the issue is more complex than that. From a research perspective, we would welcome some concrete studies on the efficacy of treatment and education programs that are under Aboriginal control. We do not accept the view, expressed in some quarters, that such research is unnecessary, for to do so is to accept, on faith alone, that Aboriginal control is the answer. The point of such research, however, would not be to undermine Aboriginal initiatives by pointing out failures, but rather to generate new data on what works and what doesn't, with an eye to improving the extent to which self-determination can make real progress and demonstrating the need for parallel initiatives in other areas, such as employment and economic development, which have a significant impact on health.

11

Aboriginal health: old ideas and current directions

This book is an account of health and health care among the Aboriginal peoples of Canada, written from the perspective of researchers working in an academic context, and based largely on published sources that represent issues deemed significant by historians and medical and social scientists working in the area of Aboriginal health. In this final chapter we review and summarize important themes and key findings from this literature, emphasizing changes in patterns of health and disease, the place of medicine within Aboriginal cultures, and the relationships between politics and health policies. We also explore popular explanations of why Aboriginal health is what it is today, illustrate them with reference to two health problems that historically have been linked with Aboriginal people – tuberculosis and alcohol – and offer our own perspective. This is only one part of the story, however. As Aboriginal organizations increasingly conduct their own research on health problems, other definitions, visions, and explanations for the health of Aboriginal communities will gain prominence.

We began this book with a general and necessarily oversimplified overview of Aboriginal history in Canada, with descriptions of the different Aboriginal cultures at the time of contact, the social and cultural changes since contact, the political and constitutional relationships with non-Aboriginal Canadians and the Canadian state, and current socio-economic conditions. Such background information is critical for the beginnings of an understanding of Aboriginal health and health care, particularly for the non-specialist. Beyond the obvious and well-known need to understand the historico-cultural context of health, it is vital to appreciate that the concept of 'Aboriginal health' is itself a convenient but ultimately false representation of the problem at hand. It masks the rich diversity of social, economic, and political circumstances that give rise to variation in health problems and healing strategies in Aboriginal communities. If nothing else, this survey should make it clear that health and health care patterns show extensive variation across the country, despite the tendency for national, regional, and provincial databases to create the impression of widespread trends and homogeneity of experience. Clearly, we need to know more about the basis for health and disease in individual communities and to get beyond traditional epidemiological measures to encompass the perspectives and concerns of Aboriginal people in the communities whose health status is being assessed.

Despite the limitations of the available evidence, a historical epidemiological approach to the problem shows how the health status of Aboriginal peoples has changed over time. Venturing into ideas about the recent past is difficult, owing to the scantiness of the information, even without the pitfalls associated with constructing images of health and disease from fragmentary remains from thousands of years ago. Although it is widely believed that Aboriginal peoples in the North American continent enjoyed good health prior to contact with Europeans, unequivocal data are generally lacking, apart from sparse palaeopathological specimens, biased observations of early explorers and traders, fading oral traditions of Aboriginal people, and inappropriate extrapolations from contemporary hunter-gatherer societies. This has not deterred scholars from attempting to reconstruct the population size and structure of pre-contact populations, their nutrition and diet, and their disease patterns. In view of the subsequent tragic post-contact state of affairs, when recurrent epidemics and famines struck Aboriginal populations with devastating impact, it is understandable that the idea of a halcyon age has remained popular. Nevertheless, it is quite evident that health problems in past populations varied, reflecting the socio-environmental conditions in which people lived and to which they responded. To suggest that there was a single health profile for pre-contact Aboriginal communities would be to deny that Aboriginal populations were as demographically and epidemiologically dynamic and capable of adjusting to their environments as populations elsewhere in the world. Certainly, epidemiological profiles have shifted in the post-contact period, and there is no reason to suspect that they were static and unchanging prior to the arrival of European explorers and settlers.

There is powerful evidence, however, that epidemics of infectious diseases played a special role in the relationship between newcomers and Aboriginal peoples in North America from the fifteenth century onward.

Conditions were created that allowed both old and new diseases to flourish, particularly after the invention and implementation of the reserve system in the late nineteenth century. The introduction of new diseases followed well-established trade routes and settlement patterns, crisscrossing regions in some cases, and burning out locally in others. Epidemics were not simply medical events but had far-reaching consequences for Aboriginal societies and the relationships between Aboriginal and non-Aboriginal peoples. In some cases, whole communities were decimated, often resulting in the merging of bands or tribes or the assimilation of one by another. Epidemics spurred on community break-up and migration, which sometimes spread the disease further and occasionally encouraged intertribal warfare. Among the survivors, the loss of a significant number of community members altered leadership roles and disrupted the existing social structure. Traditional belief systems were unable to account for the new disaster, let alone counteract it. Their weakening paved the way for the onslaught by European Christian missionaries. Still, relatively little is known about the health and disease histories of particular communities or reserves, so that the picture of health and disease up to the Second World War can be drawn in only the broadest of strokes. Once again, the lack of detail tends to create the illusion of a uniform quality to the health and disease experience.

Epidemics, especially tuberculosis, provided the impetus for the Canadian federal government to initiate and organize health services for Aboriginal peoples. Increased surveillance and new health initiatives helped to contribute to a dramatic decline in many infectious diseases in the post-Second World War era. But in their place, new epidemics of chronic, non-communicable diseases on the one hand (such as heart disease, hypertension, obesity, and diabetes), and injuries, violence, and the so-called social pathologies on the other hand, have come to the fore in biomedical categorizations. Regardless of whether infectious diseases or social pathologies predominate in epidemiological profiles, we must not lose sight of the fact that biomedical definitions of health and disease are inextricably linked to larger structures of authority and power. The ability to define and then survey such parameters as 'health status' carries with it the power to construct institutions of healing that prescribe, proscribe, and regulate behaviour. The creation of the image of Aboriginal communities as socially pathological, as 'desperate, disorganized and depressed,' in turn, provides a rationale for policies of paternalism and dependency (O'Neil 1993).

It is important to recognize that, prior to the arrival of Europeans, there were already in existence various Aboriginal medical systems, each with its theories of disease causation, its categories of practitioners, and its diagnostic and therapeutic techniques. Medicine was closely integrated with other aspects of Aboriginal culture and was often indistinguishable from spirituality. The response of biomedicine, the church, and the Canadian state towards traditional Aboriginal health care systems has ranged from dismissive (as hocus-pocus, witchcraft, unscientific, and at best placebo therapy) to outright suppression. While self-care and care by indigenous practitioners were the main sources of health care before European contact, external agents such as traders and missionaries soon provided medical assistance at times of hardship. Such care was offered both for compassionate reasons and to enhance the health of the enterprise, be it the collection of furs or the conversion of souls. In any event, from the outset, political authority was enacted through health surveillance, policy, and practice at the community level, undermining Aboriginal medical systems and driving many underground. There are healthy signs of a strong resurgence of traditional medical practice, and instances of collaboration between Aboriginal healers and biomedical institutions and practitioners, particularly in mental health, can be found across the country.

The idea that the federal government has a responsibility for Aboriginal health care slowly emerged towards the latter part of the nineteenth century, with Euro-Canadian settlement of the West and the signing of the treaties. As part of the bargain in exchange for the Indians' land, the Canadian government offered cash, farming implements, schools, and medical care. Medical care was considered something that could entice the Indians to submit to, or at least not to obstruct, non-Aboriginal settlement. What passed for medical care – literally 'a medicine chest' – was mentioned in only one treaty, Treaty Six (1876), which covered central Saskatchewan and Alberta. Is the medicine chest simply a wooden box with a few medicines and bandages? Or is it a metaphor which represents the complete array of modern medical technologies and facilities, such that the 'chest' grows and is upgraded as medicine itself advances? Court cases have been fought over this interpretation. Before the issue could be resolved once and for all, it was over taken by events: universal hospital insurance and, later, medical care insurance, established in Canada from coast to coast, rendered the issue of who pays largely irrelevant.

The forerunner of today's multimillion-dollar Aboriginal health service began to take shape only towards the end of the nineteenth century, but a chief medical officer was not appointed in the Department of Indian

Affairs until 1904. The early years of the Indian health service were marked by internal political struggles and severe budgetary constraints, indicative of the lack of commitment of the federal government to health issues, despite rhetoric to the contrary. In the immediate pre-Second World War years, there were many reports of severe hardship, of near starvation and malnutrition, and of uncontrolled epidemics in many Aboriginal communities. It was not until after the Second World War that the Indian and Northern Health Service expanded by leaps and bounds, in terms of budget, staff, and facilities. Transferred from the Department of Indian Affairs to the newly established Department of National Health and Welfare, it provided increased services under a post-war social policy dominated by government intervention in the health and social sectors.

Over the past two decades, the debate on Aboriginal health care has shifted from 'Who gets the service?' and 'Who pays for it?' to one of 'Who controls it?' Increasingly, health care is seen as part of the broader political process of self-determination. 'Devolution' has become the new buzz-word in government circles, but many Aboriginal communities remain sceptical of the process. Across the country, implementation of the transfer of control takes many forms, with varying degrees of success. One of the important consequences of the shift of control from external agencies to the level of the community is the emergence of community-based health assessment research, controlled at the local level. We can expect a number of significant consequences for understanding Aboriginal health issues to emerge from this jurisdictional realignment: increasing incorporation of Aboriginal definitions and perceptions of health and illness, a more holistic view of health that reflects Aboriginal cultures and traditional ecological knowledge, and the generation of a variety of disease profiles, as health research becomes more closely oriented towards the social, spiritual, economic, and political needs of specific communities.

BIOLOGY AND CULTURE AS EXPLANATORY MODELS FOR ABORIGINAL HEALTH

It is important to go a step farther in this summary of major trends and themes in Aboriginal health in Canada to consider why such developments occurred. Historically, biological and cultural explanatory models have tended to dominate much of the academic discussion on Aboriginal health and disease, as illustrated by the debates about alcohol use and tuberculosis.

Tuberculosis

As documented in chapters 2, 3, and 4, tuberculosis has been and continues to be a serious problem in many Aboriginal communities in Canada.
By the early twentieth century, shocking rates of morbidity and mortality
were being observed in Aboriginal groups, along with a high frequency
of acute, rapidly fatal forms (see Hutchinson 1907:624). Although there
was little systematic research into the problem, many feared that tuberculosis would 'exterminate before long whole units of the Indian race,
and deteriorate much of the remainder' (Hrdlicka 1908:480).

Tuberculosis had become a metaphor for Aboriginal-European contact
and for the presumed fate of Aboriginal people. 'The Red Man and the
White Plague' (D.A. Stewart 1936) was conceived to be 'a kind of relent-
less process of nature, like an earthquake that we could stand in awe of,
and be very sad about but do nothing to check or change' (ibid. 674).
How could this seeming inability to resist the 'White Plague' be explained? Two main competing explanatory models were offered: racial
susceptibility, and environmental exposure.

The idea of race was the predominant way of accounting for and understanding human biological variation in the nineteenth and early twentieth centuries. Racial susceptibility to specific diseases was but one aspect
of the supposition that humankind could be classified into biologically
distinct units on the basis of fundamental, observable, heritable characteristics. The inability to mount an effective immune response to particular diseases was one of the features thought to distinguish 'primitive'
from 'civilized' races.

The application of this concept to tuberculosis is exemplified by Mc-
Carthy's (1912) interpretation of tuberculosis mortality rates for the early
twentieth century[1]: 'From the apparent almost hopelessness of this disease among the Indian and negro races to a far more favourable outlook
in the Hebrew, we readily see how racial influences stand out prominently
to workers in this disease as factors in the study and control of tuberculosis' (McCarthy 1912:207). It is easy to see how confused the use of the
term 'race' was, with McCarthy's table of comparative data referring
simultaneously to groups defined in terms of religion (Hebrew), ethnicity
(Irish), nationality (Chinese), religion and nationality (Polish Jews), and
other populations of varying size and composition (Scandinavians, U.S.
Negroes, etc.).

Notions of racial superiority and inferiority have a long history in the western-European tradition but enjoyed a revival in the late nineteenth century in association with renewed European expansion overseas. Racial ideas served to justify European colonialism and provided a convenient justification for policies of genocide and intentional neglect, based on the premise that 'civilized' races would survive at the expense of the rest (Snyder 1962). Because it was considered to be a racial trait, susceptibility to tuberculosis would lead to the inevitable demise of Aboriginal peoples ('primitive races') around the world. Paradoxically, in the North American Indian context the racial explanation also fit neatly with the narrative of decline and fall from a pristine pre-contact existence (see Bruner 1986).

The alternative to the view that susceptibility to tuberculosis was an insurmountable 'racial trait' of North American Indians is the contention that the frequency of tuberculosis in any population is directly related to the extent and duration of exposure of the population to the tubercle bacillus. When viewed in this way, the high rates and prevalence of florid and severe forms of tuberculosis among Aboriginal North Americans are conceived to be the product of the short period of time that had elapsed since many populations were exposed to tuberculinized Europeans and other Aboriginal groups. As Perla and Marmorston note: 'Tuberculosis is not essentially a racial problem. It is not established that any race is more susceptible to the disease because of any inherent phylogenetic peculiarities which distinguish one race from another. All are apparently equally susceptible when first in contact with the tubercle bacillus' (Perla and Marmorston, 1941:66). This explanation locates susceptibility to tuberculosis in the opportunity for bacilli to be transferred from infected to uninfected people. In other words, it is the social environment which creates the circumstances necessary for the spread of infection. Prolonged exposure to tuberculosis over several generations eventually leads to the development of population immunity. The process is illustrated by the gradual decline in tuberculosis rates in Aboriginal Canadians. Much of this decline is due to anti-tuberculosis control efforts discussed in chapters 4 and 7, but the decline is also related to the nature of tuberculosis epidemic waves and to the process of acquired immunity.

This second facet of the environmental explanation – the trajectory of the tuberculosis epidemic wave – introduces another level of complexity to the problem. Like other epidemics of infectious disease, tuberculosis displays a steep rise in morbidity and mortality at the onset, then peaks, slows down, and gradually declines as the population acquires immunity to it. As J. Bates explains, 'There is no clear evidence of any racial susceptibility to tuberculosis apart from that best explained as phase differences in the epidemic wave' (Bates 1982:20).

Yet another facet of the tuberculosis problem relates to the conditions of life that enhance or reduce the possibility of the spread of infection and the development of frank disease of epidemic proportions. The crowded one-room cabins associated with reserve living in the late nineteenth and early twentieth centuries, the gathering of children – infected and uninfected alike – into boarding schools, poor nutrition and sanitation, destitution, and the presence of other infectious diseases all converged to create prime conditions for the spread of infection within families and the development of tubercular disease (Bryce 1907, 1922; Hrdlicka 1908; R. Ferguson 1928, 1955; P.E. Moore 1961; Wherrett 1965). The role of boarding schools in the spread of infection cannot be underestimated, for many children who were healthy upon entering them were tuberculin-positive within two years (Drink 1969,.8). These circumstances exemplify the well-known association between local socio-economic conditions and tuber culosis rates.

As we have emphasized throughout this book, there is no simple or single explanation for patterns of illness and disease in Aboriginal Canadians. The tuberculosis case illustrates how the complex intertwining of the biological cycle of tuberculosis epidemics operates in conjunction with social and other conditions that permit the disease to wax, wane, and wax again. Nevertheless, the fact that the notion of 'racial susceptibility' to tuberculosis still must be addressed and refuted indicates how deeply entrenched the idea is in the biomedical literature.

Alcohol

The controversial issue of Aboriginal alcohol use has preoccupied analysts for generations. The discourse surrounding it further demonstrates how ill-conceived and inadequate simple racial and cultural explanations for Aboriginal health are.

In the twentieth century, scientists began to examine the possibility that Aboriginal peoples might have reduced resistance to the effects of alcohol by virtue of their biological inheritance. As discussed in chapter 4, the classic and frequently cited study by Fenna and colleagues (1971) appeared to demonstrate that Indians, and especially Inuit, metabolized alcohol more slowly than other so-called racial or ethnic groups. The parallel to tuberculosis susceptibility is transparent here: the ability to metabolize alcohol could be seen to be a racial trait and it was a short step to conclude that alcohol use, too, was rooted in the evolutionary past of Aboriginal people. Methodological problems were identified in the Fenna study (Leiber 1972), however, and subsequent studies tended to be inconclusive or suggestive of no biological susceptibility (for example, Wolff 1973; Bennion and Li 1976). Indeed, it was necessary as recently as 1987 for Fisher, among others, to point out that the notion of pristine Aboriginal 'races' in the twentieth century (let alone in the pre-contact period) is fallacious. Considerable intermarriage among different Aboriginal groups and with non-Aboriginal people has altered gene pools considerably, making it virtually impossible to establish population boundaries for the purposes of these types of alcohol studies. Other researchers have argued that social deprivation and poverty (L. Dyck 1986; Fisher 1987) are better predictors of alcoholism and related health and behavioural problems.

What is left, however, is a scientifically constructed image of Aboriginal people as biologically susceptible to alcohol and alcohol abuse quite in keeping with the idea of special susceptibility to tuberculosis. This stands in stark contrast to the supposed resistance of Euro-Canadians to both. In this we see quite clearly the outlines of the discredited notion of racial traits and all that this implies about treatment policy. Equally important, the effects of this construction reach far beyond the academic domain and 'the biological explanation maintains its strongest existence in the realm of folk belief' (May 1984:15), with the potential to serve as an explanation for individual problems with alcohol abuse for Aboriginal and non-Aboriginal people who accept the idea.

A myriad of studies concerning how and why Aboriginal people drink have been carried out by social scientists for decades. Like that of their biologically oriented counterparts, the sum total of their work has been inconclusive. 'Bar ethnography,' or participant-observation studies of Aboriginal drinking patterns, are perhaps the best examples of the inherent uselessness of much of this research (for example, Hurt and Brown 1965; Kemnitzer 1972). Frequently, such studies are linked to other cultural data to provide a general explanation of intoxicated behaviour. Perhaps the best example of this in Canada would be the ethnographic work done among northern subarctic groups throughout the 1960s and 1970s which focused on the 'atomistic-type society.' In brief, this model described northern hunting societies as consisting of the nuclear family as the major and perhaps only stable social unit. According to Rubel and Kupferer (1968:189), 'Interpersonal relationships outside of the nuclear family are characterized by contention, suspiciousness, and invidiousness. Moreover, these attitudes are normative.' The tensions which underlay such societies were believed to be largely suppressed by other cultural norms, thereby ensuring a large degree of harmony. But, under the influence of alcohol, these tensions rise to the surface, resulting in arguments, fighting and violent behaviour. One researcher even argued that, among the atomistic Kutchin, people harboured 'an intense desire' to become drunk so as to free themselves from the normal behavioural constraints of their culture (Balikci 1968:197).

A cultural argument of a different sort has suggested that Aboriginal people drink as a result of the pressures of cultural contact or acculturation. Graves (1967), for instance, has argued that acculturative pressures lead to the development of new sets of personal goals which, if unattainable, may result in alcohol abuse. Acculturation also affects the traditional cultural norms and mechanisms for expressing frustration and controlling disruptive behaviour. Hamer (1980:120) has suggested that alcohol provided a means of coping with culture-contact situations, in part by providing 'a means to compensate for lost social activities' such as dances and curing ceremonies. Honigmann (1980:277) has described the northern 'frontier' culture propagated by non-Aboriginal residents and adopted by Aboriginal peoples, in which patterns of binge drinking to excess provide a means of 'identifying with the frontier culture, resisting concession of superiority to the dominant culture, and maintaining some autonomy and spontaneity ... Therefore it helps to control further assimilation.' One researcher has even suggested that alcohol consumption represents a means 'of asserting and validating Indianness,' including 'getting purposely drunk to confirm the stereotype of the drunken Indian' (Lurie 1971:315).

Related to the notion of acculturation is that of 'anomie,' a classic sociological concept first postulated by Emile Durkheim (1951). Anomie refers to a state of normlessness, or for the individual a sense of powerlessness over one's life that inevitably leads to depression and, in some instances, suicide. As Levy and Kunitz (1974:16) have suggested, anomie theory when applied to Aboriginal drinking described this behaviour as a form of retreatism in the face of culture contact and the loss of autonomy following colonization. To quote one author who employed this explanation, 'Alcoholic beverages have been the easiest and quickest way to deaden the senses and to forget the feeling of inadequacy' (Dozier 1966:76–7). The picture of the Aboriginal alcoholic as victim looms large in this scenario.

Levy and Kunitz (1974) themselves provide still another possible per-spective. They argue that drinking behaviour is learned, and hence is 'cultural.' Furthermore, they state that 'this, in turn, is largely determined by the ecological adaptation of the tribe in question.' In rejecting anomie theory, they offer that 'drinking behavior is mainly a reflection of tradi-tional forms of social organization and cultural values ...' In other words, the way a people drink is determined by their culture and social organi-zation which, in effect, predate the introduction of alcohol. Alcohol sim-ply fits into the existing cultural pattern. This explanation is tantalizing, for it allows for the fact that studies have frequently shown differences in drinking behaviour across cultures. Yet, in the end, this perspective, like the others, seems devoid of practical utility.

With respect to alcohol and Aboriginal peoples, Gerald Vizenor has best summarized these various academic perspectives:

The view that tribal people have a predisposition or genetic weakness to alcohol is a racist response to a serious national problem. The notion that tribal people drink to relive their past memories as warriors will neither explain nor mend the broken figures who blunder drunk and backslide through cigarette smoke from one generation to the next. Separations from tribal traditions through marriage or acculturation do not explain the behavior associated with drunkenness. Tribal cultures are diverse and those individuals who are studied at the bar, or on the streets, are unique, alive and troubled, not entities from museums or the note-books of culture cultists. (Vizenor 1990:307–8)

Indeed, the great deal of attention that has been paid to issues such as how Aboriginal people drink, why they drink, and whether they are biochemically susceptible to alcohol has led to very little in the way of public health policy or the development of treatment programs. Further-more, it is also clear that racial stereotypes of the terminally pathological 'drunken Indian' have detracted from pressing, non-health concerns, such as the current movement towards self-determination. Even the most the-oretically appealing explanations of the nature and genesis of alcohol problems for some Aboriginal people, that these are born of poverty and oppression, contribute little to health policy initiatives. This fact has not been lost on one leading Aboriginal alcohol treatment director, Pat Shirt of Poundmaker's Lodge, in his submission to the Royal Commission on Aboriginal Peoples: 'While acknowledging that Aboriginal peoples have been victims of colonization and cultural genocide, he said that they could not afford to waste time debating the causes of substance abuse. What is important now is to discuss how to change that victim identity to a survival identity' (Royal Commission on Aboriginal Peoples 1993:17). Shirt, like many others, rejects the notion of Aboriginal peoples as only victims. 'We emphasize ... that we are also survivors,' he states emphatically.

As we saw in chapter 10, the most successful treatment programs seem to be based on traditional healing approaches, Alcoholics Anonymous, or a combination of both. The best approach to understanding the issue, therefore, involves setting aside biological and cultural explanations and dealing with it from a public health perspective. In other words, alcoholism should be seen as a disease which affects *individuals*; the fact that some Aboriginal communities appear to be disproportionately experiencing the negative effects of alcohol abuse is not suggestive of a *cultural* or *biological* problem, but rather of the fairly uniform negative effects of poverty, racism, and marginalization stemming from colonization. In all of this, it is nevertheless essential to stress that it is only a minority of Aboriginal people who experience alcohol-related problems.

ABORIGINAL HEALTH IN PERSPECTIVE

The academic discussions of tuberculosis and alcohol illustrate how simple biological and cultural arguments fail to explain health and health care issues among Aboriginal peoples in Canada. A complex interdigitation between socio-economic and political factors, including broader historical processes and local circumstances, explain to a greater degree the current situation than do either cultural or biological factors alone.

The past emphasis on cultural or biological explanations for Aboriginal health has served primarily to reinforce existing (and erroneous) stereotypes of Aboriginal Canadians, particularly by concentrating on perceived deficiencies, vulnerabilities, and weaknesses. These approaches have contributed little either to the understanding of Aboriginal health or to effective solutions to actual health issues. Indeed, they have often empowered the analysts and health professionals while portraying the people as solely responsible for their own misfortunes. It could be argued that these theories tell us more about the normative assumptions of the researchers than about the problems they purport to explain. At the very least, neither biological nor cultural explanations encompass an Aboriginal perspective, and both support the construction of an image of Aboriginal communities as fundamentally sick and irretrievably out of control.

In examining Aboriginal health and health care, then, it is important to move beyond simplistic explanations. An approach which stresses the political economy of health seems most appropriate, given the status of the Aboriginal peoples as indigenous, colonized minorities in their homeland. This approach should address issues of culture and biology, but also carefully investigate historical events and policies, as well as socioeconomic factors and the nature of the Canadian state and Canadian society. In so doing, we not only see the victimization of Aboriginal peoples through colonization, loss of lands, and various forms of racism, but also see Aboriginal people as individuals reacting to an oppressive situation. Any approach which fails to consider Aboriginal people as active in response to their colonial situation, rather than simply as passive victims, will fail to comprehend not only the past changes in health status and health care, but more importantly the future direction that will be taken in these areas.

It is likely that the health situation of Aboriginal peoples in Canada will improve in the future, particularly if attention is paid to five basic areas. First, in all aspects of health research, administration, and clinical service delivery, a public health perspective must be adopted, one that is devoid of moral or racial undertones and refrains from viewing Aboriginal people as culturally crippled. The cooperation of health professionals, both Aboriginal and non-Aboriginal, is needed to ensure that proper health education messages are received and acted upon at the community level.

Second, there must be a greater sensitivity to Aboriginal culture in its diversity on the part of non-Aboriginal biomedical practitioners, especially to linguistic barriers and the problems engendered by the life circumstances of some Aboriginal people. Training for cultural competence is needed and is best provided by the elders, traditional healers, and other individuals designated by the specific communities where a biomedical practitioner is hired to serve. Realistically, such training will only benefit individuals who are willing and able to see beyond the blinders created by ethnocentricity and membership in an élite sector of Canadian society.

Third, there must be a continuing process of acquisition of control over health care services at the community level, so that local customs, perceptions, and definitions of health issues and initiatives are addressed. Ideally, researchers and biomedical practitioners increasingly will work as consultants in partnerships with Aboriginal communities or through a co-managed research and health care delivery process aimed at developing community-based health policy that meets local needs and is environmentally sound, sustainable, and culturally appropriate. Research into health and health care can contribute to this process through the hiring and training of Aboriginal community members (rather than non-Aboriginal outsiders) as researchers and assistants. Such initiatives will facilitate the transfer of health care to the local level, by developing a strong base of information and skills upon which Aboriginal policy makers can draw and will, at the same time, inject cash and opportunities for personal development directly into communities.

Fourth, Aboriginal peoples need to be given increased opportunities to enter and succeed in the various health professions. Affirmative action entry programs at colleges and universities, and employment equity policies at places of employment, must continue to be developed.

Finally, and most importantly, there must be an overall general improvement in the socio economic status of Aboriginal Canadians, a huge task which requires structural changes to the broader Canadian economic and political milieu, and which is generally considered to be beyond the parameters of health research and service delivery.

Ultimately, the best chance for improved health in the Aboriginal population of Canada rests in the continuation and acceleration of the process of self-determination.

Notes

CHAPTER 1 An overview of the Aboriginal peoples of Canada

1 There were 1,002,675 people with some Aboriginal ancestry: 744,845 with North American Indian origins, 43,000 with Inuit origins, 174,710 with Métis origins, and 40,120 with multiple Aboriginal origins. However, an estimated 38,000 Aboriginal people did not participate in the census (termed 'incompletely enumerated' by Statistics Canada). The share of the national population was 3.7 per cent, if the incompletely enumerated were excluded, and 3.9 per cent if they were included. The 1986 and 1991 censuses are methodologically most comparable to each other and most different from the earlier censuses, particularly in the option of multiple ethnic origins. It is for this reason that Figure 1 does not include population data from the 1986 and 1991 censuses.
2 A comprehensive source on pre-contact and early post-contact Aboriginal cultures is the *Handbook of North American Indians*, a series of twenty volumes periodically published since 1978 by the Smithsonian Institution (Sturtevant 1978–).
3 Of course there had been Aboriginal efforts prior to this to mobilize politically. For instance, in the first half of this century, Métis activist Jim Brady and Indian leaders such as John Tootoosis and F.O. Loft spent considerable parts of their lives involved in political organizing.

CHAPTER 2 Health and disease in the pre-contact period

1 Such large and dense populations are found in many more southerly parts of the United States and other parts of the Americas.
2 There is undisputed archaeological evidence for human occupation in North

and South America at the close of the Pleistocene, roughly 11,000 years BP, but some sites, such as Meadowcroft Rockshelter in Pennsylvania, may be 20,000 to 12,000 years old (Hoffecker et al. 1993).

3 Jackes (1983) makes a case for smallpox diagnosis from ossuary remains.

4 Treponemal disease is a collective term encompassing the infections of yaws, syphilis, pinta, and bejel.

5 Stable carbon isotope analysis provides evidence of the ratio of C_3 to C_4 plants in the diet. It has been instrumental in detecting plant domestication in northeastern North America. Because maize follows the C_4 photosynthetic pathway, its presence can be detected in bone through its distinctive carbon isotope signature, which differs from that of the C_3 plants which make up most of the indigenous plant cover in the temperate zones. The shifting ratios of C_3 and C_4 plants can be detected in bone and provide evidence of the transition from a diet of almost exclusively C_3 plants to one which includes increasing amounts of the C_4 plant, maize (Katzenberg 1992:111–12).

6 A salvage excavation was undertaken in 1987 when it was discovered that most of the site would have been destroyed by a housing development (Katzenberg, Saunders, and Fitzgerald 1993).

7 William Sturtevant (1985) noted that other Aboriginal populations, such as those in Australia, also suffered from introduced European diseases after contact, despite the lack of a 'cold screen' (personal communication, cited in Thornton 1987:40).

8 Anthracosis is a chronic lung disease resulting from long-term inhalation of smoke from burning seal oil.

9 This is significantly less than the average 26 per cent of carious teeth for prehistoric and contact Canadian populations (Patterson 1984, cited in Cybulski 1990).

CHAPTER 3 Contact with Europeans and infectious diseases

1 Henige (1990:185) dubs advocates of this perspective the 'high counters' and takes them to task for, among other criticisms, assuming without evidence that introduced diseases automatically became epidemic and depopulating.

2 These estimates are based on depopulation ratios 20 to 25 times the nadir populations, derived from Dobyns's (1983) estimates of mortality from infectious disease epidemics – a seriously flawed methodology (Henige 1990; Herring 1992).

3 Archaeological evidence suggests that their direct ancestors, and those of the Innu of Labrador, had met and traded with Norse explorers and immigrants around AD 1000 (McGhee 1992:13).

4 The most important resources included various species of seal, seabirds, migratory birds, salmon, and caribou (Tuck and Pastore 1985:72–4).

5 Each of the known pre-Beothuk extinctions occurred in the absence of an invading population, and at least a century separates the disappearance of one group from the appearance of the next in the archaeological record. The Indians of the Maritime Archaic disappear from the archaeological record around 3200 BP; the Groswater Palaeo-Eskimos appear to have died out around 2100 BP, as did the Dorset Palaeo-Eskimos by about AD 500 (Tuck and Pastore 1985:70–2).

6 Upton (1977:134) arrives at a population range at AD 1500 of 1,123 to 3,050 in this way, and settles for a final estimate of 2,000 Beothuk at contact.

7 The relationship between diet and disease is underscored in V. Miller's (1976, 1982) interpretation of Micmac post-contact history. Miller's reading of the earliest accounts of travellers, adventurers, and Jesuit priests led her to postulate that a change in seasonal subsistence activities produced debilitating foodborne diseases and malnutrition among the Micmac. Reliance on European foods appears to have been linked to fatal autumn and winter outbreaks of pleurisy, quinsy, and dysentery. Epidemics of dysentery broke out following the ingestion of contaminated traded foods, and a pattern of summer gorging and alcohol consumption may have contributed to fall outbreaks. Instead of carrying out the normal activities of gathering and preserving meat and plant foods for winter, the Micmac were said to have spent the summers waiting on the coast for European ships. All this led to a winter diet heavy on dried trade foods, such as hardtack. European and Micmac sources cite an increase in lung, chest, and intestinal disorders, particularly in winter (V. Miller 1976:123).

CHAPTER 5   Medical traditions in Aboriginal cultures

1 A recent volume by Hultkrantz (1992) attempts a wide-ranging discussion of the healing traditions of Aboriginal peoples in North America, but suffers from the need to overgeneralize for any given culture area. The lesson, clearly, is that individual healing traditions require in-depth, singular treatment.

2 It should be stressed here that within Aboriginal medical systems, the distinction between 'natural' and 'supernatural' is not the same as it is in Euro-Canadian cultures and the western scientific tradition. The term 'supernatural' is somewhat inappropriate to the description of Aboriginal spirituality.

3 In accepting the view that Aboriginal healers were pragmatic in their use and manipulation of such symbols, we may appear to be at odds with the

views of many respected healers, past and present, who state unequivocally that the power to heal comes from the Creator. However, it is our view that all medical systems are inherently systems of both belief and knowledge working in tandem to heal the patient and restore balance to the society.

4 One of the authors (Waldram) has participated in various Aboriginal healing ceremonies in which some participants have observed small lights, which they believed were the spirits. These ceremonies took place in environments of complete darkness.

5 Here we are adopting the broad understanding of the concept of surgery, as outlined by Fortune (1985:23), referring to 'methods beyond the usual cutting, piercing, or suturing, such as manipulation of fractures, massage of body organs, and the care of wounds, this last being traditionally in the domain of the surgeon.'

6 Note the comparison between the ritual biting of the tamananawas ceremony and that of the Spirit Dancing which was the target of legal action in 1992; see chapter 9 for a discussion of the latter.

7 In their biography of Plains Cree leader John Tootoosis, Goodwill and Sluman (1984:84) recount his view that Chief Piapot was imprisoned in Regina, allegedly for drinking (despite his claims to be an abstainer); the Chief, according to Tootoosis, believed he had been arrested because of a 'Rain Dance' which he had allowed and which involved piercing.

CHAPTER 6 Traders, whalers, missionaries, and medical aid

1 It should be noted, however, that the related concept of variolation was known in China and the Middle East before it reached Europe and Western medicine.

2 Edwards (1980:5–6) explains that 'Turlington's Balsam of Life' dated from the fifteenth or sixteenth century, and was alleged to cure at least thirty different ailments, including gout, rheumatism, coughs, colic, and other stomach problems.

3 At this time, the term 'savage,' or 'sauvage' in French, had a variety of meanings. It meant, in some cases, simply a person living in natural surroundings. It was also used to denote a non-Christian and even a non-Catholic. But the term could mean someone who was rude and primitive. As J.R. Miller (1989:28) points out, the meaning of the term must be gleaned from the context in which it was used.

CHAPTER 7 The emergence of government health services

1 T.K. Young (1979; 1988: 39,101), has published data emanating from reports

of two northern Ontario physicians on contract to the government, Dr Hanson for the Treaty Three area in 1887, and Dr Meindl for Treaty Nine in 1905. Their account books provide a glimpse into the conditions of their work and the kinds of medical problems they encountered.

2 We are indebted to Mellisa M. Layman, whose unpublished research into the rations program forms the backbone of this presentation.

3 Graham-Cumming (1967:118) reports that, 'It is a striking commentary on the state of affairs towards the end of the nineteenth century that when, in an attempt to stop the spread of the disease through the Indian Schools, the Department of Indian Affairs issued an order banning from school any child found to be infected, the ban was found to be impractical because hardly one child could be found not to be infected. In practice the ban was applied only to children severely ill, otherwise the schools would all have been empty.'

4 A contemporary of Dr Stone, Dr Wall wrote in his 1926 report on the health of the Indians in the Cochrane, Ontario–La Tuque, Quebec, region of the 'expectoration menace ... the universal Indian habit of free expectoration within the homes' which he believed easily facilitated the spread of the tuberculosis bacteria. Dr Walls' report has also been published in *Native Studies Review* 5.1 (1989). 257–74.

CHAPTER 8 The organization and utilization of contemporary health services

1 The U.S. Indian Health Service is almost paramilitary in organization, and all professional staff are commissioned officers who wear naval uniform, complete with stripes, on special occasions.

2 In bureaucratese, a person-year is one person working one year, or two persons working part-time for half a year each, etc.

3 The use of language from the corporate world, rather than from the traditionally public-sector-oriented planning lexicon, is itself revealing of the prevailing attitudes within government.

CHAPTER 9 Aboriginal medicine in the contemporary context

1 See, for instance, the critical evaluation of studies of ethnomedicine by R. Anderson (1991) for a discussion that pertains to some of these issues.

2 David Young (1993; personal communication with Waldram) reports that the herb was also partially processed to prevent the chemists from identifying it, and the chemists agreed to sign forms ensuring that they would protect the herb's identity even if they were able to ascertain it. Young notes that Willier is opposed to providing information about Aboriginal medicines to

non-Aboriginal outsiders, but requested this scientific analysis to prove that his medicines had active ingredients and were not just placebos.

3 It should be pointed out here that our argument also holds for Christian faith healers and others who practise healing outside the bounds of biomedicine.

CHAPTER 10 Self-determination and health care

1 This discussion of the Six Nations Iroquois is taken from Weaver's (1972) excellent monograph.

2 Berger was a former British Columbia Supreme Court judge who spear-headed the landmark Mackenzie Valley Pipeline Inquiry in the early 1970s, and who has been and continues to be involved in many prominent legal actions on behalf of Aboriginal groups.

3 Various aspects of the pre-transfer process are documented in Gregory and colleagues (1992) for Gull Bay, and Warry (1992) for the North Shore Tribal Council and the Whitefish Lake First Nation, all in Ontario.

4 Public health initiatives are often in conflict with existing beliefs and atti-tudes throughout the country in general. Consider as examples needle-exchange programs and the provision of condoms to prison inmates and in school washrooms, public health initiatives aimed at reducing the spread of AIDS.

5 However, IINC has not entered the health transfer debate; the association does not take a stand on the question of 'transfer' as a type of self-determina-tion. According to Jean Cuthand Goodwill (1989:120), 'we must also uphold our professional standing and maintain a healthy working relationship with the colleagues and clients whom we serve ... It will not be sufficient to leave Bands with a messy and ambiguous health-care situation and then declare that "it's out of the department's [MSB's] hands." '

6 An interesting source of viewpoints on alcohol and substance abuse among Aboriginal peoples is *Crazywater*, by Brian Maracle (1993).

CHAPTER 11 Aboriginal health: old ideas and current directions

1 There are serious problems with nineteenth-century and early twentieth-century tuberculosis statistics (see Sawchuk and Herring 1984). The exact size and ethnic homogeneity of the populations studied is generally not known; cross-sectional tuberculosis rates are usually presented for compari-son, whereas secular trend data are needed to determine whether cross-sec-tional rates are short-term responses to worsening or improving local condi-tions; data on the age and sex composition of samples are rarely available,

even though age- and sex-specific tuberculosis mortality rates change as the population moves through the epidemic wave; and, reliable ethnohistoric information for interpreting tuberculosis was rarely collected (in contrast, see R. Ferguson 1928).

References cited

Legal references are cited separately at the end of this list.

Aboriginal Nurses Association of Canada. 1993. *Traditional Aboriginal Medicine and Primary Health Care.* Submission to the Royal Commission on Aboriginal Peoples, June 1992. Ottawa. Aboriginal Nurses Association of Canada.

Achterberg, J. 1985. *Imagery in Healing: Shamanism and Modern Medicine.* London: Shambhala.

Adair, J., W. Deuschle, and W. McDermott. 1969. 'Patterns of Health and Disease among the Navajos.' In L. Lynch, ed. *The Cross-Cultural Approach to Health Behavior,* 83–110. Rutherford: Farleigh Dickinson University Press.

Adamson, J.D., J.P. Moody, and A.F. Peart. 1949. 'Poliomyelitis in the Arctic.' *Canadian Medical Association Journal* 61:339–48.

Allen, I. 1991. 'Community Health Representatives Working in Labrador Inuit Communities.' In B. Postl et al., eds. *Circumpolar Health 90: Proceedings of the 8th International Congress,* 151–2. Winnipeg: University of Manitoba Press.

Allison, M.J., ed. 1976. 'Paleopathology.' *Medical College of Virginia Quarterly* 12(2):39–86.

Allison, M.J., D. Mendoza, and A. Pezzia. 1973. 'Documentation of a Case of Tuberculosis in pre-Columbian America.' *American Review of Respiratory Disease* 107:985–91.

Anderson, J.E. 1969. 'The People of Fairty: An Osteological Analysis of an Iroquoian Ossuary.' *National Museum of Canada Bulletin 193, Contributions to Anthropology 1961–1962* (Part I), Ottawa.

Anderson, R. 1991. 'The Efficacy of Ethnomedicine: Research Methods in Trouble.' *Medical Anthropology* 13:1–17.

Anishnawbe Health Toronto. 1990. *Budget Proposal 1990–91.* Toronto: Anishnawbe Health Toronto.

Arnason, T., R. Hebda, and T. Johns. 1981. 'Use of Plants for Food and Medicine by Native Peoples of Eastern Canada.' *Canadian Journal of Botany* 59:2189–325.

Assembly of First Nations. 1979. *Brief Summary of Rights and Priorities in Indian Health*. Ottawa: National Commission of Inquiry on Indian Health, Assembly of First Nations.

– 1988. *Special Report: The National Indian Health Transfer Conference*. Ottawa: Assembly of First Nations.

Asuni, T. 1979. 'The Dilemma of Traditional Healing with Special Reference to Nigeria.' *Social Science and Medicine* 13(B):33–9.

Atcheson, D., D. Rodgers, C. Hellon, and P. Kehoe. 1969. *Survey of Mental Health Needs of the Northwest Territories*. Report to Medical Services Branch, Department of National Health and Welfare, Ottawa.

Bagley, C., M. Wood, and H. Khumar. 1990. 'Suicide and Careless Death in Young Males: Ecologic Study of an Aboriginal Population in Canada.' *Canadian Journal of Community Mental Health* 29:127–42.

Bailey, A. 1969. *The Conflict of European and Eastern Algonkian Cultures 1504–1700*. Toronto: University of Toronto Press.

Balikci, A. 1963. 'Shamanistic Behavior among the Netsilik Eskimos.' *Southwestern Journal of Anthropology* 19:380–96.

– 1968. 'Bad Friends.' *Human Organization* 27:191–9.

Barkwell, P. 1981. 'The Medicine Chest Clause in Treaty No. 6.' *Canadian Native Law Reporter* 4:1–23.

Barnes, G.E. 1979. 'Solvent Abuse: A Review.' *International Journal of Addictions* 14:1–26.

Barron, F. 1988. 'The Indian Pass System in the Canadian West, 1882–1935.' *Prairie Forum* 13(1):25–42.

Bartlett, J., C. Cook, and M. Cox. 1988. 'Special Premedical Studies Program – Student's Perspective.' *Arctic Medical Research* 47 (Suppl. 1):327–9.

Bates, C., C. Van Dam, and D.F. Horrobin. 1985. 'Plasma Essential Fatty Acids in Pure and Mixed Race American Indians on and off a Diet Exceptionally Rich in Salmon.' *Prostaglandins and Leukotrienes in Medicine* 17:77–84.

Bates, J. 1982. 'Tuberculosis: Susceptibility and Resistance.' *American Review of Respiratory Disease* 125(3):20–4.

Beardsley, G. 1941. 'Notes on Cree Medicines, Based on a Collection Made by I. Cowie in 1892.' *Michigan Academy of Science, Arts and Letters, Papers* 83–496.

Bearskin, S., and C. Dumont. 1991. 'The Cree Board of Health and Social Services of James Bay: The First Twelve Years – 1978–1990.' In B. Postl et al., eds. *Circumpolar Health 90: Proceedings of the 8th International Congress*, 123–5. Winnipeg: University of Manitoba Press.

Bell, R. 1886. 'The "Medicine-Man" or Indian and Eskimo Notions of Medicine.' *Canada Medical and Surgical Journal* 456–537.

Ben-Dor, S. 1966. *Makkovik: Eskimos and Settlers in a Labrador Community: A Contrastive Study in Adaptation.* St John's: Institute of Social and Economic Research, Memorial University of Newfoundland.

Bennion, L., and T.K. Li. 1976. 'Alcohol Metabolism in American Indians and Whites.' *New England Journal of Medicine* 294:9–13.

Berger, T. 1980. *Report of the Advisory Commission on Indian and Inuit Health Consultation.* Ottawa: Medical Services Branch, Department of National Health and Welfare.

Bird, L., and M. Moore. 1991. 'The William Charles Health Centre of Montreal Lake Band: A Case Study of Transfer.' In B. Postl et al., eds. *Circumpolar Health 90: Proceedings of the 8th International Congress*, 20–5. Winnipeg: University of Manitoba Press.

Black, F. 1966. 'Measles Endemicity in Insular Populations: Critical Community Size and Its Evolutionary Implications.' *Journal of Theoretical Biology* 11:207–11.

Black, F.L. 1990. 'Infectious Disease and Evolution of Human Populations: The Example of South American Forest Tribes.' In George J. Armelagos and Alan C. Swedlund, eds. 55–74. *Health and Disease of Populations in Transition.* New York: Bergin and Garvey.

Black, L. 1969. 'Morbidity, Mortality and Medical Care in the Keewatin Area of the Central Arctic – 1967.' *Canadian Medical Association Journal* 101:35–41.

Black-Rogers, M. 1986. 'Varieties of "Starving": Semantics and Survival in the Subarctic Fur Trade, 1750–1850.' *Ethnohistory* 33:353–83.

Boeckx, R.L., B. Postl, and F.J. Coodin. 1977. 'Gasoline Sniffing and Tetraethyl Lead Poisoning in Children.' *Pediatrics* 60:140–5.

Bonaise, A. 1989. Personal interview with Alfred Bonaise, Cultural Counsellor, Poundmaker's Lodge, by James B. Waldram.

Booz-Allen and Hamilton Canada Ltd. 1969. *Study of Health Services for Canadian Indians: Summary Report.* Ottawa: Department of National Health and Welfare.

Borah, W. 1976. 'The Historical Demography of Aboriginal and Colonial America: An Attempt at Perspective.' In W.H. Denevan, ed. *The Native Population of the Americas in 1492*, 13–34. Madison: University of Wisconsin Press.

Boyd, R. 1992. 'Population Decline from Two Epidemics on the Northwest Coast.' In J.W. Verano and D.H. Ubelaker, eds. *Disease and Demography in the Americas*, 249–55. Washington, D.C.: Smithsonian Institution.

Brassard, P., J. Hoey, J. Ismail, and F. Gosselin. 1985. 'The Prevalence of Intestinal Parasites and Enteropathogenic Bacteria in James Bay Cree Indians, Quebec.' *Canadian Journal of Public Health* 76:322–5.

Brett, H.B. 1969. 'A Synopsis of Northern Medical History.' *Canadian Medical Association Journal* 100:521–5.

Brink, G.C. [1965.] *Across the Years: Tuberculosis in Ontario.* [Toronto.]

Brizinski, P. 1989. *Knots in a String: An Introduction to Native Studies in Canada.* Saskatoon: University of Saskatchewan.

Broussard, B.A., A. Johnson, and J.H. Himes. 1991. 'Prevalence of Obesity in American Indians and Alaska Natives.' *American Journal of Clinical Nutrition* 53:1535–42S.

Brown, Jennifer. 1980. *Strangers in Blood: Fur Trade Families in Indian Country.* Vancouver: University of British Columbia Press.

Brown, J., and R. Brightman. 1988. *'The Orders of the Dreamed': George Nelson on Cree and Northern Ojibwa Religion and Myth, 1823.* Winnipeg: University of Manitoba Press.

Bruner, E. 1986. 'Ethnography as Narrative.' In V.W. Turner and E.M. Bruner, eds. *The Anthropology of Experience,* 139–55. Urbana: University of Illinois Press.

Bryans, A. 1969. 'The Summer School of Frontier Medicine, CAMSI Exchange – Inuvik 1967.' *Canadian Medical Association Journal* 100:512–15.

Bryans, A.L. 1986. 'The Prehistory of Canadian Indians.' In R. Bruce Morrison and C. Rod Wilson, eds. *Native Peoples: The Canadian Experience,* 45–72. Toronto: McClelland and Stewart.

Bryce, P. 1907. 'Report of the Chief Medical Officer.' *Sessional Papers No. 27,* 7–8 Edward VII, A, 263–77.

– 1909. 'Report of the Superintendent of Health,' *Sessional Papers No. 27,* 7–8 Edward VII, A, 273–84.

– 1914. 'The History of the American Indians in Relation to Health.' *Ontario Historical Society* 12:128–41.

– 1922. *The Story of a National Crime: An Appeal for Justice to the Indians of Canada.* Ottawa: James Hope.

Bull, W. 1934. *From Medicine Man to Medical Man: A Record of a Century and a Half of Progress in Health and Sanitation as Exemplified by Developments in Peel.* Toronto: G. McLeod.

Canada. Various years. *Public Accounts.* Ottawa: Queen's Printer.

Canada. Auditor General. Various years. *Report to the House of Commons, Fiscal Year Ended March 31, 19–.* Ottawa.

Canada, DIA (Department of Indian Affairs). 1882. *Sessional Papers, No. 5,* 195.

Canada, DIAND (Department of Indian Affairs and Northern Development). 1989. *Fire Loss Report – 1989.* Ottawa: DIAND, Technical Services.

– 1990. *Impacts of the 1985 Amendments to the Indian Act (Bill C-31): Summary Report*. Ottawa: DIAND.

Canada, DNHW (Department of National Health and Welfare). 1958. *Annual Report, 1957*, 76. Ottawa: Queen's Printer.

– 1965. *Annual Report, 1964*, 95. Ottawa: Queen's Printer.

– 1970. *Report of the Committee on Clinical Training of Nurses for Medical Services in the North* (Chair: Dorothy Kergin). Ottawa: DNHW.

– 1971. *Annual Report, 1970*, 105. Ottawa: Queen's Printer.

– 1974. *Report of the Interdepartmental Committee on the Nursing Group*. Ottawa: DNHW.

– 1975a. *Nutrition Canada: Eskimo Survey Report*. Ottawa: DNHW.

– 1975b. *Nutrition Canada: Indian Survey Report*. Ottawa: DNHW.

– 1983. *Report of the Task Force on Medical Officers* (Chair: K. Butler). Ottawa: DNHW.

1988. *Health Indicators Derived from Vital Statistics for Status Indian and Canadian Populations 1978–1986*. Ottawa: DNHW, Medical Services Branch.

– Spring 1989; Fall 1989; Special Issue 1990; Winter 1992. *Health Transfer Newsletter*.

– Joint National Committee on Aboriginal AIDS Education and Prevention. 1990a. *Findings Document*. Ottawa: DNHW.

– Joint National Committee on Aboriginal AIDS Education and Prevention. 1990b. *Recommendations for a National Strategy on Aboriginal AIDS Education and Prevention*. Ottawa: DNHW.

– 1991. *Health Status of Canadian Indians and Inuit – 1990*. Ottawa: DNHW, Medical Services Branch.

– 1993–4. *Estimates, Part III: Expenditure Plan*. Ottawa: DNHW.

Canadian Pediatric Society. 1970. *Indian and Eskimo Child Health Committee: White Paper*. (mimeo).

Canitz, B. 1989a. 'Northern Nurses: A Profession in Crisis.' *Musk-Ox* (37):175–83.

– 1989b. 'Nursing in the North: Challenge and Isolation.' In M. Crnkovich, ed. *'GOSSIP': A Spoken History of Women in the North*, 193–212. Ottawa: Canadian Arctic Resources Committee.

Cannon, A. 1993. 'Contingency and Opportunity in the Growth of Northwest Coast Maritime Economies.' Paper presented at the International Seminar on the Origins, Development, and Spread of Prehistoric North Pacific–Bering Sea Maritime Cultures, Tokai University at Honolulu, Hawaii.

– 1995. 'The Ratfish and Marine Resource Deficiencies on the Northwest Coast.' *Canadian Journal of Archaeology* 19:49–60.

Card, B., G. Hirabayashi, and C. French. 1963. *The Metis in Alberta Society*. Edmonton: University of Alberta and the Alberta Tuberculosis Association.

Cardenas, B., and J. Lucarz. 1985. 'Canadian Indian Health Service: A Model for Service.' In M. Stewart, ed. *Community Health Nursing in Canada*, 246–68. Toronto: Gage.

Cardinal, Harold. 1969. *The Unjust Society*. Edmonton: Hurtig.

Carlson, C., G. Armelagos, and A. Magennis. 1992. 'Impact of Disease on the Precontact and Early Historic Populations of New England and the Maritimes.' In J.W. Verano and D.H. Ubelaker, eds. *Disease and Demography in the Americas*, 141–54. Washington, D.C.: Smithsonian Institution.

Carter, S.A. 1990. *Lost Harvests: Prairie Indian Reserve Farmers and Government Policy*. Montreal: McGill-Queen's University Press.

Churchill, W. 1990. 'Spiritual Hucksterism.' *Z Magazine* December:94–8.

Clatworthy, S., and H. Stevens. 1987. *An Overview of the Housing Conditions of Registered Indians in Canada*. Ottawa: Department of Indian Affairs and Northern Development.

Coates, K.S. 1991. *Best Left as Indians: Native-White Relations in the Yukon Territory, 1840–1973*. Montreal: McGill-Queen's University Press.

Cohen, M.N. 1989. *Health and the Rise of Civilization*. New Haven: Yale University Press.

Cole, D., and Ira Chaikin. 1990. *An Iron Hand upon the People: The Law against the Potlatch on the Northwest Coast*. Vancouver: Douglas and McIntyre.

Connell, G., R. Flett, and P. Stewart. 1991. 'Implementing Primary Health Care through Community Control: The Experience of Swampy Cree Tribal Council.' In B. Postl et al., eds. *Circumpolar Health 90: Proceedings of the 8th International Congress*, 44–6. Winnipeg: University of Manitoba Press.

Connop, P.J. 1983. 'A Canadian Indian Health Status Index.' *Medical Care* 21:67–81.

Cook, S. 1973. 'The Significance of Disease in the Extinction of the New England Indians.' *Human Biology* 45:485–508.

Cook, S., and W. Borah. 1971. *Essays in Population History: Mexico and the Caribbean*. Berkeley: University of California Press.

Cooper, J. 1944. 'The Shaking Tent Rite among the Plains and Forest Algonquians.' *Primitive Man* 17(3):60–84.

Corrigan, C. 1946. 'Medical Practice among the Bush Indians of Northern Manitoba.' *Canadian Medical Association Journal* 54:220–3.

Crosby, A.W. 1986. *Ecological Imperialism: The Biological Expansion of Europe, 900–1900*. Cambridge: Cambridge University Press.

Cruikshank, J. 1979. 'Athapaskan Women: Lives and Legends.' *Canadian Ethnology Service Paper* No. 57. Ottawa.

Culhane Speck, Dara. 1989. 'The Indian Health Transfer Policy: A Step in the Right Direction, or Revenge of the Hidden Agenda?' *Native Studies Review* 5(1):187–213.

Cuthand Goodwill, Jean. 1989. 'Indian and Inuit Nurses of Canada.' *Canadian Woman Studies* 10 (2, 3):117–23.

Cybulski, J.S. 1977. 'Cribra Orbitalia, a Possible Sign of Anemia in Early Historic Native Populations of the British Columbia Coast.' *American Journal of Physical Anthropology* 47(1):31–40.

– 1990. 'Human Biology.' In W. Suttles, ed. *Handbook of North American Indians: Vol 7*. Northwest Coast, 52–9. Washington, D.C.: Smithsonian Institution Press.

– 1994. 'Culture Change, Demographic History, and Health and Disease on the Northwest Coast.' In C.S. Larsen and G.R. Milner, eds. *In the Wake of Contact: Biological Responses to Conquest*, 75–85. New York: Wiley-Liss.

Dailey, R. 1968. 'The Role of Alcohol among North American Indian Tribes as Reported in the Jesuit Relations.' *Anthropologica*, NS 10(1):45–80.

Daniel, R. 1987. 'The Spirit and Terms of Treaty Eight.' In Richard Price, ed. *The Spirit of the Alberta Indian Treaties*, 47–100. Montreal: Institute for Research on Public Policy.

Daniel, T.M. 1981. 'An Immunochemist's View of the Epidemiology of Tuberculosis.' In J.E. Buikstra, ed. *Prehistoric Tuberculosis in the Americas*, 221–8. Evanston, Ill.: Northwestern University Archaeological Program.

Davey, K.W. 1974. 'Dental Therapists in the Canadian North.' *Journal of the Canadian Dental Association* 40:287–91.

Dean, H.J., R.L. Mundy, and M. Moffatt. 1992. 'Non-insulin-dependent Diabetes Mellitus in Indian Children in Manitoba.' *Canadian Medical Association Journal* 147:52–7.

Decker, J. 1988. 'Tracing Historical Diffusion Patterns: The Case of the 1780–82 Smallpox Epidemic among the Indians of Western Canada.' *Native Studies Review* 4(1–2):1–24.

– 1989. '"We Should Never Be Again the Same People": The Diffusion and Cumulative Impact of Acute Infectious Diseases Affecting the Natives on the Northern Plains of the Western Interior of Canada. *1774–1839*.' PhD diss. York University, Toronto.

Delisle, H.F., and J.M. Ekoé. 1993. 'Prevalence of Non-Insulin-Dependent Diabetes Mellitus and Impaired Glucose Tolerance in Two Algonquin Communities in Québec.' *Canadian Medical Association Journal* 148:41–7.

Denevan, W. 1976. *The Native Population of the Americas in 1492*. Madison: University of Wisconsin Press.

Densmore, F. 1929. *Chippewa Customs*. Bulletin 68, Bureau of American Ethnology. Washington, D.C.: Smithsonian Institution.

Dickason, O.P. 1992. *Canada's First Nations: A History of Founding Peoples from Earliest Times*. Toronto: McClelland and Stewart.

Dickson, G. 1989. 'Iskwew: Empowering Victims of Wife Abuse.' *Native Studies Review* 5:115–35.

Dobbin, M. 1981. *The One-and-a-Half Men. The Story of Jim Brady and Malcolm Norris, Metis Patriots of the 20th Century*. Vancouver: New Star Books.

Dobyns, H. 1966. 'An Appraisal of Techniques for Estimating Aboriginal American Population with a New Hemispheric Estimate.' *Current Anthropology* 7:395–416.

– 1976. 'Scholarly Transformation: Widowing the "Virgin Land." ' *Ethnohistory* 23:161–72.

– 1983. *Their Number Become Thin*. Knoxville: University of Tennessee Press.

– 1984. 'Native American Population Collapse and Recovery.' In W.R. Swagerty, ed. *Scholars and the Indian Experience*, 17–35. Bloomington: Indiana University Press.

– 1989. 'More Methodological Perspectives on Historical Demography.' *Ethnohistory* 36(3):285–98.

– 1992. 'Native American Trade Centers as Contagious Disease Foci.' In J.W. Verano and D.H. Ubelaker, eds. *Disease and Demography in the Americas*, 215–22. Washington, D.C.: Smithsonian Institution Press.

Dorken, E., S. Grzybowski, and D.A. Enarson. 1984. 'Ten-year Evaluation of a Trial of Chemoprophylaxis against Tuberculosis in Frobisher Bay, Canada.' *Tubercle* 65:93–9.

Doucette, S. 1989. 'The Changing Role of Nurses: The Perspective of Medical Services Branch.' *Canadian Journal of Public Health* 80:92–4.

Dozier, E.P. 1966. 'Problem Drinking among American Indians: The Role of Sociocultural Deprivation.' *Quarterly Journal of Studies on Alcohol* 27:72–87.

Dressler, W.W. 1984. 'Social and Cultural Influences in Cardiovascular Disease: A Review.' *Transcultural Psychiatric Research Review* 21:5–41.

Driver, H. 1969. *Indians of North America*. 2nd. ed. Chicago: University of Chicago Press.

Duffy, R.Q. 1988. *The Road to Nunavut: The Progress of the Eastern Arctic Inuit since the Second World War*. Montreal: McGill-Queen's University Press.

Dunn, F.L. 1968. 'Epidemiological Factors: Health and Disease in Hunter-gatherers.' In Richard B. Lee and Irven DeVore, eds. *Man the Hunter*, 221–8. Chicago: Aldine.

Durkheim, E. 1951. *Suicide: A Study in Sociology*. Glencoe, Ill.: The Free Press.

Dyck, L.E. 1986. 'Are North American Indians Biochemically More Susceptible to the Effects of Alcohol?' *Native Studies Review* 2:85–9.

Dyck, N. 1986. 'An Opportunity Lost: The Initiative of the Reserve Agricultural

Programme in the Prairie West.' In F.L. Barron and James B. Waldram, eds. *1885 and After: Native Society in Transition,* 121–37. Regina: Canadian Plains Research Centre.

Dyck, R.F., and L. Tan. 1994. 'Rates and Outcomes of Diabetic End-stage Renal Disease among Registered Native People in Saskatchewan.' *Canadian Medical Association Journal* 150:203–8.

Dyerberg, J. 1989. 'Coronary Heart Disease in Greenland Inuit: A Paradox.' *Arctic Medical Research* 48:47–54.

Eaton, R.D. 1968. 'Amebiasis in Northern Saskatchewan: Epidemiological Considerations.' *Canadian Medical Association Journal* 99:706–11.

Edwards, G.T. 1980. 'Bella Coola Indian and European Medicines.' *The Beaver* Winter:5–11.

Eisenberg, D., R. Kessler, C. Foster, F. Norlock, D. Calkins, and T. Delbanco. 1993. 'Unconventional medicine in the United States.' *New England Journal of Medicine* 328: 246–52.

El-Najjar, M.Y. 1979. 'Human Treponematosis and Tuberculosis: Evidence from the New World.' *American Journal of Physical Anthropology* 51:599–618.

Ellestad-Sayed, J., F.H. Coodin, L.A. Dilling, and J.C. Haworth. 1979. 'Breast-feeding Protects against Infection in Indian Infants.' *Canadian Medical Association Journal* 120:295–8.

Enarson, D.A., and S. Grzybowski. 1986. 'Incidence of Active Tuberculosis in the Native Population of Canada.' *Canadian Medical Association Journal* 134:1149–52.

Evers, S.E., E. McCracken, and G. Deagle. 1989. 'Body Fat Distribution and Non-insulin Dependent Diabetes Mellitus in North American Indians.' *Nutrition Research* 9:977–87.

Evers, S.E., E. McCracken, I. Antone, and G. Deagle. 1987. 'Prevalence of Diabetes in Indians and Caucasians Living in Southwestern Ontario.' *Canadian Journal of Public Health* 78:240–3.

Evers, S.E., J. Orchard, and E. McCracken. 1985. 'Lower Respiratory Disease in Indian and Non-Indian Infants.' *Canadian Journal of Public Health* 76:195–8.

Evers, S.E., and C.G. Rand. 1982. 'Morbidity in Canadian Indian and Non-Indian Children in the First Year of Life.' *Canadian Medical Association Journal* 126:249–52.

– 1983. 'Morbidity in Canadian Indian and Non-Indian Children in the Second Year of Life.' *Canadian Journal of Public Health* 74:191–4.

Ewart, W. 1983. 'Causes of Mortality in a Subarctic Settlement (York Factory, Man.) 1714–1946.' *Canadian Medical Association Journal* 129:571–4.

Ewers, J. 1973. 'The Influence of Epidemics on the Indian Populations and Cultures of Texas.' *Plains Anthropologist* 18:104–15.

Favel-King, A. 1993. 'The Treaty Right to Health Care'. In Royal Commission on Aboriginal Peoples. *The Path to Healing*, 120–9. Ottawa: Royal Commission on Aboriginal Peoples.

Fecteau, R., J. Molnar, and G. Warwick. 1991. 'Iroquoian Village Ecology.' Paper presented at the 24th Annual Meeting of the Canadian Archaeology Association, St John's, Newfoundland.

Federation of Saskatchewan Indian Nations. 1986. *Suicides, Violent and Accidental Deaths among Treaty Indians in Saskatchewan: Analysis and Recommendations for Change*. Regina: Federation of Saskatchewan Indian Nations, Health and Social Development Commission.

Felton, J. 1959. 'Friend in Need.' *The Beaver* 290 (Summer): 36–8.

Fenna, D., L. Mix, O. Schaefer, and J.A. Gilbert. 1971. 'Ethanol Metabolism in Various Racial Groups.' *Canadian Medical Association Journal* 105:472–5.

Ferguson, R. 1928. *Tuberculosis among the Indians of the Great Canadian Plains*. London: Adlard and Sons Limited.

– 1955. *Studies in Tuberculosis*. Toronto: University of Toronto Press.

Ferguson, R.G., and A.B. Sime. 1949. 'BCG Vaccination of Indian Infants in Saskatchewan.' *Tubercle* 30:5–11.

Fetherstonhaugh, R. 1940. *The Royal Canadian Mounted Police*. New York: Garden City Publishing Co.

Fisher, A.D. 1987. 'Alcoholism and Race: The Misapplication of Both Concepts to North American Indians.' *Canadian Review of Sociology and Anthropology* 24:81–98.

Fisher, R. 1977. *Contact and Conflict: Indian-European Relations in British Columbia, 1774-1890*. Vancouver: University of British Columbia Press.

Flannery, Regina. 1939. 'The Shaking-Tent Rite among the Montagnais of James Bay.' *Primitive Man* 17(1):11–16.

Fleming, A. nd. *An Arctic Hospital*. Toronto: The Arctic Mission.

Fleming, R., ed. 1940. *Minutes of Council Northern Department of Rupert Land, 1821–1831*. London: The Hudson's Bay Record Society.

Ford, R. 1981. 'Ethnobotany in North America: An Historical Phytogeographic Perspective.' *Canadian Journal of Botany* 59:2178–88.

Fortuine, R. 1971. 'The Health of the Eskimos as Portrayed in the Earliest Written Accounts.' *Bulletin of the History of Medicine* 65(2):97–114.

– 1985. 'Lancets of Stone: Traditional Methods of Surgery among the Alaska Natives.' *Arctic Anthropology* 22(1):23–45.

– 1989. *Chills and Fever: Health and Disease in the Early History of Alaska*. Fairbanks: University of Alaska Press.

Foster, J. 1987. 'Indian-White Relations in the Prairie West during the Fur Trade Period: A Compact?' In Richard Price, ed. *The Spirit of the Alberta Indian Treaties*, 181–200. Montreal: Institute for Research on Public Policy.

Foulkes, R.G. 1962a. 'Medics in the North: A History of the Contributions of the Royal Canadian Air Force to the Medical Care of Civilians in the Fort Nelson Area of British Columbia. Part 1.' *Medical Services Journal of Canada* 18(7):523–50.

– 1962b. 'Medics in the North: A History of the Contributions of the Royal Canadian Air Force to the Medical Care of Civilians in the Fort Nelson Area of British Columbia. Part 3.' *Medical Services Journal of Canada* 18(9):675–86.

– 1962c. 'Medics in the North: A History of the Contributions of the Royal Canadian Air Force to the Medical Care of Civilians in the Fort Nelson Area of British Columbia. Part 4.' *Medical Services Journal of Canada* 18(10):736–52.

Fox, J., D. Manitowabi, and J.A. Ward. 1984. 'An Indian Community with a High Suicide Rate – 5 Years After.' *Canadian Journal of Psychiatry* 29:425–7.

Francis, D., and T. Morantz. 1983. *Partners in Furs: A History of the Fur Trade in Eastern James Bay, 1600–1870.* Montreal: McGill-Queen's University Press.

Franklin, J. 1969. *Narrative of a Journey to the Shore of the Polar Sea in the Years 1819, 20, 21, 22.* New York: Greenwood.

Friesen, B. 1985. 'Haddon's Strategy for Prevention: Application to Native House Fires.' In Robert Fortuine, ed. *Circumpolar Health 84: Proceedings of the 6th International Symposium,* 105–9. Seattle: University of Washington Press.

Fritz, W., and C. D'Arcy. 1982. 'Comparisons: Indian and Non-Indian Use of Psychiatric Services.' *Canadian Journal of Psychiatry* 27:194–203.

Frost, W.H. 1939. 'The Age Selection of Mortality from Tuberculosis in Successive Decades.' *American Journal of Hygiene* Section A (30):91–6.

Fry, G. 1974. 'Ovum and Parasite Examination of Saltes Cave Human Paleofeces.' In P.J. Watson, ed. *Archeology of the Mammoth Cave Area.* New York: Academic Press.

Fuchs, M., and R. Bashshur. 1975. 'Use of Traditional Indian Medicine among Urban Native Americans.' *Medical Care* 13(11):915–27.

Fumoleau, René. 1973. *As Long as the Land Shall Last.* Toronto: McClelland and Stewart.

Gagnon, Y. 1989. 'Physicians' Attitudes toward Collaboration with Traditional Healers.' *Native Studies Review* 5(1):175–86.

Gallagher, R.P., and J.M. Elwood. 1979. 'Cancer Mortality among Chinese, Japanese, and Indians in British Columbia, 1964–73.' *National Cancer Institute Monographs* 53:89–94.

Garrison, V. 1977. 'Doctor, Espiritista or Psychiatrist?: Health-seeking Behavior in a Puerto Rican Neighbourhood of New York City.' *Medical Anthropology* 1(2):65–191.

Garro, L.C. 1987. 'Cultural Knowledge about Diabetes.' In T.K. Young, ed. *Diabetes in the Canadian Native Population: Biocultural Perspectives,* 97–109. Toronto: Canadian Diabetes Association.

- 1988a. 'Culture and High Blood Pressure: Understandings of a Chronic Illness in an Ojibwa Community.' *Arctic Medical Research* 47 (Suppl. 1):70–3.
- 1988b. 'Explaining High Blood Pressure: Variation in Knowledge about Illness.' *American Ethnologist* 15:98–119.
- 1988c. 'Resort to Folk Healers in a Manitoba Ojibwa Community.' *Arctic Medical Research* 47 (Suppl. 1):317–20.
- 1988d. 'Suicides by Status Indians in Manitoba.' In H. Lindenholm, C. Backman, N. Broadbent, and I. Joelsson, eds. *Circumpolar Health 87: Proceedings of the 7th International Congress*, 590–2. Oulu, Finland: Nordic Council for Arctic Medical Research.
- 1990. 'Continuity and Change: The Interpretation of Illness in an Anishinaabe (Ojibway) Community.' *Culture, Medicine and Psychiatry* 14:417–54.
- 1991. 'Consultations with Anishinaabe (Ojibway) Healers in a Manitoba Community.' In B. Postl et al., eds. *Circumpolar Health 90: Proceedings of the 8th International Congress*, 213–16. Winnipeg: University of Manitoba Press.

Garro, L.C., and G.C. Lang. 1994. 'Explanations of Diabetes: Anishinaabe and Dakota Deliberate upon a New Illness.' In J.R. Joe and R.S. Young, eds. *Diabetes as a Disease of Civilization: The Impact of Culture Change on Indigenous Peoples*, 293–328. Berlin: Mouton de Gruyter.

Garro, L., J. Roulette, and R. Whitmore. 1986. 'Community Control of Health Care Delivery: The Sandy Bay Experience.' *Canadian Journal of Public Health* 77:281–4.

Garvin, J., ed. 1927. *Alexander Mackenzie: Voyages from Montreal*. Toronto: The Radisson Society of Canada.

Gaudette, L.A., R.-N. Gao, S. Freitag, and M. Wideman. 1993. 'Cancer Incidence by Ethnic Group in the Northwest Territories (NWT), 1969–1988.' Statistics Canada *Health Reports* 5:23–32.

George, P., and B. Nahwegahbow. 1993. 'Anishinawbe Health.' In Royal Commission on Aboriginal Peoples. *The Path to Healing*, 241–3. Ottawa: Royal Commission on Aboriginal Peoples.

Gibbons, A. 1993. 'Geneticists Trace the DNA Trail of the First Americans.' *Science* 259:312–13.

Gillis, D.C., J. Irvine, and L. Tan. 1991. 'Cancer Incidence and Survival of Saskatchewan Northerners and Registered Indians, 1967–1986.' In B.D. Postl et al., eds. *Circumpolar Health 90: Proceedings of the 8th International Congress*, 447–51. Winnipeg: University of Manitoba Press.

Glover, R., ed. 1958. *A Journey from Prince of Wales's Fort in Hudson's Bay to the Northern Ocean, 1769, 1770, 1771, 1772 by Samuel Hearne*. Toronto: Macmillan.

Goodman, J. 1981. *American Genesis*. New York: Summit Books.

Goodwill, Jean Cuthand. *See* Cuthand Goodwill.

Goodwill, J., and N. Sluman. 1984. *John Tootoosis*. Winnipeg: Pemmican.

Graburn, N. 1969. *Eskimos without Igloos: Social and Economic Development in Sugluk*. Boston: Little, Brown.

Graham-Cumming, G. 1967. 'Health of the Original Canadians, 1867–1967.' *Medical Services Journal* 23(2):115–66.

Grant, J.W. 1984. *Moon of Wintertime: Missionaries and the Indians of Canada in Encounter since 1534*. Toronto: University of Toronto Press.

Graves, T. 1967. 'Acculturation, Access, and Alcohol in a Tri-ethnic Community.' *American Anthropologist* 69:306–21.

Greenberg, J.H., C.G. Turner, II, and S.L. Zegura. 1986. 'The Settlement of the Americas: A Comparison of the Linguistic, Dental, and Genetic Evidence.' *Current Anthropology* 27(5):477–98.

Gregory, D. 1989. 'Traditional Indian Healers in Northern Manitoba: An Emerging Relationship with the Health Care System.' *Native Studies Review* 5(1):163–74.

Gregory, D., C. Russell, J. Hurd, J. Tyance, and J. Sloan. 1992. 'Canada's Indian Health Transfer Policy: The Gull Bay Band Experience.' *Human Organization* 51(3):214–22.

Grigg, E. 1958. 'The Arcana of Tuberculosis.' *American Review of Respiratory Disease* 78:151–72, 583–603.

Grinnell, G. 1972. *Blackfoot Lodge Tales: The Story of a Prairie People*. Williamstown, Mass.: Corner House. (Original publication 1892.)

Grygier, P.S. 1994. *A Long Way from Home: The Tuberculosis Epidemic among the Inuit*. Montreal and Kingston: McGill-Queen's University Press.

Hackett, C. 1983. 'Problems in the Paleopathology of the Human Treponematosis.' In Gerald D. Hart, ed. *Diseases in Ancient Man*, 106–28. Toronto: Clarke Irwin.

Hackett, F. 1991. *The 1819–20 Measles Epidemic: Its Origin, Diffusion and Mortality Effects upon the Indians of the Petit Nord*. MA diss., University of Manitoba.

Hader, J. 1990. *The Effect of Tuberculosis on the Indians of Saskatchewan, 1926–1965*. MA diss., University of Saskatchewan.

Hagey, N.J., G. Larocque, and C. McBride. 1989. *Highlights of Aboriginal Conditions 1981–2001: Part I – Demographic Trends; Part II – Social Conditions; Part III – Economic Conditions*. Ottawa: Department of Indian Affairs and Northern Development.

Hagey, Rebecca. 1984. 'The Phenomenon, the Explanations and the Responses: Metaphors Surrounding Diabetes in Urban Canadian Indians.' *Social Science and Medicine* 18:265–72.

Hallowell, A.I. 1942. *The Role of Conjuring in Saulteaux Society*. Philadelphia: University of Pennsylvania Press.

– 1963. 'Ojibwa World View and Disease.' In Iago Galdston, ed. *Man's Image in*

Medicine and Anthropology, 258–315. New York: International Universities Press.

Hamer, J. 1980. 'Acculturation Stress and the Functions of Alcohol among the Forest Potawatomi.' In J. Hamer, and J. Steinbring, eds. *Alcohol and Native Peoples of the North*, 107–53. Washington, D.C.: University Press of America.

Hamer, J., and J. Steinbring. 1980. 'Alcohol and the North American Indian: Examples from the Subarctic.' In J. Hamer, and J. Steinbring, eds. *Alcohol and Native Peoples of the North*, 1–29. Washington, D.C.: University Press of America.

Hamilton, M.K. 1990. 'The Health and Activity Limitation Survey: Disabled Aboriginal Persons in Canada.' Statistics Canada *Health Reports* 2:279–87.

Hammond, G.W., B.E. Rutherford, R. Malazdrewicz, and N. MacFarlane. 1988. 'Haemophilus Influenzae Meningitis in Manitoba and the Keewatin District, NWT: Potential for Mass Vaccination.' *Canadian Medical Association Journal* 139:743–7.

Harmon, D. 1911. *A Journal of Voyages and Travels in the Interior of North America.* Toronto: Courier Press.

Hartney, P.C. 1981. 'Tuberculous Lesions in a Prehistoric Population Sample from southern Ontario.' In J.E. Buikstra, ed. *Prehistoric Tuberculosis in the Americas*, 141–60. Evanston, Ill.: Northwestern University Archaeological Program.

Hauschild, A.H., and L. Gauvreau. 1985. 'Food-born Botulism in Canada, 1971–84.' *Canadian Medical Association Journal* 133:1141–6.

Heagerty, J.J. 1928. *Four Centuries of Medical History in Canada.* Toronto: Macmillan.

Health Status Research Unit. 1989. *Health Status of the Saskatchewan Population: Risk Factors and Health Promotion Priorities.* Saskatoon: Department of Community Health and Epidemiology, University of Saskatchewan.

Hellson, J. 1974. 'Ethnobotany of the Blackfoot Indians.' *Canadian Ethnology Service Paper* No. 19, National Museum of Canada, Ottawa.

Helm, J. 1980. 'Female Infanticide, European Diseases and Population Levels among Mackenzie Dene.' *American Ethnologist* 7:259–85.

Henderson, J. 1987. 'Factors Determining the State of Preservation of Human Remains.' In A. Boddington, A.N. Garland, and R.C. Janaway, eds. *Death, Decay and Reconstruction: Approaches to Archaeology and Forensic Sciences*, 43–54. Manchester: Manchester University Press.

Henige, D. 1990. 'Their Numbers Become Thick: Native American Historical Demography as Expiation.' In James A. Clifton, ed. *The Invented Indian: Cultural Fictions and Government Policies*, 169–91. London: Transaction Publications.

Henry, Alexander. 1976. *Travels and Adventures in Canada and the Indian Territo-*

ries between the Years 1760 and 1776. New York: Garland. (Original publication 1809.)

Herring, D.A. 1992. 'Toward a Reconsideration of Disease and Contact in the Americas.' *Prairie Forum* 17(2):153–65.

– 1993. ' "There Were Young People and Old People and Babies Dying Every Week": The 1918–1919 Influenza Pandemic at Norway House.' *Ethnohistory* 41(1):73–105.

– 1994. 'The 1918 Influenza Epidemic in the Central Canadian Subarctic.' In A. Herring and L. Chan, eds. *Strength in Diversity: A Reader in Physical Anthropology*, 365–84. Toronto: Canadian Scholars' Press.

Hildes, J.A., and O. Schaefer. 1973. 'Health of Igloolik Eskimos and Change with Urbanization.' *Journal of Human Evolution* 2:241–6.

– 1984. 'The Changing Picture of Neoplastic Disease in the Western and Central Canadian Arctic (1950–1980).' *Canadian Medical Association Journal* 130:25–33.

Hislop, T.G., M. Deschamps, P.R. Band, J.M. Smith, and H.F. Clarke. 1992. 'Participation in the British Columbia Cervical Cytology Screening Program by Native Indian Women.' *Canadian Journal of Public Health* 83:344–5.

Hislop, T.G., W.J. Threlfall, R.P. Gallagher, and P.R. Band. 1987. 'Accidental and Intentional Violent Deaths among British Columbia Native Indians.' *Canadian Journal of Public Health* 78:271–4.

Hoffecker, J.F., W.R. Powers, and T. Goebel. 1993. 'The Colonization of Beringia and the Peopling of the New World.' *Science* 259:46–53.

Holcomb, R.C. 1940. 'Syphilis of the Skull among Aleuts, and the Asian and North American Eskimo about Bering and Arctic Seas.' *U.S. Naval Medical Bulletin* 38:177–92.

Honigmann, J.J. 1980. 'Perspectives on Alcohol Behaviour.' In J. Hamer and J. Steinbring, eds. *Alcohol and Native Peoples of the North*, 267–85. Washington, D.C.: University Press of America.

Hood, E., S.A. Malcolmsonm, L.T. Young, and S.Abbey. 1993. 'Psychiatric Consultation in the Eastern Canadian Arctic. I. Development and Evolution of the Baffin Psychiatric Consultation Service.' *Canadian Journal of Psychiatry* 38:23–7.

Hopwood, V., ed. 1971. *David Thompson: Travels in Western North America, 1784–1812.* Toronto: Macmillan.

Houston, S., A. Fanning, C.L. Soskolne, and N. Fraser. 1990. 'The Effectiveness of Bacille Calmette-Guérin (BCG) Vaccination against Tuberculosis.' *American Journal of Epidemiology* 131:340–8.

Howard, J. 1977. *The Plains-Ojibwa or Bungi: Hunters and Warriors of the Northern*

Prairies with Special Reference to the Turtle Mountain Band. Lincoln, Nebr.: J. and L. Reprint Co. Reprints in Anthropology, vol. 7.

Hrdlicka, A. 1908. 'Contribution to the Study of Tuberculosis in the Indian.' *Transactions of the Sixth International Congress on Tuberculosis, Washington.* Vol. III, Section V, 480–93. Philadelphia: William F. Fell Co.

Hultkrantz, A. 1992. *Shamanic Healing and Ritual Drama: Health and Medicine in Native North American Religious Traditions.* New York: Crossroad.

Hurlich, M. 1983. 'Historical and Recent Demography of the Algonkians of Northern Ontario.' In A.T. Steegmann, Jr, ed. *Boreal Forest Adaptations: The Northern Algonkians,* 143–200. New York: Plenum.

Hurt, W.R., and R.M. Brown. 1965. 'Social Drinking Patterns of the Yankton Sioux.' *Human Organization* 24:222–30.

Hutchens, Alma. 1973. *Indian Herbalogy of North America.* Windsor: Merco.

Hutchison, W. 1907. 'Varieties of Tuberculosis According to Race and Social Condition.' *International Record of Medicine* 86:624–9.

Imrie, R., and R. Warren. 1988. 'Health Promotion Survey in the Northwest Territories.' *Canadian Journal of Public Health* 79:16–24.

Indian Association of Alberta. 1970. *Citizens Plus.* Edmonton: Indian Association of Alberta.

Innis, S.M., and H.V. Kuhnlein. 1987. 'The Fatty Acid Composition of Northern Canadian Marine and Terrestrial Mammals.' *Acta Medica Scandinavica* 222:105–9.

Irvine, J., D.C. Gillis, and L. Tan. 1991. 'Lung, Breast, and Cervical Cancer Incidence and Survival in Saskatchewan Northerners and Registered Indians (1967–86).' In B.D. Postl et al., eds. *Circumpolar Health 90: Proceedings of the 8th International Congress,* 452–6. Winnipeg: University of Manitoba Press.

Irving, W.N. 1985. 'Context and Chronology of Early Man in the Americas.' *Annual Review of Anthropology* 14:529–55.

Jackes, M. 1983. 'Osteological Evidence of Smallpox: A Possible Case from Seventeenth Century Ontario.' *American Journal of Physical Anthropology* 60:75–81.

– 1986. 'The Mortality of Ontario Archaeological Populations.' *Canadian Journal of Anthropology* 5(2):33–47.

– 1988. *The Osteology of the Grimsby Site.* Edmonton, Alberta: Department of Anthropology, University of Alberta.

– 1994. 'Bones and Birth Rates.' In A. Herring and L. Chan, eds. *Strength in Diversity: A Reader in Physical Anthropology,* 155–85. Toronto: Canadian Scholars' Press.

Jarvis, G.K., and M. Boldt. 1982. 'Death Styles among Canada's Indians.' *Social Science and Medicine* 16:1345–52.

Jenkins, D. 1977. 'Tuberculosis: The Native Indian Viewpoint on Its Prevention, Diagnosis, and Treatment.' *Preventive Medicine* 6:545–55.

Jenness, D. 1938. *The Sarcee Indians of Alberta*. Ottawa: National Museum of Canada. Bulletin 90.

– 1972. *Eskimo Administration: II. Canada*. Arctic Institute of North America Technical Paper No. 14. (Original publication 1964.)

Jilek, W.G. 1978. 'Native Renaissance: The Survival and Revival of Indigenous Therapeutic Ceremonials among North American Indians.' *Transcultural Psychiatric Research Review* 15:117–47.

– 1982a. 'Altered States of Consciousness in North American Indian Ceremonials.' *Ethos* 10:326–43.

– 1982b. *Indian Healing: Shamanic Ceremonialism in the Pacific Northwest Today*. Surrey, B.C.: Hancock House.

– 1991. 'Traditional Medicine and Mental Health Care.' In B. Postl et al., eds. *Circumpolar Health 90: Proceedings of the 8th International Congress*, 303–8. Winnipeg: University of Manitoba Press.

Jilek, W.G., and L. Jilek-Aall. 1982. 'Shamanic Symbolism in Salish Indian Rituals.' In I. Rossi, ed. *The Logic of Culture*, 127–36. South Hadley, Mass.: J.F. Bergen Publishers.

– 1991. 'Traditional Medicine and Mental Health Care.' In B. Postl et al., eds. *Circumpolar Health 90: Proceedings of the 8th International Congress*, 303–8. Winnipeg: University of Manitoba Press.

Jilek, W.G., and C. Roy. 1976. 'Homicide Committed by Canadian Indians and Non-Indians.' *International Journal of Offender Therapy Comparative Criminology* 20:201–16.

Jilek-Aall, L. 1981. 'Acculturation, Alcoholism and Indian-style Alcoholics Anonymous.' *Journal of Studies in Alcoholism* Suppl. 9:143–58.

Johansson, S. 1982. 'The Demographic History of the Native Peoples of North America: A Selected Bibliography.' *Yearbook of Physical Anthropology* 25:133–52.

Johnson, J., and F. Johnson. 1993. 'Community Development, Sobriety and After-care at Alkali Lake Band.' In Royal Commission on Aboriginal Peoples. *The Path to Healing*, 227–30. Ottawa: Royal Commission on Aboriginal Peoples.

Joraleman, D. 1982. 'New World Depopulation and the Case of Disease.' *Journal of Anthropological Research* 38(1):108–27.

Katzenberg, M.A. 1989. 'Stable Isotope Analysis of Archaeological Faunal Remains from Southern Ontario.' *Journal of Archaeological Science* 16(3):319–30.

– 1992. 'Changing Diet and Health in Pre- and Proto-historic Ontario.' *MASCA Research Papers in Science and Archaeology* 9:23–31.

Katzenberg, M.A., S.R. Saunders, and W.R. Fitzgerald. 1993. 'Age Differences in Stable Carbon and Nitrogen Isotope Ratios in a Population of Prehistoric Maize Horticulturalists.' *American Journal of Physical Anthropology* 90(3):267–81.

Katzenberg, M.A., and J.P. Schwarcz. 1986. 'Paleonutrition in Southern Ontario: Evidence from Strontium and Stable Isotopes.' *Canadian Journal of Anthropology* 5(2):15–21.

Kaufert, J., and W. Koolage. 1985. 'Culture Brokerage and Advocacy in Urban Hospitals: The Impact of Native Language Interpreters.' *Santé Culture Health* 3(2):3–8.

Keenleyside, A. 1990. 'Euro-American Whaling in the Canadian Arctic: Its Effects on Eskimo Health.' *Arctic Anthropology* 27(1):1–19.

– 1993. 'Skeletal Evidence of Health and Disease in Pre-contact and Contact Period Alaskan Eskimos and Aleuts.' Paper presented at the 62nd Annual Meeting of the American Association of Physical Anthropologists, Toronto, Ontario.

– 1994. *Skeletal Evidence of Health and Disease in Pre- and Postcontact Alaskan Eskimos and Aleuts.* PhD diss., McMaster University.

Keewatin Regional Health Board. 1992. *Report on the 1991 Epidemic of E. coli 0157:H7 Gastroenteritis in the Keewatin.* Rankin Inlet, N.W.T.: Keewatin Regional Health Board.

Kemnitzer, L.S. 1972. 'The Structure of Country Drinking Parties on Pine Ridge Reservation, South Dakota.' *Plains Anthropologist* 17:134–42.

Kennedy, D. 1984. 'The Quest for a Cure: A Case Study in the Use of Health Care Alternatives.' *Culture* 4(2):21–31.

Kidd, G. 1946. 'Trepanation among the Early Indians of British Columbia.' *Canadian Medical Association Journal* 55:513–15.

Kleinman, A. 1980. *Patients and Healers in the Context of Culture.* Berkeley: University of California Press.

Kralt, J. 1990. 'Ethnic Origins in the Canadian Census, 1871–1986.' In S.S. Halli, F. Trovato, and L. Driedger, eds. *Ethnic Demography: Canadian Immigrant, Racial and Cultural Variations,* 13–29. Ottawa: Carleton University Press.

Krech, S., III. 1983a. 'Disease, Starvation, and Northern Athapaskan Social Organization.' *American Ethnologist* 5:710–32.

– 1983b. 'The Influence of Disease and the Fur Trade on Arctic Drainage Lowlands Dene, 1800–1850.' *Journal of Anthropological Research* 39(1):123–46.

Kroeber, A.L. 1934. 'Native American Population.' *American Anthropologist* 36:1–25.

Kunitz, S.J. 1990. 'Public Policy and Mortality among Indigenous Populations of Northern America and Australasia.' *Population Development Review* 16:647–72.

Lamoureux, M., ed. 1991. *Domestic Violence in Aboriginal Communities: Reference Manual*. Quebec: Ministère de la Santé et des Services sociaux.

LaPointe, K. 1986. 'Bureaucratic Bungling Separated Inuit.' Saskatoon *Star-Phoenix*, 23 September 1986, B:4.

Larocque, R. 1991. 'The Detection of Epidemics on Human Skeletal Remains: An Example from Huronia.' Paper presented at the 1991 Canadian Association for Physical Anthropology meeting, Hamilton, Ontario, Canada.

Larsen, C.S. 1994. 'In the Wake of Columbus: Native Population Biology in the Postcontact Americas.' *Yearbook of Physical Anthropology* 37:109–54.

Larsen, C.S., and G.R. Milner, eds. 1994. *In the Wake of Contact: Biological Responses to Conquest*. New York: Wiley-Liss.

Latulippe-Sakamoto, C. 1971. *Estimation de la mortalité des indiens du Canada, 1900 1968*. MA diss., University of Ottawa.

Laughlin, W., A. Harper, and D. Thompson. 1979. 'New Approaches to the Pre- and Post-contact History of Arctic peoples.' *American Journal of Physical Anthropology* 51:579–88.

LaViolette, F. 1973. *The Struggle for Survival: Indian Cultures and the Protestant Ethic in British Columbia*. Toronto: University of Toronto Press.

Leacy, F.H., ed. 1983. *Historical Statistics of Canada*. 2nd ed. Ottawa: Statistics Canada.

Lederman, J.M., A.C. Wallace, and J.A. Hildes. 1962. 'Arteriosclerosis and Neoplasms in Canadian Eskimos.' In *Biological Aspects of Aging: Proceedings of the Fifth International Congress on Gerontology*, 201–7. New York: Columbia University Press.

Leiber, C.S. 1972. 'Metabolism of Ethanol and Alcoholism: Racial and Acquired Factors.' *Annals of Internal Medicine* 76:326–7

Leighton, A. 1985. *Wild Plant Use by the Woods Cree of East-Central Saskatchewan*. Ottawa: National Museum of Canada, Ethnology Service Paper No. 101.

Levine, S., M. Eastwood, and Q. Rae-Grant. 1974. 'Psychiatry Service to Northern Indians: A University Project.' *Canadian Psychiatric Association Journal* 19:343–9.

Levy, J.E., and S. Kunitz. 1974. *Indian Drinking: Navajo Practices and Anglo-American Theories*. New York: Wiley and Sons.

Long, J., and C. Merbs. 1981. 'Coccidioidomycosis: A Primate Model.' In J.E. Buikstra, ed. *Prehistoric Tuberculosis in the Americas*, 69–83. Evanston, Ill.: Northwestern University Archaeological Program.

Long, R., J. Manfreda, L. Mendella, J. Wolfe, S. Parker, and E. Hershfield. 1993. 'Antituberculous Drug Resistance in Manitoba from 1980–1989.' *Canadian Medical Association Journal* 148:1489–95.

Longclaws, L., G.E. Barnes, L. Grieve, and R. Dumoff. 1980. 'Alcohol and Drug Use among the Brokenhead Ojibwa.' *Journal of Studies in Alcohol* 41:21–36.

Lopatin, I. 1960. 'Origin of the Native American Steam Bath.' *American Anthropologist* 62:977–93.

Lucier, C., J. VanStone, and D. Keats. 1971. 'Medical Practice and Human Anatomical Knowledge among the Noatak Eskimos.' *Ethnology* 10(3):251–64.

Lurie, N.O. 1971.'The World's Oldest On-going Protest Demonstration: North American Indian Drinking Patterns.' *Pacific Historical Review* 40:311–32.

Lux, M. 1992. 'Prairie Indians and the 1918 Influenza Epidemic.' *Native Studies Review* 8(1):23–33.

Lynch, G.I. 1991. 'Movement toward Professional Excellence – Medical Services Branch Indian Health.' In B. Postl et al., eds. *Circumpolar Health 90: Proceedings of the 8th International Congress*, 173–6. Winnipeg: University of Manitoba Press.

Macaulay, A.C., and N. Hanusaik. 1988. 'Diabetic Education Program in the Mohawk Community of Kahnawake, Quebec.' *Canadian Family Physician* 34:1591–3.

Macaulay, A.C., L.T. Montour, and N. Adelson. 1988. 'Prevalence of Diabetic and Atherosclerotic Complications among Mohawk Indians of Kahnawake, PQ.' *Canadian Medical Association Journal* 139:221–4.

McCarthy, F. 1912. 'The Influence of Race in the Prevalence of Tuberculosis.' *Boston Medical and Surgical Journal* 166:207–13.

McClure, L., M. Boulanger, J. Kaufert, and S. Forsyth. 1992. *First Nations Urban Health Bibliography: A Review of the Literature and Exploration of Strategies.* Winnipeg: Northern Health Research Unit, Department of Community Health Sciences, University of Manitoba.

McGhee, R. 1992. 'Before Columbus: Early European Visitors to the Shores of the "New World".' *The Beaver* 72(3):6–23.

McGrath, J. 1988. 'Social Networks of Disease Spread in the Lower Illinois Valley: A Simulation Approach.' *American Journal of Physical Anthropology* 77:483–96.

– 1991. 'Biological Impact of Social Disruption Resulting from Epidemic Disease.' *American Journal of Physical Anthropology* 84:407–20.

McIntyre, L., and C.P. Shah. 1986. 'Prevalence of Hypertension, Obesity and Smoking in Three Indian Communities in Northwestern Ontario.' *Canadian Medical Association Journal* 134:345–9.

McKennan, R. 1965. *The Chandalar Kutchin.* Edmonton: Arctic Institute of North America. Technical Paper No. 17.

Mackenzie, Alexander. 1971. *Voyages from Montreal on the River St. Laurence through the Continent of North America to the Frozen and Pacific Oceans in the Years 1789–1793.* Edmonton: Hurtig.

McKeown, T. 1988. *The Origins of Human Disease.* Oxford: Blackwell.

McLean, John. 1889. *The Indians of Canada: Their Manners and Customs*. Toronto: William Briggs.

McMillan, A.D. 1988. *Native Peoples and Cultures of Canada: An Anthropological Overview*. Vancouver: Douglas and McIntyre.

McNab, Claire. 1993. Personal interview with Claire McNab, National Native Access Program to Nursing, University of Saskatchewan, by James B. Waldram, 18 February 1993.

McNeill, W.H. 1976. *Plagues and Peoples*. New York: Penguin.

Mandelbaum, D.G. 1935. Unpublished Field Notebooks. Saskatchewan Archives Board, Regina.

– 1979. *The Plains Cree: An Ethnographic, Historical, and Comparative Study*. Regina: Canadian Plains Research Centre.

Mao, Y., B.W. Moloughney, R. Semenciw, and H. Morrison. 1992. 'Indian Reserve and Registered Indian Mortality in Canada.' *Canadian Journal of Public Health* 83:350–3.

Mao, Y., H. Morrison, R. Semenciw, and D. Wigle. 1986. 'Mortality on Canadian Indian Reserves 1976–1983.' *Canadian Journal of Public Health* 77:263–8.

Marchand, J.F. 1943. 'Tribal Epidemics in the Yukon.' *Journal of the American Medical Association* 123:1019–20.

Marshall, I. 1977. 'An Unpublished Map Made by John Cartwright between 1768–1773 Showing Beothuk Indian Settlements and Artifacts and Allowing a New Population Estimate.' *Ethnohistory* 24(3):223–49.

– 1981. 'Disease as a Factor in the Demise of the Beothuk Indians.' *Culture* 1(1):71–7.

Martens, T., B. Daily, and M. Hodgson. 1988. *Characteristics and Dynamics of Incest and Child Sexual Abuse, with a Native Perspective*. Edmonton: Nechi Institute.

Maundrell, C. 1942. *Indian Health: 1867–1940*. MA diss., Queen's University.

Mausner, J., and A. Bahn. 1974. *Epidemiology*. Boston: Little, Brown.

May, P.A. 1984. 'Explanations of Native American Drinking: A Literature Review.' In R. Hornby and R. Dana, eds. *Mni Wakan and the Sioux: Respite, Release and Recreation*, 13–27. Brandon: Justin Publishing.

Mayhall, J.T. 1992. 'Techniques for the Study of Dental Morphology.' In S.R. Saunders and M.A. Katzenberg, eds. *Skeletal Biology of Past Peoples: Research Methods*, 59–78. New York: Wiley-Liss.

Meerovitch, E., and R.D. Eaton. 1965. 'Outbreak of Amebiasis among Indians in Northwestern Saskatchewan, Canada.' *American Journal of Tropical Medicine and Hygiene* 14:719–23.

Meister, C. 1976. 'Demographic Consequences of Euro-American Contact on

Selected American Indian Populations and Their Relationship to the Demographic Transition.' *Ethnohistory* 23(2):161–72.

Meltzer, H., L. Kovacs, T. Orford, and M. Matas. 1956. 'Echinococcosis in North American Indians and Eskimos.' *Canadian Medical Association Journal* 75:121–8.

Merbs, C.F. 1963. 'Patterns of Pathology in Eskimos and Aleuts.' *American Journal of Physical Anthropology* 19(1):103 (abstract).

– 1992. 'A New World of Infectious Disease.' *Yearbook of Physical Anthropology* 35:3–42.

Merbs, C.F., and W. Wilson. 1960. 'Anomalies and Pathologies of the Sadlermiut Eskimo Vertebral Column.' *National Museum of Canada Bulletin, Contributions to Anthropology, Part 1*, 154–80.

Merbs, C.F., W. Wilson, and W.S. Laughlin. 1961. 'The Vertebral Column of the Sadlermiut Eskimos.' *American Journal of Physical Anthropology* 19(1):103 (abstract).

Millar, W.J. 1982. 'Mortality Patterns in a Canadian Indian Population.' *Canadian Studies in Population* 9:17–31.

– 1990. 'Smoking Prevalence in the Canadian Arctic.' *Arctic Medical Research* 49 (Suppl. 2):23–8.

Millar, W.J., and J. Peterson, 1989. *Tobacco Use by Youth in the Canadian Arctic.* Ottawa: Health and Welfare Canada, Health Services and Promotion Branch.

Miller, J.R. 1989. *Skyscrapers Hide the Heavens: A History of Indian-White Relations in Canada.* Toronto: University of Toronto Press.

Miller, V. 1976. 'Aboriginal Micmac Population: A Review of the Evidence.' *Ethnohistory* 23(2):117–27.

– 1982. 'The Decline of Nova Scotia Micmac Population, AD 1600–1850.' *Culture* 2(3):107–20.

Moerman, D.E. 1983. 'Physiology and Symbols: The Anthropological Implications of the Placebo Effect.' In L. Romanucci-Ross, D. Moreman, and L. Tancredi, eds. *The Anthropology of Medicine: From Culture to Method*, 156–67. New York: Praeger.

– 1986. *Medicinal Plants of North America.* Ann Arbor: University of Michigan Museum of Anthropology. Technical Reports, No. 19.

Moffatt, M. 1987. 'Land Settlements and Health Care: The Case of the James Bay Cree.' *Canadian Journal of Public Health* 78:223–7.

Molto, J.E. In press. 'A Treponematosis "Endemic" to the Precontact Population of the Cape Region of Baja California Sur.' In O. Dutour, G. Pálfi, J. Bérato, and J-P Brun, eds. *L'Origine de la Syphilis en Europe. Avant ou après 1493?*, 176–84. Paris: Editions Errance.

Molto, J.E., and F.J. Melbye. 1984. 'Treponemal Disease from Two Seventeenth

Century Iroquois Sites in Southern Ontario.' Paper presented at the 1984 Paleopathology Association meeting, Philadelphia, Pennsylvania.

Montour, L.T., A.C. Macaulay, and N. Adelson. 1989. 'Diabetes Mellitus in Mohawks of Kahnawake, PQ: A Clinical and Epidemiologic Description.' *Canadian Medical Association Journal* 141:549–52.

Mooney, J. 1928. 'The Aboriginal Population of America North of Mexico.' In J.R. Swanton, ed. *Smithsonian Miscellaneous Collections* 80(7). Washington, D.C.: Smithsonian Institution.

Moore, M., H. Forbes, and L. Henderson. 1990. 'The Provision of Primary Health Services under Band Control: The Montreal Lake Case.' *Native Studies Review* 6(1):153–64.

Moore, P.E. 1946. 'Indian Health Services.' *Canadian Journal of Public Health* 37:140–2.

- 1956. 'Medical Care of Canada's Indians and Eskimos.' *Canadian Journal of Public Health* 47(6):227–36.

- 1961. 'No Longer Captain: A History of Tuberculosis and Its Control amongst Canadian Indians.' *Canadian Medical Association Journal* 84:1012–16.

- 1974. 'The Modern Medicine Man.' In M. Van Steensel, ed. *People of Light and Dark*, 132–6. Ottawa. Department of Indian Affairs and Northern Development.

Moore, P.E., H.D. Kruse, F.F. Tisdall, and R.S. Corrigan. 1946. 'Medical Survey of Nutrition among the Northern Manitoba Indian.' *Canadian Medical Association Journal* 54:223–33.

Morice, A. 1900–1. 'Dene Surgery.' *Transactions of the Canadian Institute* 7:15–27.

Morris, A. 1880. *The Treaties of Canada with the Indians.* Repr. 1979. Toronto: Coles.

Morrison, H.I., R.M. Semenciw, Y. Mao, and D. Wigle. 1986. 'Infant Mortality on Canadian Indian Reserves, 1976–1983.' *Canadian Journal of Public Health* 77:269–73.

Morrison, W. 1985. *Showing the Flag: The Mounted Police and Canadian Sovereignty in the North, 1894–1925.* Vancouver: University of British Columbia Press.

Morse, S.S. 1993. 'Examining the Origins of Emerging Viruses.' In S.S. Morse, ed. *Emerging Viruses*, 10–28. Oxford: Oxford University Press.

Munro, J. 1983. Speech given to 'National Indian and Inuit Health Conference.'

Murray, R. 1990. *Future Directions for Health Care in Saskatchewan. Report of the Saskatchewan Commission on Directions in Health Care.* Regina: Government of Saskatchewan.

Myers, T., M.C. Liviana, R. Cockerill, W.M. Victor, and S.L. Bullock. 1993. *Ontario First Nations AIDS and Health Lifestyle Survey.* Toronto: University of Toronto, Department of Health Administration.

Neel, J.V. 1982. 'Infectious Disease among Amerindians.' *Medical Anthropology* 6(1):47–55.

New Democrats' Task Force on Northern Health Issues. 1989. *First Come, Last Served: Native Health in Northern Ontario.* Toronto: New Democratic Party of Ontario.

Newman, M.T. 1976. 'Aboriginal New World Epidemiology and Medical Care, and the Impact of Old World Disease Imports.' *American Journal of Physical Anthropology* 45:667–72.

Norris, M.J. 1990. 'The Demography of Aboriginal People in Canada.' In S.S. Hallis, F. Trovato, and L. Driedger, eds. *Ethnic Demography: Canadian Immigrant, Racial and Cultural Variations,* 33–59. Ottawa: Carleton University Press.

Nuttall, R.N. 1982. 'The Development of Indian Boards of Health in Alberta.' *Canadian Journal of Public Health* 73:300–3.

O'Neil, J.D. 1985. 'Community Control over Health Problems: Alcohol Prohibition in a Canadian Inuit Village.' In R. Fortuine, ed. *Circumpolar Health 84: Proceedings of the 6th International Symposium,* 340–3. Seattle: University of Washington Press.

– 1986. 'The Politics of Health in the Fourth World: A Northern Canadian Example.' *Human Organization* 45:119–28.

– 1988. 'Referrals to Traditional Healers: The Role of Medical Interpreters.' In D. Young, ed. *Health Care Issues in the Canadian North,* 29–38. Edmonton: Boreal Institute for Northern Studies.

– 1990. 'The Impact of Devolution on Health Services in the Baffin Region, NWT: A Case Study.' In G. Dacks, ed. *Devolution and Constitutional Development in the Canadian North,* 157–93. Ottawa: Carleton University Press.

– 1991. 'Regional Health Boards and the Democratization of Health Care in the Northwest Territories.' In B. Postl et al., eds. *Circumpolar Health 90: Proceedings of the 8th International Congress,* 20–5. Winnipeg: University of Manitoba Press.

– 1993. 'Aboriginal Health Policy for the Next Century: A Discussion Paper for the Royal Commission on Aboriginal People.' In Royal Commission on Aboriginal Peoples. *The Path to Healing: Report of the National Round Table on Aboriginal Health and Social Issues.* Ottawa: Royal Commission on Aboriginal Peoples.

Ontario. Ministry of Health. 1994. *New Directions: Aboriginal Health Policy for Ontario.* Toronto.

Oosten, J.G. 1986. 'Male and Female in Inuit Shamanism.' *Études Inuit Studies* 10(1–2):115–31.

Ortiz, Roxanne Dunbar. 1984. *Indians of the Americas.* London: Zed Books.

Ortner, D.J. 1992. 'Skeletal Paleopathology: Probabilities, Possibilities, and Impossibilities.' In J.W. Verano and D.H. Ubelaker, eds. *Disease and Demography in the Americas*, 5–13. Washington, D.C.: Smithsonian Institution Press.

Osgood, C. 1931. *The Ethnography of the Great Bear Lake Indians*. Ottawa: National Museum of Canada. Bulletin No. 70.

– 1936. *Contributions to the Ethnography of the Kutchin*. New Haven: Yale University Press.

Palkovich, A. 1981. 'Demography and Disease Patterns in a Protohistoric Plains Group: A Study of the Mobridge Site (39 WW 1).' *Plains Anthropologist* 26 (Memoir 17):71–84.

Pastore, R. 1987. 'Fishermen, Furriers, and Beothuks: The Economy of Extinction.' *Man in the Northeast* 33:47–62.

– 1989. 'The Collapse of the Beothuk World.' *Acadiensis* 19(1):52–71.

Patterson, D.K. 1984. *A Diachronic Study of Dental Palaeopathology and Attritional Status of Prehistoric Ontario Pre-Iroquois and Iroquois Populations*. Mercury Series, Archaeological Survey of Canada Paper 122. Ottawa: National Museum of Man.

Peart, A.F., and F.P. Nagler. 1954. 'Measles in the Canadian Arctic, 1952.' *Canadian Journal of Public Health* 45:146–57.

Pelz, M., H. Merskey, C. Brant, P.G.R. Patterson, and G.F.D. Heseltine. 1981. 'Clinical Data from a Psychiatric Service to a Group of Native People.' *Canadian Journal of Psychiatry* 26: 345–8.

Penner, Keith (Chair). 1983. *Indian Self Government in Canada: Report of the Special Committee on Indian Self-Government*. Ottawa: House of Commons.

Perla, D., and J. Marmorston. 1941. *Natural Resistance and Clinical Medicine*, 66–83 Boston: Little, Brown.

Pettipas, K. 1994. *Severing the Ties That Bind: Government Repression of Indigenous Religious Ceremonies on the Prairies*. Winnipeg: University of Manitoba Press.

Pfeiffer, S. 1984. 'Paleopathology in an Iroquoian Ossuary, with Special Reference to Tuberculosis.' *American Journal of Physical Anthropology* 65:181–9.

– 1986. 'Morbidity and Mortality in the Uxbridge Ossuary.' *Canadian Journal of Anthropology* 5(2):23–31.

– 1991. 'Is Paleopathology a Relevant Predictor of Contemporary Health Patterns?' In D.J. Ortner and A.C. Aufderheide, eds. *Human Paleopathology: Current Syntheses and Future Options*, 12–17. Washington, D.C.: Smithsonian Institution Press.

Pfeiffer, S., and S.I. Fairgrieve. 1994. 'Evidence from Ossuaries: The Effect of Contact on the Health of Iroquoians.' In C.S. Larsen, and G.R. Milner, eds. *In the Wake of Contact: Biological Responses to Conquest*, 47–61. New York: Wiley-Liss.

Pfeiffer, S., and P. King. 1983. 'Cortical Bone Formation and Diet among Proto-historic Iroquoians.' *American Journal of Physical Anthropology* 60:23–8.

Piché, V., and M.V. George. 1973. 'Estimates of Vital Rates for the Canadian Indians, 1960–1970.' *Demography* 10(3):367–82.

Pocklington, T. 1991. *The Government and Politics of the Alberta Metis Settlements.* Regina: Canadian Plains Research Centre.

Pollitzer, W.S. 1994. 'Ethnicity and Human Biology.' *American Journal of Human Biology* 6:3–11.

Press, I. 1969. 'Urban Illness: Physicians, Curers and Dual Use in Bogota.' *Journal of Health and Social Behavior* 10:209–18.

Preston, R. 1975. 'Cree Narrative: Expressing the Personal Meanings of Events.' Ottawa: National Museums of Canada, Canadian Ethnology Service Paper No. 30.

Price, J.A. 1975. 'An Applied Analysis of North American Indian Drinking Patterns.' *Human Organization* 34:17–26.

Price, W.A. 1934. 'Why Dental Caries with Modern Civilizations? VIII. Field Studies on Modernized Indians in Twenty Communities of the Canadian and Alaskan Pacific Coast.' *Dental Digest* 40:81–4.

Ramenofsky, A.F. 1987. *Vectors of Death: The Archaeology of European Contact.* Albuquerque: University of New Mexico Press.

Ray, A.J. 1974. *Indians in the Fur Trade: Their Role as Hunters, Trappers and Middlemen in the Lands Southwest of Hudson Bay, 1660–1870.* Toronto: University of Toronto Press.

– 1975. 'Smallpox: The Epidemic of 1837–38.' *The Beaver* 306(2):8–13.

– 1976. 'Diffusion of Diseases in the Western Interior of Canada, 1830–1950.' *Geographical Review* 66(2):139–57.

– 1984. 'William Todd: Doctor and Trader for the Hudson's Bay Company, 1816–51.' *Prairie Forum* 9(1):13–26.

– 1990. *The Canadian Fur Trade in the Industrial Age.* Toronto: University of Toronto Press.

Read, J., and F.L. Strick. 1969. 'Medical Education and the Native Canadian: An Example of Mutual Symbiosis.' *Canadian Medical Association Journal* 100:515–20.

Reed, T.E. 1985. 'Ethnic Differences in Alcohol Use, Abuse, and Sensitivity: A Review with Genetic Interpretation.' *Social Biology* 32:195–209.

Reed, T.E., H. Kalant, R.J. Gibbins, B.M. Kapur, and J.G. Rankin. 1976. 'Alcohol and Acetaldehyde Metabolism in Caucasians, Chinese and Amerinds.' *Canadian Medical Association Journal* 115:851–5.

Reff, D. 1991. *Disease, Depopulation and Culture Change in Northwestern New Spain, 1518–1764.* Salt Lake City: University of Utah Press.

Remington, G., and B.F. Hoffman. 1984. 'Gas Sniffing as a Form of Substance Abuse.' *Canadian Journal of Psychiatry* 29:31–5.

Revised Statutes of Canada. 1886. c.43, S.115.

– 1906. c.81, S.8.

Rheinhard, K. 1992. 'Parasitology as an Interpretive Tool in Archaeology.' *American Antiquity* 57:231–45.

Rheinhard, K., J. Ambler, and M. McGuffie. 1985. 'Diet and Parasitism in Dust Devil Cave.' *American Antiquity* 50:819–24.

Rich, E. 1951–2. *Cumberland and Hudson House Journals, 1775–1782.* London: Hudson's Bay Record Society.

Rich, E., ed. 1938. *Journal of Occurrences in the Athabasca Department by George Simpson, 1820 and 1821, and Report.* London: The Hudson's Bay Record Society.

– 1949. *James Isham's Observations on Hudson's Bay, 1743 and Notes and Observations on a Book Entitled 'A Voyage to Hudson's Bay in the Dobbs Galley, 1749.'* London: The Hudson's Bay Record Society.

Riley, T.J. 1993. 'Ascarids, American Indians, and the Modern World: Parasites and the Prehistoric Record of a Pharmacological Tradition.' *Perspectives in Biology and Medicine* 36:369–75.

Ritzenthaler, R. 1963. 'Primitive Therapeutic Practices among the Wisconsin Chippewa.' In I. Galdston, ed. *Man's Image in Medicine and Anthropology,* 316–34. New York: International Universities Press.

Robb, J.C. 1988. 'Legal Impediments to Traditional Indian Medicine.' In D. Young, ed. *Health Care Issues in the Canadian North,* 134–9. Edmonton: Boreal Institute for Northern Studies.

Roberts, E. 1991. 'Community Development. How Can Education and Training Have an Impact?' In B. Postl et al., eds. *Circumpolar Health 90: Proceedings of the 8th International Congress,* 138–40. Winnipeg: University of Manitoba Press.

Robinson, E.J. 1988. 'The Health of the James Bay Cree.' *Canadian Family Physician* 34:1606–13.

Robinson, E.J., and M.E. Moffatt. 1985. 'Outbreak of Rotavirus Gastroenteritis in a James Bay Cree Community.' *Canadian Journal of Public Health* 76:21–4.

Robitaille, N., and R. Choinière. 1985. *An Overview of Demographic and Socioeconomic Conditions of the Inuit in Canada.* Ottawa: Research Branch, Corporate Policy, Department of Indian and Northern Affairs.

Rode, A., and R.J. Shephard. 1992. *Fitness and Health of an Inuit Community: 20 Years of Cultural Change.* Ottawa: Department of Indian and Northern Affairs, Circumpolar and Scientific Affairs Directorate, Publ. No. 92–05.

Rogan, P.K., and S.E. Lentz. 1994. 'Molecular Genetic Evidence Suggesting

Treponematosis in Pre-Columbian, Chilean Mummies.' *American Journal of Physical Anthropology.* Supplement 18:171 (abstract).

Romaniuk, A., and V. Piché. 1972. 'Natality Estimates for the Canadian Indians by Stable Population Models, 1900–1969.' *Canadian Journal of Sociology and Anthropology* 9:1–20.

Ross, C.A., and B. Davis. 1986. 'Suicide and Parasuicide in a Northern Canadian Native Community.' *Canadian Journal of Psychiatry* 31:331–4.

Ross, W.G. 1977. 'Whaling and the Decline of Native Populations.' *Arctic Anthropology* 14(2):138–59.

– 1984. *An Arctic Whaling Diary: The Journal of Captain George Comer in Hudson Bay, 1903–1905.* Toronto: University of Toronto Press.

Roth, E. 1981. 'Sedentism and Changing Fertility Patterns in a Northern Athapascan Isolate.' *Journal of Human Evolution* 10:413–25.

Rothschild, B.M. 1992. 'Advances in Detecting Disease in Earlier Human Populations.' In S.R. Saunders and M.A. Katzenberg, eds. *Skeletal Biology of Past Peoples: Research Methods,* 131–52. New York: Wiley-Liss.

Rothschild, B.M., and W. Turnbull. 1987. 'Treponemal Infection in a Pleistocene Bear.' *Nature* 329:61–2.

Royal Commission on Aboriginal Peoples. 1993a. *Exploring the Options: Overview of the Third Round.* Ottawa: Royal Commission on Aboriginal Peoples.

– 1993b. *The Path to Healing: Report of the National Round Table on Aboriginal Health and Social Issues.* Ottawa: Royal Commission on Aboriginal Peoples.

Rubel, A.J., and H.J. Kupferer. 1968. 'Perspectives on the Atomistic-type Society: Introduction.' *Human Organization* 27:189-90.

Ruderman, P., and G. Weller. 1981. 'Health Services for the Keewatin Inuit in a Period of Transition: The View from 1980.' *Études Inuit Studies* (5):49–62.

Salisbury, R.F. 1986. *A Homeland for the Cree: Regional Development in James Bay, 1971-1981.* Montreal and Kingston: McGill-Queen's University Press.

Salo, W.L., A.C. Aufderheide, J. Buikstra, and T.A. Holcomb. 1994. 'Identification of *Mycobacterium tuberculosis* DNA in a Pre-Columbian Peruvian Mummy.' *Proceedings of the National Academy of Science* 91:2091–4.

Salter, E.M. 1984. *Skeletal Biology of Cumberland Sound, Baffin Island, N.W.T.* PhD diss., University of Toronto.

Saunders, S.R. 1988. *The MacPherson Site: Human Burials, a Preliminary Descriptive Report.* Hamilton, Ont.: Department of Anthropology, McMaster University.

Saunders, S.R., and A. Herring, eds. 1995. *Grave Reflections: Portraying the Past through Cemetery Studies.* Toronto: Canadian Scholars' Press.

Saunders, S.R., and F.J. Melbye. 1990. 'Subadult Mortality and Skeletal Indicators of Health in Late Woodland Ontario Iroquois.' *Canadian Journal of Archaeology* 14:1–14.

Saunders, S.R., P.G. Ramsden, and D.A. Herring. 1992. 'Transformation and Disease: Precontact Ontario Iroquoians.' In J. Verano and D. Ubelaker, eds. *Disease and Demography in the America*, 117–26. Washington, D.C.: Smithsonian Institution Press.

Sawchuk, L.A., and D.A. Herring. 1984. 'Respiratory Tuberculosis Mortality among the Sephardic Jews of Gibraltar.' *Human Biology* 56:291–306.

Schaefer, O. 1959. 'Medical Observations and Problems in the Canadian Arctic.' *Canadian Medical Association Journal* 81:248–53.

– 1977. 'Are Eskimos More or Less Obese than other Canadians? A Comparison of Skinfold Thickness and Ponderal Index in Canadian Eskimos.' *American Journal of Clinical Nutrition* 30:1623–8.

Schaefer, O., J.A. Hildes, L.M. Medd, and D.G. Cameron. 1975. 'The Changing Pattern of Neoplastic Disease in Canadian Eskimos.' *Canadian Medical Association Journal* 112:1399–404.

Schaefer, O., J.F. Timmermans, R.D. Eaton, and A.R. Mathews. 1980. 'General and Nutritional Health in Two Eskimo Populations at Different Stages of Acculturation.' *Canadian Journal of Public Health* 71:397–405.

Schaeffer, C. 1969. *Blackfoot Shaking Tent*. Calgary: Glenbow Museum. Occasional Paper No. 5.

Schindler, D.L. 1985. 'Anthropology in the Arctic: A Critique of Racial Typology and Normative Theory.' *Current Anthropology* 26:475-500.

Schwarcz, H.P., F.J. Melbye, M.A. Katzenberg, and M. Knyf. 1985. 'Stable Isotopes in Human Skeletons of Southern Ontario: Reconstructing Paleodiet.' *Journal of Archaeological Science* 12:187–206.

Schwartz, L. 1969. 'The Hierarchy of Resort in Curative Practices: The Admiralty Islands, Melanesia.' *Journal of Health and Social Behavior* 10:201–9.

Scott, K.A., and A.M. Myers. 1988. 'Impact of Fitness Training on Native Adolescents' Self-evaluations and Substance Use.' *Canadian Journal of Public Health* 79:424–9.

Scott-McKay-Bain Health Panel. 1989a. *Companion Documents*. Toronto.

Scott-McKay-Bain Health Panel. 1989b. *From Here to There, Steps Along the Way: Achieving Health for All in the Sioux Lookout Zone*. Toronto.

Seaby, S. 1983. *Native Healer Program, Lake of the Woods Hospital, Kenora. Evaluation Report* (unpublished).

Shadomy, H. 1981. 'The Differential Diagnosis of Various Fungal Pathogens and Tuberculosis in the Prehistoric Indians.' In J.E. Buikstra, ed. *Prehistoric Tuberculosis in the Americas*, 25–34. Evanston, Ill.: Northwestern University Archaeological Program.

Shaw, W. 1923. 'Medical Experiences among the Kwquithlih Indians along Discovery Passage.' *Canadian Medical Association Journal* 13:657–9.

Sherley-Spiers, S.K. 1989. 'Dakota Perceptions of Clinical Encounters with Western Health Care Providers.' *Native Studies Review* 5(1):41–51.

Sioui, G.E. 1992. *For an Amerindian Autohistory.* Montreal: McGill-Queen's University Press.

Skinner, M., and A.H. Goodman. 1992. 'Anthropological Uses of Developmental Defects of Enamel.' In S.R. Saunders and M.A. Katzenberg, eds. *Skeletal Biology of Past Peoples: Research Methods*, 153–74. New York: Wiley-Liss.

Smith, D. 1973. *Inkonze: Magico-Religious Beliefs of Contact-Traditional Chipewyan Trading at Fort Resolution, NWT, Canada.* Ottawa: National Museum of Canada. Ethnology Division Paper No. 6.

Smith, D.G. 1993. 'The Emergence of "Eskimo Status": An Examination of the "Eskimo Disk List System" and Its Social Consequences, 1925–1970.' In J.B. Waldram and Noel Dyck, eds. *Anthropology, Public Policy and Native Peoples in Canada*, 41–74. Montreal: McGill-Queen's University Press.

Snow, D. 1992. 'Diseases and Population Decline in the Northeast.' In J.W. Verano and D.H. Ubelaker, eds. *Disease and Demography in the Americas*, 177–86. Washington, D.C.: Smithsonian Institution Press.

Snow, D., and K. Lanphear. 1987. 'European Contact and Indian Depopulation in the Northeast: The Timing of the First Epidemics.' *Ethnohistory* 35:15–35.

Snyder, L.L. 1962. *The Idea of Racialism: Its Meaning and History.* Toronto: D. Van Nostrand.

Sole, T.D., and N. Croll. 1980. 'Intestinal Parasites in Man in Labrador, Canada.' *American Journal of Tropical Medicine and Hygiene* 29:364–8.

Southern, B. 1990. 'An Assessment of Bone Quality and Age-related Patterns of Bone Loss among Iroquoian Populations.' Paper presented at the Canadian Archaeological Association Meetings, Whitehorse, Yukon.

Southesk, Earl of. 1875. *Saskatchewan and the Rocky Mountains. A Diary and Narrative of Travel, Sport, and Adventure during a Journey through the Hudson's Bay Company's Territories, in 1859–1860.* Toronto: James Campbell and Son.

Speck, Dara Culhane. *See* Culhane Speck.

Starna, W.A., G.R. Hammell, and W.L. Butts. 1984. 'Northern Iroquoian Horticulture and Insect Infestation: A Cause for Village Removal.' *Ethnohistory* 31(3):197–207.

Statistics Canada. 1987. *General Social Survey Analysis Series: Health and Social Support,* 1985. Ottawa: Statistics Canada, Cat. No. 11-612E, No.1.

– 1989. *A Data Book on Canada's Aboriginal Population from the 1986 Census of Canada.* Ottawa: Statistics Canada, Aboriginal Peoples Output Program.

– 1990. *The Health and Activity Limitation Survey. Highlights: Disabled Persons in Canada.* Ottawa: Statistics Canada, Cat. No. 82-602.

– 1993a. *Age and Sex: 1991 Aboriginal Data.* Ottawa: Statistics Canada, Cat. No. 94-327.
– 1993b. *Language, Tradition, Health, Lifestyle and Social Issues: 1991 Aboriginal Peoples Survey.* Ottawa: Statistics Canada, Cat. No. 89-533.
– 1993c. *Schooling, Work and Related Activities, Income, Expenses and Mobility: 1991 Aboriginal Peoples Survey.* Ottawa: Statistics Canada, Cat. No. 89-534.
– 1994. *1-Disability; 2-Housing: 1991 Aboriginal Peoples Survey.* Ottawa: Statistics Canada, Cat. No. 89-535 Occasional.
Statistics Canada and Health and Welfare Canada. 1981. *The Health of Canadians: Report of the Canada Health Survey.* Ottawa: Statistics Canada, Cat. No. 82-538E.
Statutes of Canada. 1884. 'The Indian Act,' 47 Vic., c.27.
Steinbock, R. 1976. *Paleopathological Diagnosis and Interpretation.* Springfield, Ill.: Charles C. Thomas.
Stephens, M. 1991. 'The Special Premedical Studies Program – Review of Ten Years of Experience.' In B. Postl et al., eds. *Circumpolar Health 90: Proceedings of the 8th International Congress,* 134–7. Winnipeg: University of Manitoba Press.
Stern, E.W., and A.E. Stern. 1945. *The Effect of Smallpox on the Destiny of the Amerindian.* Boston: Bruce Humphries Inc.
Stewart, D.A. 1936. 'The Red Man and the White Plague.' *Canadian Medical Association Journal* 35:674–6.
Stewart, T.D. 1932. 'The Vertebral Column of the Eskimos.' *American Journal of Physical Anthropology* 17:123–36.
– 1973. *The People of America.* New York: Charles Scribner's Sons.
1979. 'Patterning of Skeletal Pathologies and Epidemiology.' In William S. Laughlin and Albert B. Harper, eds. *The First Americans: Origins, Affinities and Adaptations,* 257–74. New York: Gustav Fischer.
Stini, W.A. 1975. 'Adaptive Strategies of Human Populations under Nutritional Stress.' In E.S. Watts, F.E. Johnston, and G.W. Lasker, eds. *Biosocial Interrelations in Population Adaptation,* 19–42. The Hague: Mouton.
Stone, E.L. 1925a. 'Health and Disease at the Norway House Indian Agency.' Repr. in *Native Studies Review* 5(1):237–56, 1989.
– 1925b. 'Tuberculosis among the Indians of the Norway House Agency.' *The Public Health Journal* 16(2):76–81.
– 1935. 'Canadian Indian Medical Services.' *Canadian Medical Association Journal* 33:82–5.
Storey, R. 1992. *Life and Death in the Ancient City of Teotihuacan: A Modern Paleodemographic Synthesis.* Tuscaloosa: University of Alabama Press.
Stuart-Macadam, P. 1992. 'Porotic Hyperostosis: A New Perspective.' *American Journal of Physical Anthropology* 87:39–47.

Sturtevant, W.C., general ed. Various years since 1978. *Handbook of North American Indians*. Washington, D.C.: Smithsonian Institution.

Suttles, W. 1968. 'Coping with Abundance: Subsistence on the Northwest Coast.' In Richard B. Lee and Irven DeVore. *Man the Hunter*, 56–68. Chicago: Aldine.

Swartz, L. 1988. 'Healing Properties of the Sweatlodge Ceremony.' In David E. Young, ed. *Health Care Issues in the Canadian North*, 102–7. Edmonton: Boreal Institute for Northern Studies.

Szathmary, E.J. 1985. 'Peopling of North America: Clues from Genetic Studies'. In R. Kirk and E. Szathmary, eds. *Out of Asia: Peopling of the Americas and the Pacific*, 79–104. Canberra: The Journal of Pacific History.

– 1993. 'Genetics of Aboriginal North Americans.' *Evolutionary Anthropology* 1:202–20.

Szathmary, E.J., and N. Holt. 1983. 'Hyperglycemia in Dogrib Indians of the NWT, Canada: Association with Age and a Centripetal Distribution of Body Fat.' *Human Biology* 55:493–515.

Szathmary, E.J., and N.S. Ossenberg. 1978. 'Are the Biological Differences between North American Indians and Eskimos Truly Profound?' *Current Anthropology* 19:673–701.

Tanner, C.E., M. Staudt, and R. Adamowski. 1987. 'Seroepidemiological Study for Five Different Zoonotic Parasites in Northern Quebec.' *Canadian Journal of Public Health* 78:262–6.

Thistle, P.C. 1986. *Indian-European Trade Relations in the Lower Saskatchewan River Region to 1840*. Winnipeg: University of Manitoba Press.

Thomlinson, E., D. Gregory, and J. Larsen. 1991. 'A Northern Bachelor of Nursing Program: One Solution to Problems in Health Care Provision.' In B. Postl et al., eds, *Circumpolar Health 90: Proceedings of the 8th International Congress*, 145–8. Winnipeg: University of Manitoba Press.

Thomson, M., and J. Philion. 1991. 'Children's Respiratory Hospitalizations and Air Pollution.' *Canadian Journal of Public Health* 82:203–4.

Thornton, R. 1987. *American Indian Holocaust and Survival. A Population History since 1492*. Norman: University of Oklahoma Press.

Thornton, R., T. Miller, and J. Warren. 1991. 'American Indian Population Recovery Following Smallpox Epidemics.' *American Anthropologist* 93(1):28–45.

Thorpe, E.L.M. 1989. *The Social Histories of Smallpox and Tuberculosis in Canada*. University of Manitoba Anthropology Papers, No. 30. Winnipeg: University of Manitoba.

Thouez, J.-P., P. Foggin, and A. Rannou. 1990. 'Correlates of Health-care Use: Inuit and Cree of Northern Quebec.' *Social Science and Medicine* 30(1):25–34.

Timpson, J. 1984. 'Indian Mental Health: Changes in the Delivery of Care in Northwestern Ontario.' *Canadian Journal of Psychiatry* 29:234–41.

Titley, E. 1986. *A Narrow Vision: Duncan Campbell Scott and the Administration of Indian Affairs in Canada*. Vancouver: University of British Columbia Press.

Titley, K.C. 1973. 'Sioux Lookout Dental Care Project: A Progress Report.' *Journal of the Canadian Dental Association* 39:793-6.

Titley, K.C., and D.H. Bedard. 1986. 'An Evaluation of a Dental Care Program for Indian Children in the Community of Sandy Lake: Sioux Lookout Zone, 1973-1983.' *Journal of the Canadian Dental Association* 52:923-8.

Tobias, J.L. 1976. 'Protection, Civilization, Assimilation: An Outline History of Canada's Indian Policy.' *Western Canadian Journal of Anthropology* 6(2):13-30.

Torbert, K.W. 1990. 'Dental Therapists in Canada.' *Canadian Journal of Community Dentistry* February: 10-11.

Trigger, B.G. 1985. *Natives and Newcomers: Canada's 'Heroic Age' Reconsidered*. Montreal: McGill-Queen's University Press.

Trimble, J., S. Manson, N. Dinges, and B. Medicine. 1984. 'American Indian Concepts of Mental Health: Reflections and Directions.' In P. Pederson, N. Sartorius, and A. Marsella, eds. *Mental Health Services: The Cross-Cultural Context*, 199-220. Beverly Hills: Sage.

Trott, L., G. Barnes, and R. Dumoff. 1981. 'Ethnicity and Other Demographic Characteristics as Predictors of Sudden Drug-related Deaths.' *Journal of Studies in Alcohol* 42:564-78.

Trowell, H.C., and D.P. Burkitt, eds. 1981. *Western Diseases: Their Emergence and Prevention*. Cambridge, Mass.: Harvard University Press.

Tuck, J.A. 1971a. 'A Current Summary of Newfoundland Prehistory.' *Newfoundland Quarterly* 57:17-25.

- 1971b. 'Newfoundland Prehistory since 1950.' *Man in the Northeast* 1:27-34.

- 1976. *Newfoundland and Labrador Prehistory*. Ottawa: National Museum of Man.

Tuck, J.A., and R.T. Pastore. 1985. 'A Nice Place to Visit, but ... Prehistoric Human Extinctions on the Island of Newfoundland.' *Canadian Journal of Archaeology* 9(1):69-80.

Turner, D.G., II. 1985. 'The Dental Search for Native American Origins.' In R. Kirk and E. Szathmary, eds. *Out of Asia: Peopling of the Americas and the Pacific*, 31-78. Canberra: The Journal of Pacific History.

Ubelaker, D.H. 1976. 'Prehistoric New World Population Size: Historical Review and Current Appraisal of North American Estimates.' *American Journal of Physical Anthropology* 45:661-5.

- 1988. 'North American Indian Population Size, A.D. 1500 to 1985.' *American Journal of Physical Anthropology* 77: 289-94.

- 1992. 'North American Indian Population Size: Changing Perspectives.' In J.W. Verano and D.H. Ubelaker, eds. *Disease and Demography in the Americas*, 169-76. Washington, D.C.: Smithsonian Institution Press.

Upton, L. 1977. 'The Extermination of the Beothuks of Newfoundland.' *Canadian Historical Review* 58(2):133–53.

Van Kirk, S. 1980. *'Many Tender Ties': Women in Fur-Trade Society, 1670–1870.* Winnipeg: Watson and Dwyer.

van Rooyen, C. 1968. 'Serologic Surveys of Arctic Populations and Some Virus Diseases of Interest.' *Archives of Environmental Health* 17:547–54.

Vanast, W.J. 1991a. 'The Death of Jennie Kanajuq: Tuberculosis, Religious Competition and Cultural Conflict in Coppermine, 1929–31.' *Études Inuit Studies* 15(1):75–104.

– 1991b. ' "Hastening the Day of Extinction": Canada, Quebec, and the Medical Care of Ungava's Inuit, 1867–1967.' *Études Inuit Studies* 15(2):55–84.

Vecsey, C. 1983. *Traditional Ojibwa Religion and Its Historical Changes.* Philadelphia: American Philosophical Society.

Verano, J.W., and D.H. Ubelaker, eds. 1992. *Disease and Demography in the Americas.* Washington, D.C.: Smithsonian Institution Press.

Vivian, R.P., C. McMillan, and P.E. Moore. 1948. 'The Nutrition and Health of the James Bay Indian.' *Canadian Medical Association Journal* 59:505–18.

Vizenor, G. 1990. *Crossbloods: Bone Courts, Bingo, and Other Reports.* Minneapolis: University of Minnesota Press.

Vogel, V. 1970. *American Indian Medicine.* Norman: University of Oklahoma Press.

Waldram, J.B. 1980. *Relocation and Social Change among the Swampy Cree and Metis of Easterville, Manitoba.* MA diss., University of Manitoba.

– 1990a. 'Access to Traditional Medicine in a Western Canadian City.' *Medical Anthropology* 12:325–48.

– 1990b. 'The Persistence of Traditional Medicine in Urban Areas: The Case of Canada's Indians.' *American Indian and Alaska Native Mental Health Research* 4(1):9–29.

– 1990c. 'Physician Utilization and Urban Native People in Saskatoon, Canada.' *Social Science and Medicine* 30(5):579–89.

– 1992. *Aboriginal Offenders at the Regional Psychiatric Centre.* Unpublished report prepared for the Correctional Service of Canada.

– 1993. 'Aboriginal Spirituality: Symbolic Healing in Canadian Prisons.' *Culture, Medicine and Psychiatry* 17:345–62.

Wall, D. 1926. *Report of Medical Service to Indians Located along the Line of the Canadian National Railways from Cochrane, Ont., to La Tuque, Quebec, June to October.* Repr. in *Native Studies Review* 5(1):257–75, 1989.

Wallace, D.C., K. Garrison, and W.C. Knowler. 1985. 'Dramatic Founder Effects in Amerindian Mitochondrial DNAs.' *American Journal of Physical Anthropology* 68(2):149–56.

Wallace, D.C., and A. Torroni. 1992. 'American Indian Prehistory as Written in the Mitochondrial DNA: A Review.' *Human Biology* 64:403–16.

Ward, J.A., and J. Fox. 1977. 'A Suicide Epidemic on an Indian Reserve.' *Canadian Psychiatric Association Journal* 22:423–6.

Ward, R.H., A. Redd, D. Valencia, B.L. Frazier, B. Matsumara, and M. Santos. 1992. 'Molecular Evolution and Linguistic Differentiation in the Americas'. *American Journal of Physical Anthropology* Suppl. 14:170–1.

Warry, W. 1992. 'The Eleventh Thesis: Applied Anthropology as Praxis.' *Human Organization* 51(2):155–63.

Warwick, G. 1984. *Reconstructing Ontario Iroquoian Village Organization*. Ottawa: National Museum of Man, Mercury Series, Archaeological Survey of Canada Papers 124: vi–180.

Warwick, O.H., and A.J. Phillips. 1954. 'Cancer among Canadian Indians.' *British Journal of Cancer* 8.223–30.

Watson, T.G., R.S. Freeman, and M. Staszak. 1979. 'Parasites in Native Peoples of the Sioux Lookout Zone, Northwestern Ontario.' *Canadian Journal of Public Health* 70:179–82.

Way, J.E., III. 1978. *An Osteological Analysis of a Late Thule / Early Historic Labrador Eskimo Population*. PhD diss., University of Toronto.

Weaver, S.M. 1972. *Medicine and Politics among the Grand River Iroquois: A Study of the Non-Conservatives*. Ottawa: National Museums of Canada.

– 1981. *Making Canadian Indian Policy: The Hidden Agenda, 1968–1970.* Toronto: University of Toronto Press.

– 1986. 'Indian Policy in the New Conservative Government, Part I: The Nielsen Task Force of 1985.' *Native Studies Review* 2(1):1–43.

Welsch, R. 1983. 'Traditional Medicine and Western Medical Options among the Ningerum of Papua-New Guinea.' In L. Romanicci-Ross, D. Moerman, and L. Tancredi, eds. *The Anthropology of Medicine: From Culture to Method*, 32–53. South Hadley, Mass.: J.F. Bergen.

Wherrett, G.J. 1965. *Tuberculosis in Canada*. Ottawa: Queen's Printer.

Whitmore, T. 1992. *Disease and Death in Early Colonial Mexico: Simulating Amerindian Depopulation*. Boulder, Colo.: Westview Press.

Widmer, L., and A.J. Perzigian. 1981. 'Skeletal Lesions in Prehistoric Populations from North America.' In J.E. Buikstra, ed. *Prehistoric Tuberculosis in the Americas*, 99–113. Evanston, Ill.: Northwestern University Archaeological Program.

Wiebe, J. 1970. 'Health Service Delivery Problems in Northern Canada.' *Canadian Journal of Public Health* 61:481–7.

Wigmore, M., and D. McCue. 1991. 'No Information on a Forgotten People: How Healthy are Native People in Canada When They Live Off Reserve?' In

B.D. Postl et al., eds. *Circumpolar Health 90: Proceedings of the 8th International Congress*, 90–3. Winnipeg: University of Manitoba Press.

Williams, G., ed. 1969. *Andrew Graham's Observations on Hudson's Bay 1767–91*. London: Hudson's Bay Historical Society.

Williams, R.C., A.G. Steinberg, H. Gerschowitz, P.H. Bennett, et al. 1985. 'GM Allotypes in Native Americans: Evidence for Three Distinct Migrations across the Bering Land Bridge.' *American Journal of Physical Anthropology* 66(1):1–19.

Willms, D.G., P. Lange, D. Bayfield, M. Beardy, E.A. Lindsay, D.C. Cole, and N.A. Johnson. 1992. 'A Lament by Women for "The People, the Land" [Nishnawbi-Aski Nation]: An Experience of Loss.' *Canadian Journal of Public Health* 83:331–4.

Wilson, R., L.H. Krefting, P. Sutcliffe, and L. VanBussel. 1992. 'Incidence and Prevalence of End-stage Renal Disease among Ontario's James Bay Cree.' *Canadian Journal of Public Health* 83:143–6.

Wolff, P.H. 1973. 'Vasomotor Sensitivity to Alcohol in Diverse Mongoloid Populations.' *American Journal of Human Genetics* 25:193–9.

Wolfgang, R.W. 1954. 'Indian and Eskimo Diphyllobothriasis.' *Canadian Medical Association Journal* 70:536–9.

Wood, J.W., G.R. Milner, H.C. Harpending, and K.M. Weiss. 1992. 'The Osteological Paradox: Problems of Inferring Prehistoric Health from Skeletal Samples.' *Current Anthropology* 33(4):343–70.

Woods, C. 1977. 'Alternative Curing in a Changing Medical Situation.' *Medical Anthropology* 1(3):25–54.

World Health Organization. 1978. *Primary Health Care: Report of the International Conference on Primary Health Care, Alma-Ata, USSR, 6-12 September, 1978*. Geneva: World Health Organization.

Wotton, K. 1985. 'Mortality of Labrador Innu and Inuit, 1971–1982.' In R. Fortuine, ed. *Circumpolar Health 84: Proceedings of the 6th International Symposium*, 139–42. Seattle: University of Washington Press.

York, G. 1989. *The Dispossessed: Life and Death in Native Canada*. London: Vintage U.K.

Young, D.E., G. Ingram, and L. Swartz. 1988. 'A Cree Healer Attempts to Improve the Competitive Position of Native Medicine.' *Arctic Medical Research* 47 (Suppl. 1):313–16.

– 1989. *Cry of the Eagle: Encounters with a Cree Healer*. Toronto: University of Toronto Press.

Young, D.E., L. Swartz, G. Ingram, and J. Morse. 1988. 'The Psoriasis Research Project: An Overview.' In D.E. Young, ed. *Health Care Issues in the Canadian North*, 76–88. Edmonton: Boreal Institute for Northern Studies.

Young, D.E., and L.L. Smith. 1992. *The Involvement of Canadian Native Communities in Their Health Care Program: A Review of the Literature since the 1970's.* Edmonton: Canadian Circumpolar Institute, University of Alberta.

Young, T.K. 1979. 'Changing Patterns of Health and Sickness among the Cree-Ojibwa of Northwestern Ontario.' *Medical Anthropology* 3:191–223.

– 1981. 'Primary Health Care for Isolated Indians in Northwestern Ontario.' *Public Health Reports* 96:391–7.

– 1983. 'Mortality Pattern of Isolated Indians in Northwestern Ontario: A 10-year Review.' *Public Health Reports* 98:467–75.

– 1984. 'Indian Health Services in Canada: A Sociohistorical Perspective.' *Social Science and Medicine* 18(3):257–64.

– 1988. *Health Care and Cultural Change: The Indian Experience in the Central Subarctic.* Toronto: University of Toronto Press.

– 1991. 'Prevalence and Correlates of Hypertension in a Subarctic Indian Population.' *Preventive Medicine* 20:474–85.

– 1993. 'Diabetes Mellitus among Native Americans in Canada and the United States: An Epidemiologic Review.' *American Journal of Human Biology* 5:399–413.

– 1994. *The Health of Native Americans: Toward a Biocultural Epidemiology.* New York: Oxford University Press.

Young, T.K., and I. Casson. 1988. 'The Decline and Persistence of Tuberculosis in a Canadian Indian Population: Implications for Control.' *Canadian Journal of Public Health* 79:302–6.

Young, T.K., and N.W. Choi. 1985. 'Cancer Risks among Residents of Manitoba Indian Reserves, 1970–79.' *Canadian Medical Association Journal* 132:1269–72.

Young, T.K., and J.W. Frank. 1983. 'Cancer Surveillance in a Remote Indian Population in Northwestern Ontario.' *American Journal of Public Health* 73:515–20.

Young, T.K., and E.S. Hershfield. 1986. 'A Case-control Study to Evaluate the Effectiveness of Mass BCG Vaccination among Canadian Indians.' *American Journal of Public Health* 76:783–6.

Young, T.K., J.M. Kaufert, J.K. McKenzie, et al. 1989. 'Excessive Burden of End-stage Renal Disease among Canadian Indians: A National Survey.' *American Journal of Public Health* 79:756–8.

Young, T.K., L.L. McIntyre, J. Dooley, and J. Rodriguez. 1985. 'Epidemiologic Features of Diabetes Mellitus among Indians in Northwestern Ontario and Northeastern Manitoba.' *Canadian Medical Association Journal* 132:793–7.

Young, T.K., M.E. Moffatt, and J.D. O'Neil. 1993. 'Cardiovascular Diseases in a Canadian Arctic Population.' *American Journal of Public Health* 83:881–7.

Young, T.K., C.D. Schraer, E.V. Shubnikoff, E.J. Szathmary, and Y.P. Nikitin.
1992. 'Prevalence of Diagnosed Diabetes in Circumpolar Indigenous Populations.' *International Journal of Epidemiology* 21:730–6.

Young, T.K., and G. Sevenhuysen. 1989. 'Obesity in Northern Canadian Indians: Patterns, Determinants, and Consequences.' *American Journal of Clinical
Nutrition* 49:786–93.

Young, T.K., G. Sevenhuysen, N. Ling, and M.E.K. Moffatt. 1990. 'Determinants
of Plasma Glucose Levels and Diabetes in a Northern Canadian Indian Population.' *Canadian Medical Association Journal* 142:821–30.

Young, T.K., E.J. Szathmary, S. Evers, and B. Wheatley. 1990. 'Geographical
Distribution of Diabetes among the Native Population of Canada: A National
Survey.' *Social Science and Medicine* 31:129–39.

Zegura, S. 1985. 'The Initial Peopling of the Americas: An Overview.' In R. Kirk
and E. Szathmary, eds. *Out of Asia: Peopling of the Americas and the Pacific*,
1–18. Canberra: The Journal of Pacific History.

Zimmerly, D. 1975. *Cain's Land Revisited: Culture Change in Central Labrador,
1775–1972*. St John's: Institute of Social and Economic Research, Memorial
University of Newfoundland.

Zimmerman, M.R., and A.C. Aufderheide. 1984. 'The Frozen Family of Utqi-
agvik: The Autopsy Findings.' *Arctic Anthropology* 21(1):53–64.

Zimmerman, M.R., and G.S. Smith. 1975. 'A Probable Case of Accidental Inhu-
mation of 1600 Years Ago.' *Bulletin of the New York Academy of Medicine* 51
(2nd ser.):828–37.

Zimmerman, M.R., E. Trinkaus, and M. LeMay, et al. 1981. 'The Paleopathology
of an Aleutian Mummy.' *Archives of Pathology and Laboratory Medicine*
105(12):638–41.

Zimmerman, M.R., M.R. Yeatman, H. Sprinz, and W. Titterington, et al. 1971.
'Examination of an Aleutian Mummy.' *Bulletin of New York Academy of Medicine* 47(1):80–103.

LEGAL REFERENCES

Manitoba Hospital Commission v. Klein and Spence (1969), 67 W.W.R. 440 (Man.
Q.B.).

R. v. Johnston (1966), 56 D.L.R. (2d) 749 (Sask. C.A.).

R. v. Swimmer (1971), 1 W.W.R. 756 (Sask. C.A.).

Thomas v. Norris et al. (1992), 2 C.N.L.R., 139–63.

Guide to resources

A large literature exists on the health status and health care of Aboriginal peoples in Canada. Most of the published literature can be accessed through such on-line search services as MEDLINE and CITATION INDEX. A large 'grey' literature also exists, consisting of reports by government agencies and Aboriginal organizations. Relatively untapped are several archives with particularly rich collections of materials related to Aboriginal health. This guide provides a list of Canadian contributions to this literature. Journal articles and chapters in books are too numerous to include, those that are cited can be found in the 'References Cited.' Works listed here are included in 'References Cited' only if they have been cited in the text.

1 BIBLIOGRAPHIES

In addition to sections on health in some general bibliographies of Aboriginal peoples in Canada, the following are devoted exclusively to health:

Barrow, M.V., J.D. Niswander, and R. Fortuine, comps. 1972. *Health and Disease of American Indians North of Mexico: A Bibliography, 1800–1969.* Gainesville: University of Florida Press.
Fortuine, R., comp. 1968. *The Health of the Eskimos: A Bibliography, 1857–1967.* Hanover, N.H.: Dartmouth College Libraries.
Fortuine, R., J. Braun-Allen, J. Alward, L. Andress, and J. van den Top, comps. 1993. *The Health of the Inuit of North America: A bibliography from the earliest times through 1990.* Suppl. 8, vol. 52, of *Arctic Medical Research.*
Justice, J.J., comp. 1987. *Bibliography of Health and Disease: North American Indians, Eskimos, and Aleuts: 1969–1979.* Tucson: University of Arizona, Native American Research and Training Center. Monograph Series No. 8.

Lavallée, C., and E. Robinson, eds. 1993. *The Health of the Eastern James Bay Cree: Annotated Bibliography.* Montreal: Northern Quebec Module, Montreal General Hospital.

McCardle, B., ed. 1981. *Bibliography of the History of Canadian Indian and Inuit Health.* Edmonton: Treaty and Aboriginal Rights Research of the Indian Association of Alberta.

Meiklejohn, C., and D.A. Rokala, comps. 1986. *The Native Peoples of Canada: An Annotated Bibliography of Population Biology, Health and Illness.* Ottawa: National Museums of Canada (Canadian Museum of Civilisation Mercury Series, Archaeological Survey of Canada Paper No. 134).

Sproat, B., and J. Feather, eds. 1990. *Northern Saskatchewan Health Research Bibliography.* Second Edition. Saskatoon: Department of Community Health and Epidemiology, University of Saskatchewan.

2 BOOKS

Barbeau, M. 1958. *Medicine-Men on the North Pacific Coast.* Ottawa: National Museum of Canada. Bulletin No. 152, Anthropological Series No. 42.

Brown, J.S., and R. Brightman. 1988. *The Order of the Dreamed: George Nelson on Cree and Northern Ojibwa Religion and Myth.* Winnipeg: University of Manitoba Press.

Culhane Speck, D.C. 1987. *An Error in Judgement: The Politics of Medical Care in an Indian/White Community.* Vancouver: Talonbooks.

Dufour, R. 1983. *Femme et enfantement: Sagesse dans la culture Inuit.* Québec: Editions Papyrus.

Jilek, W.G. 1982. *Indian Healing: Shamanic Ceremonialism in the Pacific Northwest Today.* Surrey, B.C.: Hancock House.

Kuhnlein, H.V., and N.J. Turner. 1991. *Traditional Plant Foods of Canadian Indigenous Peoples: Nutrition, Botany and Use.* Philadelphia: Gordon and Breach.

Martens, T., B. Daily, and M. Hodgson. 1988. *The Spirit Weeps: Characteristics and Dynamics of Incest and Child Sexual Abuse.* Edmonton: Nechi Institute.

Shkilnyk, A.M. 1985. *A Poison Stronger than Love: The Destruction of an Ojibwa Community.* New Haven: Yale University Press.

Weaver, S.M. 1972. *Medicine and Politics among the Grand River Iroquois.* Ottawa: National Museums of Canada. Publications in Ethnology No. 4.

Young, D., G. Ingram, and L. Swartz. 1989. *Cry of the Eagle: Encounters with a Cree Healer.* Toronto: University of Toronto Press.

Young, T.K. 1988. *Health Care and Cultural Change: The Indian Experience in the Central Subarctic.* Toronto: University of Toronto Press.

- 1994. *The Health of Native Americans: Toward a Biocultural Epidemiology.* New York: Oxford University Press.

3 MONOGRAPHS / RESEARCH REPORTS

Atkinson, H.B., and G. Magonet, eds. 1990. *The James Bay Experience: A Guide for Health Professionals Working among the Cree of Northern Québec.* Québec: Ministère de la Santé et des Services sociaux.

Feather, J., ed. 1991. *Social Health in Northern Saskatchewan.* Saskatoon: Northern Medical Services, University of Saskatchewan.

Labbé, J. 1987. *Les Inuit du nord québécois et leur santé.* Québec: Ministère de la Santé et des Services Sociaux.

Myers, T., L.M. Calzavara, R. Cockerill, V.W. Marshall, and S.L. Bullock. 1993. *Ontario First Nations AIDS and Healthy Lifestyle Survey.* Toronto: University of Toronto, Department of Health Administration.

Normandeau, L., and V. Piché, eds. 1984. *Les Populations amérindiennes et inuit du Canada: Aperçu démographique.* Montréal: Les presses de l'Université de Montréal.

Waldram, J.B., and M.M. Layman. 1989. *Health Care in Saskatoon Inner City: A Comparative Study of Native and Non-Native Utilization Patterns.* Winnipeg: Institute of Urban Studies, University of Winnipeg.

Young, T.K, ed. 1987. *Diabetes in the Canadian Native Population: Biocultural Perspectives.* Toronto: Canadian Diabetes Association.

Young, T.K., L. Bruce, J. Elias, J.D. O'Neil, and A. Yassi. 1991. *The Health Effects of Housing and Community Infrastructure on Canadian Indian Reserves.* Ottawa: Department of Indian Affairs and Northern Development.

The **Canadian Circumpolar Institute** (formerly the Boreal Institute for Northern Studies), University of Alberta, Edmonton, publishes a monograph series, the following of which are concerned with health issues:

Spady, D.W., F.C. Covill, C.W. Hobart, O. Schaefer, and R.S. Tasker. 1982. *Between Two Worlds: The Report of the Northwest Territories Perinatal and Infant Mortality and Morbidity Study.* Occasional Publ. No. 16.

Young, D.E., ed. 1988. *Health Care Issues in the Canadian North.* Occasional Publ. No. 26.

Young, D.E., and L.L. Smith. 1992. *The Involvement of Canadian Native Communities in Their Health Care Programs: A Review of the Literature since the 1970s.* Northern Reference Series No. 2.

The **Northern Health Research Unit** of the University of Manitoba publishes a monograph series specifically on Aboriginal health.

Young, T.K. 1990. *Cardiovascular Diseases and Risk Factors among North American Indians.* No. 1.

O'Neil, J.D., and P. Gilbert, eds. 1990. *Childbirth in the Canadian North: Epidemiological, Clinical and Cultural Perspectives.* No. 2.

Postl, B.D., ed. 1990. *Epidemiology and Control of Haemophilus Influenzae Infection in Northern Populations.* No. 3.

Rokala, D.A., S.G. Bruce, and C. Meiklejohn, eds. 1991. *Diabetes Mellitus in Native Populations of North America: An Annotated Bibliography.* No. 4.

McClure, L., M. Boulanger, J. Kaufert, and S. Forsyth, eds. 1992. *First Nations Urban Health Bibliography: A Review of the Literature and Exploration of Strategies.* No. 5.

Schaefer, O., ed. 1993. *Health Problems and Health Care Delivery in the Canadian North: Selected Papers of J.A. Hildes and O. Schaefer.* No. 6.

4 SPECIAL JOURNAL ISSUES

Cuthand Goodwill, J., and J. Demay, eds. 1988. *Indian Health. Saskatchewan Indian Federated College Journal* (Regina) 4(1).

Waldram, J.B., and J.D. O'Neil, eds. 1989. *Native Health Research in Canada. Native Studies Review* (Saskatoon) 5(1).

5 CONFERENCE PROCEEDINGS

The proceedings of the triennial International Circumpolar Health Congresses have a high Canadian Aboriginal content.

Selected papers presented at the First International Symposium on Circumpolar Health, held in Fairbanks, Alaska, in 1967, can be found in *Archives of Environmental Health* 18:1969.

Proceedings of the Second International Symposium on Circumpolar Health, Oulu, Finland, June 21–24, 1971. Suppl. 6, 1972, of *Acta Socio-medica Scandinavica.*

Shephard, R.J., and S. Itoh, eds. 1976. *Circumpolar Health: Proceedings of the 3rd International Symposium, Yellowknife, NWT, 1974.* Toronto: University of Toronto Press.

The Fourth International Symposium on Circumpolar Health was held in Novosibirsk, USSR, in 1978. The proceedings were not published.

Harvald, B., and J.P.H. Hansen, eds. 1982. *Circumpolar Health 81: Proceedings of the 5th International Symposium, Copenhagen, 9–13 August 1981.* Oulu: Nordic Council for Arctic Medical Research.

Fortuine, R., ed. 1985. *Circumpolar Health 84: Proceedings of the 6th International*

Symposium, Anchorage, Alaska (13–18 May 1984). Seattle: University of Washington Press.

Linderholm, H., C. Backman, N. Broadbent, and I. Joelsson, eds. 1988. *Circumpolar Health 87: Proceedings of the 7th International Congress, Umea, Sweden, June 8–12, 1987*. Oulu: Nordic Council for Arctic Medical Research. Suppl. 1, vol. 47, of Arctic Medical Research.

Postl, B.D., P. Gilbert, J. Goodwill, M.E.K. Moffatt, J.D. O'Neil, P. Sarsfield, and T.K. Young, eds. 1991. *Circumpolar Health 90: Proceedings of the 8th International Congress, Whitehorse, Yukon, May 20–25, 1990*. Winnipeg: University of Manitoba Press.

6 STATISTICAL DATA

The Nutrition Canada Survey of 1972 remains the only national survey involving clinical examinations and laboratory tests which has data from Indian and Inuit communities across the country. Several reports are available.

Canada, Department of National Health and Welfare. 1975. *Nutrition Canada: Eskimo Survey Report*. Ottawa.

Canada, Department of National Health and Welfare. 1975. *Nutrition Canada: Indian Survey Report*. Ottawa.

Canada, Department of National Health and Welfare. 1980. *Nutrition Canada: Anthropometry Report*. Ottawa.

The Medical Services Branch of Health and Welfare Canada has published several reviews of health statistics of the Indian and Inuit populations it serves.

Canada, Department of National Health and Welfare, Medical Services Branch. 1988. *Health Status of Canadian Indians and Inuit: Update 1987*. Ottawa.

Canada, Department of National Health and Welfare, Medical Services Branch. 1991. *Health Status of Canadian Indians and Inuit – 1990*. Ottawa.

The Department of Indian Affairs and Northern Development, Management Information and Analysis Branch, Quantitative Analysis and Socio-demographic Research Section, publishes occasional statistical reviews of demographic and socio-economic data on registered Indians, both nationally and by individual regions.

Published reports and custom tabulations from the 1986 and 1991 censuses as well as the 1991 Aboriginal Peoples Survey can be obtained from Statistics Canada.

Statistics Canada. 1989. *A Data Book on Canada's Aboriginal Population from the 1986 Census of Canada*. Ottawa: Statistics Canada, Aboriginal Peoples Output Program.

Statistics Canada. 1993. *Age and Sex: 1991 Aboriginal Data.* Ottawa: Statistics
  Canada, Cat. No. 94-327.
Statistics Canada. 1993. *Language, Tradition, Health, Lifestyle and Social Issues:
  1991 Aboriginal Peoples Survey.* Ottawa: Statistics Canada, Cat. No. 89-533.
Statistics Canada. 1993. *Schooling, Work and Related Activities, Income, Expenses
  and Mobility: 1991 Aboriginal Peoples Survey.* Ottawa: Statistics Canada, Cat.
  No. 89-534.
Statistics Canada. 1994. *1-Disability; 2-Housing: 1991 Aboriginal Peoples Survey.*
  Ottawa: Statistics Canada, Cat. No. 89-535 Occasional.

7 DISSERTATIONS

Many dissertations dealing with Aboriginal health issues in Canada have been
defended in universities in Canada and overseas. Up-to-date listings can be
found in directories available in most reference libraries.

8 JOURNALS AND NEWSLETTERS

There are many journals in the biomedical and social sciences which have published articles on various aspects of Aboriginal health in Canada. Examples include the *Canadian Journal of Public Health,* the *Canadian Medical Association Journal,* and *Native Studies Review. Arctic Medical Research,* the official journal of the
International Union for Circumpolar Health and the Nordic Council for Arctic
Medical Research, has frequent contributions on Canadian Aboriginal and
northern health topics. The National Center for American Indian and Alaska
Native Mental Health in Denver, Colorado, publishes a journal called *American
Indian and Alaska Native Mental Health Research.*

9 ARCHIVAL MATERIALS

Those wishing to conduct archival research on Aboriginal health in Canada
should investigate the holdings of the National Archives of Canada. For a guide
to records relating to Indian Affairs in the National Archives, see: Public Archives of Canada. 1975. *Records Relating to Indian Affairs (RG 10).* Ottawa, Public
Records Division, General Inventory Series.
    The Hudson's Bay Company (HBC) Archives in Winnipeg, Manitoba, is a
particularly rich source of information on health, disease, and health care in
Aboriginal communities engaged in the fur trade. Much of this information is
scattered in files from various departments. Especially useful are the annual
reports of the district officers (*District Reports*), which often mention illnesses,

deaths, or living conditions that interfered with the fur trade at specific locations in the district. Careful scrutiny of the *Post Journals* often turns up information on illness, medical services, social conditions, the progress of epidemics, and sometimes the names and death dates of individuals who died at the post during bouts of disease or in childbirth. The correspondence files of the governors of the HBC (inward and outward) also contain narrative detail on conditions at the posts. The records of the Development Department (1925–40) provide information on the HBC attitudes and policies towards Aboriginal welfare in the early twentieth century (Series A.94 to A.97).

The records of various church missions (Methodist [now United Church of Canada], Church of England [now Anglican Church of Canada], Presbyterian, Oblate, and other Roman Catholic orders, etc.) are an invaluable and underutilized source of information on health, disease, and living conditions. Over and above the parish records for specific locations, these archives house correspondence, unpublished memoirs of clergymen and their wives, reports on living conditions, and census data, all of which mention (sometimes at length) health issues, methods of treatment, and attitudes towards disease and health care.

Most government document depository libraries in university libraries in Canada should contain recent annual reports of various government departments and agencies (such as Health and Welfare, Indian Affairs, Auditor General), as well as the *Public Accounts of Canada,* which provides details of expenditures by the federal government. Annual reports on Indian Affairs from the early years of Confederation are particularly rich in narrative reports of Indian agents, correspondences, expenditures, and occasional remarks on health conditions. These can be found in the House of Commons' *Sessional Papers.*

The Royal Commission on Aboriginal Peoples conducted extensive hearings, contracted research, and received submissions from many individuals and organizations. A large archive has been accumulated and should become available to individual researchers in the future. Of particular relevance to health are:

Royal Commission on Aboriginal Peoples. 1993. *The Path to Healing: Report of the National Round Table on Aboriginal Health and Social Issues.* Ottawa: Royal Commission on Aboriginal Peoples.

Canadian Medical Association. 1994. *Bridging the Gap: Promoting Health and Healing for Aboriginal Peoples in Canada.* Ottawa: Canadian Medical Association.

Index